Pharmacological and Psychosocial Treatments in Schizophrenia

Pharmacological and Psychosocial Treatments in Schizophrenia

Edited by Willey Campbell

hayle
medical

New York

Hayle Medical,
750 Third Avenue, 9th Floor,
New York, NY 10017, USA

Visit us on the World Wide Web at:
www.haylemedical.com

ISBN: 978-1-63241-461-8

Printed in China.

Cataloging-in-Publication Data

Pharmacological and psychosocial treatments in schizophrenia / edited by Willey Campbell.
p. cm.
Includes bibliographical references and index.
ISBN 978-1-63241-461-8
1. Schizophrenia. 2. Schizophrenia--Treatment. 3. Schizophrenia--Chemotherapy.
4. Psychotherapy. I. Campbell, Willey.

RC514 .P43 2017
616.898--dc23

Table of Contents

Preface

Schizophrenia is a mental disorder that causes long-term damage to a person's mind. Hallucinations, delusions, altered states of perception and confusion are common symptoms of this disease. This book on schizophrenia deals with the medication and psychological treatment that are available in the treatment of schizophrenia. Cognitive behavioral therapy, antipsychotic medication, etc. are effective treatments against this disease. This book, with its detailed analyses and data, will prove immensely beneficial to professionals and students involved in this area at various levels. A number of latest researches have been included to keep the readers up-to-date with the global concepts in this area of study. It is a vital tool for all researching and studying this field.

Significant researches are present in this book. Intensive efforts have been employed by authors to make this book an outstanding discourse. This book contains the enlightening chapters which have been written on the basis of significant researches done by the experts.

Finally, I would also like to thank all the members involved in this book for being a team and meeting all the deadlines for the submission of their respective works. I would also like to thank my friends and family for being supportive in my efforts.

Editor

1

Age-Related Increase in the Number of Oligodendrocytes Is Dysregulated in Schizophrenia and Mood Disorders

Victor Vostrikov and Natalya Uranova

Laboratory of Clinical Neuropathology, Mental Health Research Center, Moscow 115522, Russia

Correspondence should be addressed to Victor Vostrikov, vostrikovvm@mail.ru

Academic Editor: Haiyun Xu

The postnatal maturation of the human prefrontal cortex is associated with substantial increase of number of oligodendrocytes. Previously, we reported decreased numerical density of oligodendrocytes in the prefrontal cortex in schizophrenia and mood disorders. To gain further understanding of the role oligodendrocytes in pathogenesis of schizophrenia and mood disorders, we examined the effect of the age on the number of oligodendrocytes in the prefrontal cortex in schizophrenia, bipolar disorder, and major depressive disorder. We revealed the age-related increase in numerical density of oligodendrocytes in layer VI and adjacent white matter of BA10 and BA 9 in normal controls but not in schizophrenia, bipolar disorder, and major depressive disorder. The absence of normal increase in the number of oligodendrocytes in gray and white matter with age in schizophrenia and mood disorders suggests that age-related process of oligodendrocyte increase is dysregulated in schizophrenia and mood disorders.

1. Introduction

Disconnection among different brain regions is believed to contribute to the abnormal functioning of neural networks and has been postulated to be central to the pathophysiology of schizophrenia [1–3]. The neurobiological substrate of these connectivity abnormalities remains unknown, but recent evidence suggests that abnormalities in myelination and altered oligodendrocyte number and function may be prominent contributors to schizophrenia. Indirect evidence for disturbed structural connectivity in schizophrenia has been obtained from functional neuroimaging and electrophysiologic studies. Imaging and postmortem studies provide converging evidence that patients with schizophrenia have a dysregulated process of frontal lobe myelination.

With growing evidence of disturbed connectivity in schizophrenia, myelin pathology has been a target of recent postmortem studies. As oligodendrocytes are essential for the production of myelin, disturbed myelination might be caused by dysfunctional oligodendrocytes or a reduced number of oligodendroglial cells. Many postmortem studies are focusing on the investigation of numerical density of oligodendroglial cells and structural alterations of myelin sheets. Evidence for the involvement of oligodendrocytes and myelin in the pathophysiology of schizophrenia has come from analysis of postmortem tissue subjects with schizophrenia using protein [4, 5] and gene expression studies [5–11], light, and electron microscopic studies [12–14], and in vivo neuroimaging studies [15–19].

The first direct evidence of oligodendrocyte deficit in schizophrenia was obtained from a series of studies performed in our laboratory [12, 13, 20].

We used the Stanley brain collection to estimate Nv of oligodendrocytes in the prefrontal cortex (BA9) in schizophrenia, bipolar disorder and major depression and our own Mental Health Research Center brain collection to estimate numerical density (Nv) of oligodendrocytes in the prefrontal cortex (BA10) in schizophrenia. Reduced Nv of oligodendrocytes was detected in BA9 in layer VI in schizophrenia, bipolar disorder and major depression [13] and in layer VI of BA10 and in adjacent white matter in schizophrenia [21]. Similarly, conducting a stereologic analysis of numbers, densities, and spatial distribution of oligodendrocytes, Hof et al. [22] also found a decrease in total number in cortical layer III and white matter in the superior frontal gyrus in schizophrenics compared to control cases.

In another morphometric study, we demonstrated decreased number of pericapillary oligodendrocytes in layer V BA10 of prefrontal cortex in schizophrenia [23]. We also found that the number of pericapillary oligodendrocytes per unit capillary length positively and significantly correlated with age in control group but not in schizophrenic group [23].

There are only few data on the effect of age on Nv of oligodendrocytes in normal controls and mental illnesses. Byne et al. [24] using the Stanley brain collection demonstrated a significant deficit of oligodendrocytes in thalamic nuclei in schizophrenia and in bipolar disorder. Both psychiatric groups compared to normal controls exhibited an attenuation of an age-related increase in the number of oligodendrocytes.

There is an apparent temporal relationship between myelination and the onset of schizophrenia. Myelination in the frontal and temporal lobes, brain regions consistently implicated in the pathophysiology of schizophrenia, occurs during late adolescence to early adulthood corresponding closely to the peak incidence of schizophrenia onset [25–30].

We hypothesized that the effect of age on Nv of oligodendrocytes might be different in controls and psychiatric groups. The aim of the study was to reveal the effect of age on numerical density of oligodendrocytes in the prefrontal cortex in two brain collections—Stanley Foundation Neuropathology Consortium (SFNC) and Mental Health Research Center (MHRC) collections to learn more about the origin of previously found deficit of oligodendroglial cells in the prefrontal cortex in major psychiatric disorders.

2. Methods

The SFNC consisted of 60 subjects: 15 schizophrenia, 15 bipolar disorder, 15 major depression, and 15 unaffected controls. Clinical records were obtained and DSM-IV diagnoses were made by psychiatrists from the SFNC. Routine neuropathological examinations were also conducted on each case by neuropathologists from the SFNC. Demographic data are given in Table 1.

The MHRC brain collection consisted of 64 subjects: 32 schizophrenia and 32 normal controls subjects matched by age, gender, and postmortem delay. Brains for this collection were obtained within short postmortem delay (mean 6 h). Ethical considerations in obtaining and using human autopsy material were informed by the Ethics Committee of the MHRC, the Russian Academy of Medical Sciences. Consent for autopsy and research was taken from family members. Demographic data are given in Table 2. Clinical records were obtained, and ICD-10 diagnoses were made by psychiatrists from MHRC. Causes of death in the schizophrenia group were the same as those in controls: coronary vascular disease, pulmonary embolism, myocardial infarction, pneumonia, and cardiac failure. Brains were excluded from the study if there was evidence of neurological damage, stroke, substantial drug, or alcohol abuse, or if there were changes characteristic of Alzheimer's disease or Parkinson's disease. Only the left hemispheres of brains were taken for study.

For estimation Nv of oligodendrocytes in BA9 and BA10 paraffin sections of 10 μm thickness were obtained from each case using systematic random sampling [31]. Sections were Nissl stained according to the standard method. BA9 and BA10 were verified by us using the morphological criteria established by Rajkowska and Goldman-Rakic [32]. Layer VI was identified by its location between layer V, which contains large pyramidal neurons, and adjacent white matter. Oligodendroglial cells were identified as profiles with a small round nucleus, with densely and homogenously staining and a narrow rim of cytoplasm [33]. In a similar study [22], close agreement was found between such profiles and immunocytochemically identified oligodendrocytes. Ten sections from each brain were used for estimation of the Nv of oligodendrocytes in layer VI and adjacent white matter. Nv of oligodendrogliocytes was estimated by optical dissector method [34]. Sections were viewed using a Carl Zeiss Axio Imager M1 light microscope with 100 × (N.A. = 1.40) oil immersion objective lens, which was connected via AxioCam MRc5 digital camera to a video monitor. Optical sectioning by AxioVision Module Z-stack was used for creation series Z-stack images. An unbiased sampling frame (frame size 0.05×0.065 mm $= 0.00325$ mm^2)was superimposed on the images of layer VI and of adjacent white matter with random start, 10 fields with equal interval (three frames) between fields were counted from each section, and 100 fields per each case were counted. One hundred dissectors were counted per layer VI and 100 dissectors per white matter per case. The thickness of the counting brick was 0.75 μm, and the total depth of the optical dissector was 6.75 μm with guards above and bellow ~0.5 μm.

Numerical density (Nv) of oligodendroglial cells was estimated using the formula: $\mathrm{Nv} = Q/v$ (dis), where Q is the average number of cell nuclei counted per dissector and v(dis) is the volume of the disector: $v(\mathrm{dis}) = a[\mathrm{frame}] \times h$, where "$a$" is area of frame and "$h$" is dissector height. Nv of oligodendroglial cells was estimated as number of oligodendroglial cells in 0.001 mm^3. Values for coefficient of error of the oligodendroglial density estimates in layer VI and adjacent white matter were consistently low, with group mean scores of <2.5% for layer VI and <1% for white matter.

For estimation of number of pericapillary oligodendrocytes in BA10 (layer V) the 30 paraffin sections of 20 mm thickness were prepared from each case. Ten sections from the series were sampled in systematic random manner for analysis. These sections were stained with Luxol-fast blue and cresyl violet for visualization of capillaries and of pericapillary oligodendrocytes. BA10 was verified, and layer V was identified as containing large pyramidal neurons. A Carl Zeiss Axio Image M1 light microscope with a 25/0.45 objective, which was connected via AxioCam MRc5 digital camera to a video monitor, was used. Ten rectilinear capillary segments from layer V were systematically random sampled from each section. In this manner, 100 rectilinear capillary segments were sampled per brain, and a total of 3200 capillary segments per group were sampled. The length of each segment was measured, the number of oligodendrocytes visible alongside each segment was counted, and

TABLE 1: Demographic data of SFNC brain collection.

	Schizophrenia $n = 15$	Bipolar disorder $n = 15$	Major depression $n = 15$	Normal controls $n = 15$
Age (mean ± SD)	44.5 ± 13.1	42.3 ± 11.7	46.5 ± 9.3	48.1 ± 10.7
Gender	9M, 6F	9M, 6F	9M, 6F	9M, 6F
Duration of disease (years) (mean ± SD)	20.6 ± 11.6	20.9 ± 10.2	12.7 ± 11.1	0
Age of onset (mean ± D)	23.2 ± 7.9	21.5 ± 8.3	33.9 ± 13.3	
PMI (h) (mean ± SD)	33.7 ± 14.6	32.5 ± 16.1	27.5 ± 10.6	23.7 ± 9.9
Side of brain	6R, 9L	8R, 7L	6R, 9L	7R, 8L
TF (m) (mean ± SD)	11.2 ± 8.4	9.6 ± 3.6	8.4 ± 6.6	4.4 ± 3.8

M: male; F: female; W: white; B: Black; A: Asian; PMI: postmortem interval in hours; L: left; R: right; TF: time in formalin in months.

TABLE 2: Demographic data of MHRC brain collection.

	Controls ($n = 32$)	Schizophrenia ($n = 32$)
Age (mean ± SD)	55.9 ± 15.2	51.4 ± 13.9
Gender	16M, 16F	19M, 13F
Duration of disease (years) (mean ± SD)	—	24.9 ± 10.5
Age of onset (mean ± SD)	—	26.7 ± 10.6
PMI (h) (mean ± SD)	6.0 ± 0.9	10.1 ± 7.7
TF (m) (mean ± SD)	1.3 ± 0.3	1.3 ± 0.4

M: male; F: female; PMI: postmortem interval in hours; TF: time in formalin in months.

oligodendrocyte densities were expressed as the number of oligodendrocytes per 0.01 mm of capillary length.

Statistical analysis was performed using STATISTICA 6 software package for Windows (StatSoft. Inc, Tusla, Okla, USA). Comparisons of number of oligodendrocytes to age in schizophrenia and normal controls were performed using multiple linear regression analysis. Statistical group comparisons between patients and the control groups were made using one-way analysis of variance (ANOVA).

3. Results and Discussion

Regression analyses examining the relationship between age and Nv of oligodendrocytes showed in controls a significant diagnosis by age interaction in layer VI of BA9 ($F = 10.05$, $df = 1.13$, $P = .007$) and in adjacent white matter ($F = 5.48$, $df = 1.13$, $P = .03$). In contrast, none of age-related changes were showed in schizophrenia, bipolar disorder, and major depression (all $P > .05$) (Table 3) (Figure 1).

Regression analyses of the relationship between neuroleptics dosage and Nv of oligodendrocytes in schizophrenic cases showed no significant neuroleptics by age interaction in layer VI of BA9 ($F = 0.6$, $df = 1.12$, $P = .5$) and in adjacent white matter ($F = 0.15$, $df = 1.12$, $P = .7$). Also, there was no significant neuroleptics by age interaction in bipolar disorder in layer VI of BA9 ($F = 0.01$, $df = 1.10$, $P = .9$) and in adjacent white matter ($F = 3.44$, $df = 1.10$, $P = .09$).

Regression analyses examining the relationship between age and Nv of oligodendrocytes showed in controls a significant diagnosis by age interaction in layer VI of BA10 ($F = 6.55$, $df = 1.30$, $P = .015$) and adjacent white matter ($F = 20.44$, $df = 1.30$, $P < .001$). In contrast, none of meaningful age-related change showed in schizophrenia ($F = 0.02$, $P = .9$, $F = 0.90$, $P = .34$, resp.) (Table 4) (Figure 2).

TABLE 3: Regression of Nv of oligodendrocytes on age in BA9.

	F	df	P
Controls			
layer VI	10.05	1.13	.007
white matter	5.48	1.13	.03
Schizophrenia			
layer VI	2.15	1.13	.16
white matter	0.14	1.13	.7
Bipolar disorder			
layer VI	0.51	1.13	.5
white matter	4.63	1.13	.051
Major depression			
layer VI	0.01	1.13	.9
white matter	1.34	1.13	.26

Regression analyses examining the relationship between neuroleptics dosage and Nv of oligodendrocytes in schizophrenia showed no significant neuroleptics by age interaction in layer VI of BA10 ($F = 3.15$, $df = 1.30$, $P = .09$) and in adjacent white matter ($F = 0.18$, $df = 1.30$, $P = .7$).

Comparisons of young (<50 years) and elderly patient subgroups (>50 years) with young and elderly controls showed that only elderly patients with schizophrenia had

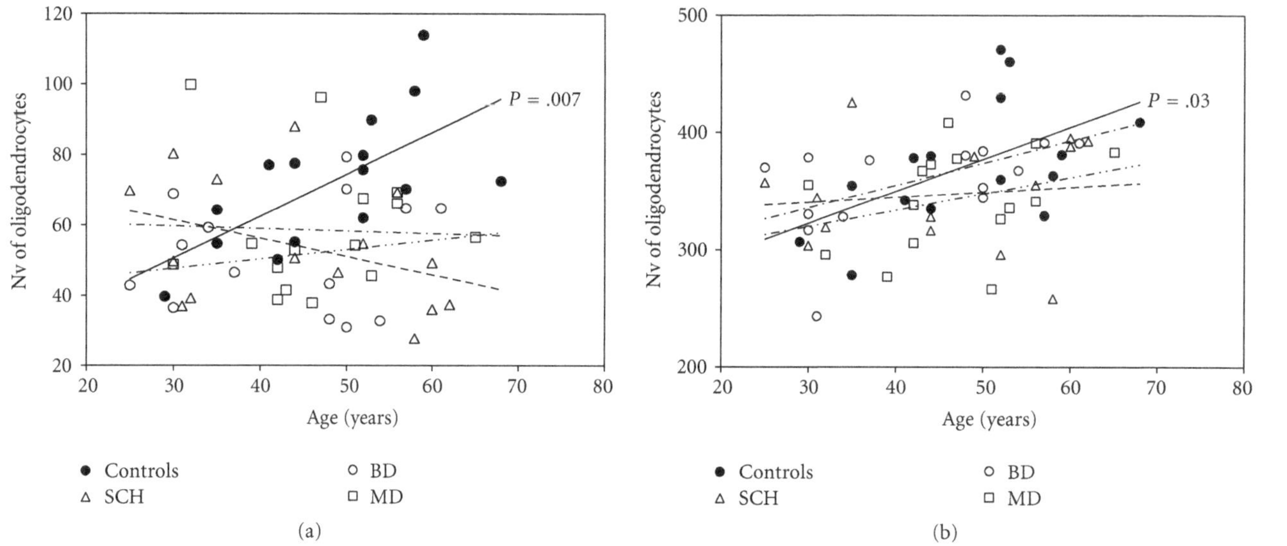

FIGURE 1: Plots summarizing results of regression analysis in BA9. There is a significant positive correlation between Nv of oligodendrocytes and age in controls in layer VI ($P = .007$) (a) and in adjacent white matter ($P = .03$) (b) but no significant correlations in schizophrenia, bipolar disorder, and major depression.

TABLE 4: Regression of Nv of oligodendrocytes on age in BA10.

	F	*df*	*P*
Controls			
layer VI	6.55	1.30	.015
white matter	20.44	1.30	<.001
Schizophrenia			
layer VI	0.02	1.30	.9
white matter	0.90	1.30	.34

significantly lower oligodendrocyte number as compared to elderly controls (in BA10 layer VI ($F = 26.78$, $df = 1.36$, $P < .001$)), in adjacent white matter ($F = 51.24$, $df = 1.36$, $P < .001$), in BA9 layer VI ($F = 7.28$, $df = 1.12$, $P = .02$) (Figures 3(a), 3(b) and 3(c)).

Significant reduction of oligodendrocyte density only was found in young patients with bipolar disorder as compared to young controls ($F = 11.30$, $df = 1.14$, $P = .005$) (Figure 3(d)).

Results of our study revealed a significant age-related increase in Nv of oligodendrocytes in layer VI and in white matter both in BA9 and BA10 in control groups. It is of interest to note that previously the age-related increase number of pericapillary oligodendrocytes in layer V in BA10 was also revealed in controls [23]. Of note, such an increase was not observed in age-matched psychiatric groups.

Our results obtained in normal control groups are consistent with the results of imaging studies on myelination of normal subjects. Bartzokis et al. [19] reported that the normal age-related development of the frontal and temporal lobes in adulthood is dysregulated in adults with schizophrenia primary due to a lack of normal myelination. van Haren et al. [35] proposed that cerebral gray matter volume loss in patients with schizophrenia was characterized by the absence of the normal curved trajectory of volume change with age that was present in healthy subjects. These data together with the results of postmortem studies suggest that age-related increase in oligodendrocyte number and progressive myelination that are evidenced in normal controls may be disrupted in psychiatric patients. A significant age-associated reduction in fractional anisotropy, progressive decrement of white matter volume in frontal lobe, and the relationships between white matter alterations and severity of symptoms were found in patients with schizophrenia in contrast to controls [36–39]. Our results are also in agreement with the data obtained in the monkey neocortex [40] where a substantial increase in the numbers of oligodendrocytes was found over the monkey's life span. An increase in the number of oligodendrocyte with aging has been also reported in the optic nerve, in the visual cortex [41, 42]. Severity of age-related myelin alterations in visual cortex correlated significantly with cognitive impairment index due to reduced conduction velocity along the affected nerve fibers [42, 43].

The increase of oligodendrocytes number and extensive myelination of the human brain makes myelin maintenance and repair especially critical for supporting our high cognitive processing speed [19, 44]. Importantly, that reduction of fractional anisotropy in different white matter

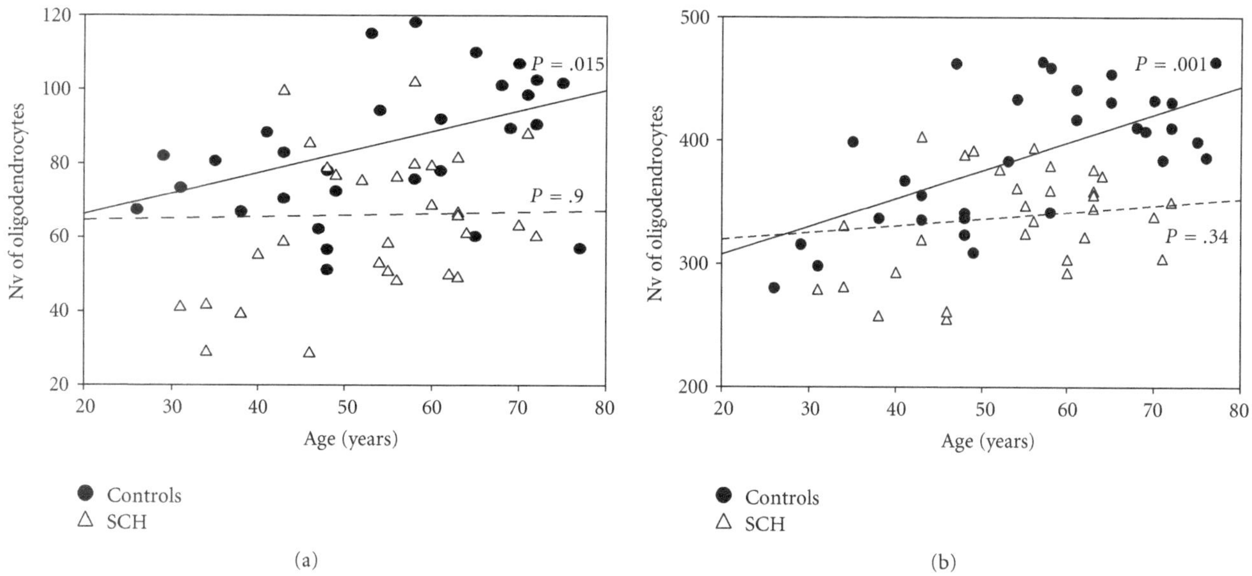

FIGURE 2: Plots summarizing results of regression analysis in BA10. There is a significant positive correlation between Nv of oligodendrocytes and age in controls in layer VI ($P = .015$) (a) and adjacent white matter ($P = .001$) (b) but no significant correlations in schizophrenia.

tracts was associated with cognitive deficits [45–49]. Thus, these data together with our results suggest that reduced oligodendrocyte density might be associated with cognitive dysfunction in schizophrenia and in bipolar disorder.

In the present study, only elderly patients with schizophrenia had significantly lower oligodendrocyte number as compared to elder controls. Elderly schizophrenia patients frequently develop more severe cognitive disturbances that younger ones. In these subjects reported reduced fractional anisotropy in frontotemporal clusters associated with frontal gray matter reduction and "frontal" cognitive deficits [50], though Frisoni et al. [51] found that orbitofrontal/cingulate region had low gray matter volume in elderly schizophrenia patients not associated with cognitive abnormalities. Neuroimaging studies demonstrated lower prefrontal gray matter volume in schizophrenia in chronic but not in first episode schizophrenia patients [52]. Patients with chronic schizophrenia showed widespread cortical thinning that particularly affected the prefrontal cortex [53–56], decreased fractional anisotropy in thalamofrontal white matter [57], lower levels of glutamate/glutamine and N-acetylaspartate compared to healthy controls and first-episode patients [58], abnormally expressed NMDA receptor subunits in elderly schizophrenia patients [59], and hypoperfusion of the prefrontal cortex [60].

On the contrary, gray and white matter volumes of prefrontal cortex were significantly smaller only in young adulthood bipolar disorder patients relative to healthy control subjects [61–64]. Decreased N-acetylaspartate was detected in the dorsolateral prefrontal cortex of young bipolar patients [65]. These findings suggest that prefrontal white matter abnormalities are present early in bipolar disorder and may consist largely of axonal disorganization, and white matter pathology may represent an early marker of bipolar disorder [66].

Our results that significant reduction of oligodendrocyte density was found in young patients with bipolar disorder as compared to young controls are in agreement with these in vivo data. They are also in line with the data obtained from other postmortem studies reported that patients with bipolar disorder demonstrated decreased neuronal size in the orbitofrontal cortex [67] and reductions in oligodendrocyte density in the prefrontal cortex [13, 14] and the number, size, and density of glial cells [68–70].

Maturity of oligodendrocytes is influenced by genetic and epigenetic factors. DNA microarray analysis repeatedly demonstrated downregulation of oligodendrocyte- and myelin-related genes [6, 8]. Most of these data were obtained on Mount Sinai and Stanley collections containing mostly elderly subjects. On the other side, Mitkus et al. [71] using brain collection containing younger cases of schizophrenia and controls did not confirmed downregulation of oligodendrocyte-related genes, but they found that individuals carrying risk-associated alleles in oligodendrocyte-related genes had relatively lower transcript levels. DTI studies of subjects at increased risk for bipolar disorder showed reduced fractional anisotropy in the superior frontal tracts [72] and decreased gray matter density. Bipolar disorder and schizophrenia share common chromosomal susceptibility loci and many risk-promoting genes. Thus, these data illustrate the importance of genetic factors in oligodendrocyte abnormalities in schizophrenia and in bipolar disorder.

Recently, epigenetic mechanisms facilitating oligodendrocyte development, maturation, and aging have been reported [73]. It is of interest to note that Iwamoto et al. [10] in BA10 of the prefrontal cortex of the Stanley brain collection detected reduced expression of SOX 10, an oligodendrocyte-specific transcription factor, and correlation between DNA methylation status of SOX 10 with its downregulation and oligodendrocyte dysfunction

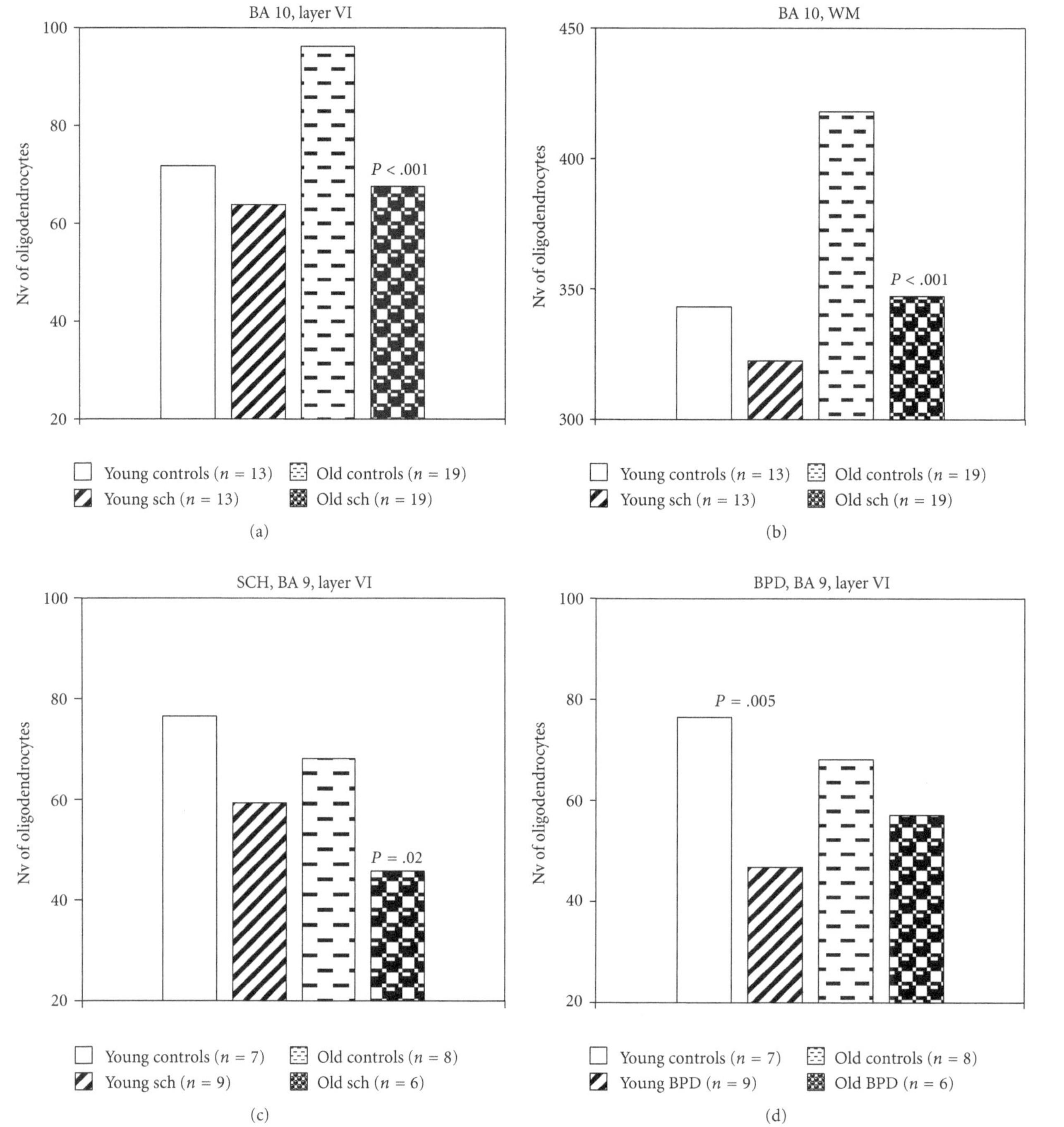

FIGURE 3: Plots summarizing results of comparisons of young and elderly patient subgroups with young and elderly controls.

in schizophrenia. It is known that oligodendrocytes are very sensitive to oxidative stress [69, 74, 75] and glutamate toxicity [69, 76]. Excess release of glutamate was found in schizophrenia patients [77] and especially in schizophrenic patients with cognitive impairment and negative symptoms [78]. Many genes modified in the brains of patients with schizophrenia are associated with glutathione and oxidative stress pathways [79]. The data provide evidence for epigenetic and intrinsic factors on oligodendrocyte dysfunction in schizophrenia.

Frontal and temporal lobe white matter volumes continue to increase in humans throughout the first five decades of life [80–82]. The convergence of natural and genetic risk factors on this area in schizophrenia and bipolar disorder may help to explain the apparent vulnerability of oligodendrocytes in these disorders [69]. Recent studies suggest that abnormal development of oligodendrocytes is involved in the pathophysiology of schizophrenia. Katsel et al. [83] suggest that oligodendroglial deficit in schizophrenia might be associated with disruption of normal patterns of cell cycle gene and protein expression. Barley et al. [84] found that genes expressed after the terminal differentiation of oligodendrocytes tended to have lower levels of mRNA expression in subjects with schizophrenia compared to normal controls. Kern et al. [85] reported deficits in the expression of oligodendrocyte and myelin genes associated with a reduction in the number of oligodendrocytes and with abnormalities of cell cycle markers in some brain regions in schizophrenia.

Some of studies indicate that chronic treatment with antipsychotics may affect brain morphology [86–88]. However, we found no effect of neuroleptic treatment on Nv of oligodendrocytes in schizophrenia and bipolar disorder groups and revealed a lack of age-related increase in this parameter in major depression group without neuroleptic treatment. On the other hand, protective effects of neuroleptics on oligodendrocytes have been reported [89, 90]. Thus, we suggest that reported reductions in oligodendrocyte density in schizophrenia and mood disorder are related to the disease.

Oligodendrocytes form after wave of neurogenesis, and they show a selective vulnerability to cell death stimuli depending on their stage of development [91]. Gritti et al. [92] found age- and region-dependent quantitative changes in the cell composition of neural stem cells progeny (decreased quantity of neurons and oligodendrocytes; increased amount of astroglial cells). Aging had an effect on the morphological feature, number, and developmental regulation of oligodendroglial progenitors in rat CNS [93]. It is of interest to note that neural stem cell proliferation is decreased in schizophrenia, but not in depression [94], and haloperidol stimulate proliferation of oligodendrocytes precursors [90]. Benes [95] suggested delayed myelination in the prefrontal cortex in patients with schizophrenia. Akbarian et al. [96, 97] reported a maldistribution of the interstitial neurons in both prefrontal and temporal white matter in schizophrenia. The data suggested that neurodevelopmental abnormalities were present in at least a subgroup of psychiatric patients. Since young schizophrenia patients in the present study demonstrated decrease in Nv of oligodendrocytes, though no significant, we suppose that the deficit of oligodendrocytes might start during brain development and continue to become significant in elderly patients with schizophrenia.

Several limitations of the study must be noted. First, mean age in bipolar disorder was less than in schizophrenia group. Second, samples need to be comprised of both males and females, as there is clear evidence to suggest that the timing, course, and clinical features of schizophrenia are manifested quite differently in males and females, and this may be related to brain differences. Future studies will also need to include an evaluation of first episode psychotic patients, so as to provide a sample of patients who have limited exposure to psychotropic medications. It will also be important to evaluate a representative sample of normal controls across age, as white matter changes with age, and such changes may be quite different in pathological populations such as schizophrenia. Future DTI studies need also to include other imaging techniques, which highlight white matter pathologies, such as proton spectroscopy, magnetization transfer techniques, and relaxation times measurements. Moreover, such studies should be conducted in concert with functional MRI and PET imaging in order to characterize and to understand more fully both functional and structural abnormalities in schizophrenia. Although gender ratios were not precisely matched, previous studies have failed to correlate gender and measures of diffusion tensor imaging.

4. Conclusion

In conclusion, the study highlights the importance of inclusion of age effects in imaging and postmortem studies for further studies of white matter abnormalities in major psychiatric disorders.

Conflict of Interests

The authors have no conflict of interest with any commercial or other associations in connection with the submitted article.

Acknowledgment

The authors express their gratitude to the Stanley Medical Research Institute for support of this work.

References

[1] D. R. Weinberger and B. K. Lipska, "Cortical maldevelopment, anti-psychotic drugs, and schizophrenia: a search for common ground," *Schizophrenia Research*, vol. 16, no. 2, pp. 87–110, 1995.

[2] V. Haroutunian and K. L. Davis, "Introduction to the special section: Myelin and oligodendrocyte abnormalities in schizophrenia," *International Journal of Neuropsychopharmacology*, vol. 10, no. 4, pp. 499–502, 2007.

[3] K. L. Davis, D. G. Stewart, J. I. Friedman et al., "White matter changes in schizophrenia evidence for myelin-related dysfunction," *Archives of General Psychiatry*, vol. 60, no. 5, pp. 443–456, 2003.

[4] S. W. Flynn, D. J. Lang, A. L. Mackay et al., "Abnormalities of myelination in schizophrenia detected in vivo with MRI, and post-mortem with analysis of oligodendrocyte proteins," *Molecular Psychiatry*, vol. 8, no. 9, pp. 811–820, 2003.

[5] S. Dracheva, K. L. Davis, B. Chin, D. A. Woo, J. Schmeidler, and V. Haroutunian, "Myelin-associated mRNA and protein expression deficits in the anterior cingulate cortex and hippocampus in elderly schizophrenia patients," *Neurobiology of Disease*, vol. 21, no. 3, pp. 531–540, 2006.

[6] Y. Hakak, J. R. Walker, C. Li et al., "Genome-wide expression analysis reveals dysregulation of myelination-related genes in chronic schizophrenia," *Proceedings of the National Academy of Sciences of the United States of America*, vol. 98, no. 8, pp. 4746–4751, 2001.

[7] S. Bahn, "Gene expression in bipolar disorder and schizophrenia: new approaches to old problems," *Bipolar Disorders*, vol. 4, no. 1, pp. 70–72, 2002.

[8] D. Tkachev, M. L. Mimmack, M. M. Ryan et al., "Oligodendrocyte dysfunction in schizophrenia and bipolar disorder," *The Lancet*, vol. 362, no. 9386, pp. 798–805, 2003.

[9] C. Aston, L. Jiang, and B. P. Sokolov, "Microarray analysis of postmortem temporal cortex from patients with schizophrenia," *Journal of Neuroscience Research*, vol. 77, no. 6, pp. 858–866, 2004.
[10] K. Iwamoto, M. Bundo, K. Yamada et al., "DNA methylation status of SOX10 correlates with its downregulation and oligodendrocyte dysfunction in schizophrenia," *Journal of Neuroscience*, vol. 25, no. 22, pp. 5376–5381, 2005.
[11] P. Katsel, K. L. Davis, and V. Haroutunian, "Variations in myelin and oligodendrocyte-related gene expression across multiple brain regions in schizophrenia: a gene ontology study," *Schizophrenia Research*, vol. 79, no. 2-3, pp. 157–173, 2005.
[12] N. Uranova, D. Orlovskaya, O. Vikhreva et al., "Electron microscopy of oligodendroglia in severe mental illness," *Brain Research Bulletin*, vol. 55, no. 5, pp. 597–610, 2001.
[13] N. A. Uranova, V. M. Vostrikov, D. D. Orlovskaya, and V. I. Rachmanova, "Oligodendroglial density in the prefrontal cortex in schizophrenia and mood disorders: a study from the Stanley Neuropathology Consortium," *Schizophrenia Research*, vol. 67, no. 2-3, pp. 269–275, 2004.
[14] V. M. Vostrikov, N. A. Uranova, and D. D. Orlovskaya, "Deficit of perineuronal oligodendrocytes in the prefrontal cortex in schizophrenia and mood disorders," *Schizophrenia Research*, vol. 94, no. 1–3, pp. 273–280, 2007.
[15] M. S. Buchsbaum, C. Y. Tang, S. Peled et al., "MRI white matter diffusion anisotropy and PET metabolic rate in schizophrenia," *NeuroReport*, vol. 9, no. 3, pp. 425–430, 1998.
[16] K. O. Lim, M. Hedehus, M. Moseley, A. de Crespigny, E. V. Sullivan, and A. Pfefferbaum, "Compromised white matter tract integrity in schizophrenia inferred from diffusion tensor imaging," *Archives of General Psychiatry*, vol. 56, no. 4, pp. 367–374, 1999.
[17] J. Foong, M. Maier, G. J. Barker, S. Brocklehurst, D. H. Miller, and M. A. Ron, "In vivo investigation of white matter pathology in schizophrenia with magnetisation transfer imaging," *Journal of Neurology Neurosurgery and Psychiatry*, vol. 68, no. 1, pp. 70–74, 2000.
[18] J. Foong, M. R. Symms, G. J. Barker et al., "Neuropathological abnormalities in schizophrenia: evidence from magnetization transfer imaging," *Brain*, vol. 124, no. 5, pp. 882–892, 2001.
[19] G. Bartzokis, K. H. Nuechterlein, P. H. Lu, M. Gitlin, S. Rogers, and J. Mintz, "Dysregulated brain development in adult men with schizophrenia: a magnetic resonance imaging study," *Biological Psychiatry*, vol. 53, no. 5, pp. 412–421, 2003.
[20] D. D. Orlovskaya, V. M. Vostrikov, V. I. Rachmanova, and N. A. Uranova, "Decreased numerical density of oligodendroglial cells in postmortem prefrontal cortex in schizophrenia, bipolar affective disorder, and major depression. (Abstracts of the "X biennial winter workshop on schizophrenia", Davos, Switzerland, 2000)," *Schizophrenia Research*, vol. 41, pp. 105–106, 2000.
[21] V. M. Vostrikov, N. A. Uranova, V. I. Rakhmanova, and D. D. Orlovskaia, "Lowered oligodendroglial cell density in the prefrontal cortex in schizophrenia," *Zhurnal Nevrologii i Psikhiatrii Imeni S.S. Korsakova*, vol. 104, no. 1, pp. 47–51, 2004.
[22] P. R. Hof, V. Haroutunian, V. L. Friedrich et al., "Loss and altered spatial distribution of oligodendrocytes in the superior frontal gyrus in schizophrenia," *Biological Psychiatry*, vol. 53, no. 12, pp. 1075–1085, 2003.
[23] V. Vostrikov, D. Orlovskaya, and N. Uranova, "Deficit of pericapillary oligodendrocytes in the prefrontal cortex in schizophrenia," *World Journal of Biological Psychiatry*, vol. 9, no. 1, pp. 34–42, 2008.
[24] W. Byne, A. Tatusov, G. Yiannoulos, G. S. Vong, and S. Marcus, "Effects of mental illness and aging in two thalamic nuclei," *Schizophrenia Research*, vol. 106, no. 2-3, pp. 172–181, 2008.
[25] P. R. Huttenlocher, "Synaptic density in human frontal cortex: developmental changes and effects of aging," *Brain Research*, vol. 163, no. 2, pp. 195–205, 1979.
[26] R. D. Terry, R. DeTeresa, and L. A. Hansen, "Neocortical cell counts in normal human adult aging," *Annals of Neurology*, vol. 21, no. 6, pp. 530–539, 1987.
[27] F. M. Benes, S. L. Vincent, and J. P. San Giovanni, "High resolution imaging of receptor binding an analyzing neurospychiatric diseases," *BioTechniques*, vol. 7, no. 9, pp. 970–978, 1989.
[28] F. M. Benes, M. Turtle, Y. Khan, and P. Farol, "Myelination of a key relay zone in the hippocampal formation occurs in the human brain during childhood, adolescence, and adulthood," *Archives of General Psychiatry*, vol. 51, no. 6, pp. 477–484, 1994.
[29] P. S. Qoldman-Rakic and L. D. Selemon, "Functional and anatomical aspects of prefrontal pathology in schizophrenia," *Schizophrenia Bulletin*, vol. 23, no. 3, pp. 437–458, 1997.
[30] J. N. Giedd, N. O. Jeffries, J. Blumenthal et al., "Childhood-onset schizophrenia: progressive brain changes during adolescence," *Biological Psychiatry*, vol. 46, no. 7, pp. 892–898, 1999.
[31] H. J. Gundersen and E. B. Jensen, "The efficiency of systematic sampling in stereology and its prediction," *Journal of Microscopy*, vol. 147, p. 3, 1987.
[32] G. Rajkowska and P. S. Goldman-Rakic, "Cytoarchitectonic definition of prefrontal areas in the normal human cortex: I. Remapping of areas 9 and 46 using quantitative criteria," *Cerebral Cortex*, vol. 5, no. 4, pp. 307–322, 1995.
[33] M. Polak, W. Haymaker, J. E. Johnson, and F. D'Amelio, "Neuroglia and their reactions," in *Histology and Histopathology of the Nervous System*, W. Haymaker and R. D. Adams, Eds., pp. 363–480, Charles C. Thomas, Springfield, Ill, USA, 1982.
[34] H. J. G. Gundersen, T. F. Bendtsen, L. Korbo et al., "Some new, simple and efficient stereological methods and their use in pathological research and diagnosis," *APMIS*, vol. 96, no. 5, pp. 379–394, 1988.
[35] N. E. M. van Haren, W. Cahn, H. E. Hulshoff Pol, and R. S. Kahn, "Schizophrenia as a progressive brain disease," *European Psychiatry*, vol. 23, no. 4, pp. 245–254, 2008.
[36] B. C. Ho, N. C. Andreasen, P. Nopoulos, S. Arndt, V. Magnotta, and M. Flaum, "Progressive structural brain abnormalities and their relationship to clinical outcome: a longitudinal magnetic resonance imaging study early in schizophrenia," *Archives of General Psychiatry*, vol. 60, no. 6, pp. 585–594, 2003.
[37] L. R. Skelly, V. Calhoun, S. A. Meda, J. Kim, D. H. Mathalon, and G. D. Pearlson, "Diffusion tensor imaging in schizophrenia: relationship to symptoms," *Schizophrenia Research*, vol. 98, no. 1–3, pp. 157–162, 2008.
[38] E. A. Hazlett, M. S. Buchsbaum, M. M. Haznedar et al., "Cortical gray and white matter volume in unmedicated schizotypal and schizophrenia patients," *Schizophrenia Research*, vol. 101, no. 1–3, pp. 111–123, 2008.
[39] G. Rosenberger, M. Kubicki, P. G. Nestor et al., "Age-related deficits in fronto-temporal connections in schizophrenia: a diffusion tensor imaging study," *Schizophrenia Research*, vol. 102, no. 1–3, pp. 181–188, 2008.
[40] A. Peters, "The effects of normal aging on myelinated nerve fibers in monkey central nervous system," *Frontiers in Neuroanatomy*, vol. 3, p. 11, 2009.

[41] J. H. Sandell and A. Peters, "Effects of age on the glial cells in the rhesus monkey optic nerve," *Journal of Comparative Neurology*, vol. 445, no. 1, pp. 13–28, 2002.
[42] A. Peters and C. Sethares, "Oligodendrocytes, their progenitors and other neuroglial cells in the aging primate cerebral cortex," *Cerebral Cortex*, vol. 14, no. 9, pp. 995–1007, 2004.
[43] A. Peters, M. B. Moss, and C. Sethares, "Effects of aging on myelinated nerve fibers in monkey primary visual cortex," *Journal of Comparative Neurology*, vol. 419, no. 3, pp. 364–376, 2000.
[44] G. Bartzokis, M. Beckson, P. H. Lu et al., "Cortical gray matter volumes are associated with subjective responses to cocaine infusion," *American Journal on Addictions*, vol. 13, no. 1, pp. 64–73, 2004.
[45] M. Kubicki, C. F. Westin, P. G. Nestor et al., "Cingulate fasciculus integrity disruption in schizophrenia: a magnetic resonance diffusion tensor imaging study," *Biological Psychiatry*, vol. 54, no. 11, pp. 1171–1180, 2003.
[46] K. O. Lim, B. A. Ardekani, J. Nierenberg, P. D. Butler, D. C. Javitt, and M. J. Hoptman, "Voxelwise correlational analyses of white matter integrity in multiple cognitive domains in schizophrenia," *American Journal of Psychiatry*, vol. 163, no. 11, pp. 2008–2010, 2006.
[47] K. H. Karlsgodt, T. G. M. van Erp, R. A. Poldrack, C. E. Bearden, K. H. Nuechterlein, and T. D. Cannon, "Diffusion tensor imaging of the superior longitudinal fasciculus and working memory in recent-onset schizophrenia," *Biological Psychiatry*, vol. 63, no. 5, pp. 512–518, 2008.
[48] P. G. Nestor, M. Kubicki, M. Niznikiewicz, R. J. Gurrera, R. W. McCarley, and M. E. Shenton, "Neuropsychological disturbance in schizophrenia: a diffusion tensor imaging study," *Neuropsychology*, vol. 22, no. 2, pp. 246–254, 2008.
[49] P. R. Szeszko, D. G. Robinson, M. Ashtari et al., "Clinical and neuropsychological correlates of white matter abnormalities in recent onset schizophrenia," *Neuropsychopharmacology*, vol. 33, no. 5, pp. 976–984, 2008.
[50] I. Spoletini, A. Cherubini, M. Di Paola et al., "Reduced fronto-temporal connectivity is associated with frontal gray matter density reduction and neuropsychological deficit in schizophrenia," *Schizophrenia Research*, vol. 108, no. 1–3, pp. 57–68, 2009.
[51] G. B. Frisoni, A. Prestia, A. Adorni et al., "In vivo neuropathology of cortical changes in elderly persons with schizophrenia," *Biological Psychiatry*, vol. 66, no. 6, pp. 578–585, 2009.
[52] V. Molina, J. Sanz, F. Sarramea, C. Benito, and T. Palomo, "Lower prefrontal gray matter volume in schizophrenia in chronic but not in first episode schizophrenia patients," *Psychiatry Research*, vol. 131, no. 1, pp. 45–56, 2004.
[53] G. R. Kuperberg, M. R. Broome, P. K. McGuire et al., "Regionally localized thinning of the cerebral cortex in schizophrenia," *Archives of General Psychiatry*, vol. 60, no. 9, pp. 878–888, 2003.
[54] P. Lopez-Garcia, H. J. Aizenstein, B. E. Snitz, R. P. Walter, and C. S. Carter, "Automated ROI-based brain parcellation analysis of frontal and temporal brain volumes in schizophrenia," *Psychiatry Research*, vol. 147, no. 2-3, pp. 153–161, 2006.
[55] D. C. Glahn, A. R. Laird, I. Ellison-Wright et al., "Meta-analysis of gray matter anomalies in schizophrenia: application of anatomic likelihood estimation and network analysis," *Biological Psychiatry*, vol. 64, no. 9, pp. 774–781, 2008.
[56] Z. Kikinis, J. H. Fallon, M. Niznikiewicz et al., "Gray matter volume reduction in rostral middle frontal gyrus in patients with chronic schizophrenia," *Schizophrenia Research*, vol. 123, no. 2-3, pp. 153–159, 2010.
[57] J. S. Oh, M. Kubicki, G. Rosenberger et al., "Thalamo-frontal white matter alterations in chronic schizophrenia: a quantitative diffusion tractography study," *Human Brain Mapping*, vol. 30, no. 11, pp. 3812–3825, 2009.
[58] C. Y. Tang, J. Friedman, D. Shungu et al., "Correlations between diffusion tensor imaging (DTI) and magnetic resonance spectroscopy (H MRS) in schizophrenic patients and normal controls," *BMC Psychiatry*, vol. 7, article 25, 2007.
[59] S. Dracheva, S. A. E. Marras, S. L. Elhakem, F. R. Kramer, K. L. Davis, and V. Haroutunian, "N-methyl-D-aspartic acid receptor expression in the dorsolateral prefrontal cortex of elderly patients with schizophrenia," *American Journal of Psychiatry*, vol. 158, no. 9, pp. 1400–1410, 2001.
[60] N. Kanahara, E. Shimizu, Y. Sekine et al., "Does hypofrontality expand to global brain area in progression of schizophrenia? A cross-sectional study between first-episode and chronic schizophrenia," *Progress in Neuro-Psychopharmacology and Biological Psychiatry*, vol. 33, no. 3, pp. 410–415, 2009.
[61] H. P. Blumberg, J. H. Krystal, R. Bansal et al., "Age, rapid-cycling, and pharmacotherapy effects on ventral prefrontal cortex in bipolar disorder: a cross-sectional study," *Biological Psychiatry*, vol. 59, no. 7, pp. 611–618, 2006.
[62] J. R. C. Almeida, A. Mechelli, S. Hassel, A. Versace, D. J. Kupfer, and M. L. Phillips, "Abnormally increased effective connectivity between parahippocampal gyrus and ventromedial prefrontal regions during emotion labeling in bipolar disorder," *Psychiatry Research*, vol. 174, no. 3, pp. 195–201, 2009.
[63] A. C. van der Schot, R. Vonk, R. M. Brouwer et al., "Genetic and environmental influences on focal brain density in bipolar disorder," *Brain*, vol. 133, no. 10, pp. 3080–3092, 2010.
[64] J. Savitz and W. C. Drevets, "Bipolar and major depressive disorder: neuroimaging the developmental-degenerative divide," *Neuroscience and Biobehavioral Reviews*, vol. 33, no. 5, pp. 699–771, 2009.
[65] R. B. Sassi, J. A. Stanley, D. Axelson et al., "Reduced NAA levels in the dorsolateral prefrontal cortex of young bipolar patients," *American Journal of Psychiatry*, vol. 162, no. 11, pp. 2109–2115, 2005.
[66] C. M. Adler, J. Adams, M. P. DelBello et al., "Evidence of white matter pathology in bipolar disorder adolescents experiencing their first episode of mania: a diffusion tensor imaging study," *American Journal of Psychiatry*, vol. 163, no. 2, pp. 322–324, 2006.
[67] G. Rajkowska, "Cell pathology in bipolar disorder," *Bipolar Disorders*, vol. 4, no. 2, pp. 105–116, 2002.
[68] D. Öngür, W. C. Drevets, and J. L. Price, "Glial reduction in the subgenual prefrontal cortex in mood disorders," *Proceedings of the National Academy of Sciences of the United States of America*, vol. 95, no. 22, pp. 13290–13295, 1998.
[69] C. J. Carter, "EIF2B and oligodendrocyte survival: where nature and nurture meet in bipolar disorder and schizophrenia?" *Schizophrenia Bulletin*, vol. 33, no. 6, pp. 1343–1353, 2007.
[70] D. Cotter, L. Hudson, and S. Landau, "Evidence for orbitofrontal pathology in bipolar disorder and major depression, but not in schizophrenia," *Bipolar Disorders*, vol. 7, no. 4, pp. 358–369, 2005.
[71] S. N. Mitkus, T. M. Hyde, R. Vakkalanka et al., "Expression of oligodendrocyte-associated genes in dorsolateral prefrontal cortex of patients with schizophrenia," *Schizophrenia Research*, vol. 98, no. 1–3, pp. 129–138, 2008.
[72] J. A. Frazier, J. L. Breeze, G. Papadimitriou et al., "White matter abnormalities in children with and at risk for bipolar disorder," *Bipolar Disorders*, vol. 9, no. 8, pp. 799–809, 2007.

[73] S. Copray, J. L. Huynh, F. Sher, P. Casaccia-Bonnefil, and E. Boddeke, "Epigenetic mechanisms facilitating oligodendrocyte development, maturation, and aging," *Glia*, vol. 57, no. 15, pp. 1579–1587, 2009.

[74] S. P. Mahadik and R. E. Scheffer, "Oxidative injury and potential use of antioxidants in schizophrenia," *Prostaglandins Leukotrienes and Essential Fatty Acids*, vol. 55, no. 1-2, pp. 45–54, 1996.

[75] S. Y. Yao, A. Ljunggren-Rose, N. Chandramohan, W. O. Whetsell, and S. Sriram, "In vitro and in vivo induction and activation of nNOS by LPS in oligodendrocytes," *Journal of Neuroimmunology*, vol. 229, no. 1-2, pp. 146–156, 2010.

[76] C. Matute, "Interaction between glutamate signalling and immune attack in damaging oligodendrocytes," *Neuron Glia Biology*, vol. 3, no. 4, pp. 281–285, 2007.

[77] L. Tebartz van Elst, G. Valerius, M. Büchert et al., "Increased prefrontal and hippocampal glutamate concentration in schizophrenia: evidence from a magnetic resonance spectroscopy study," *Biological Psychiatry*, vol. 58, no. 9, pp. 724–730, 2005.

[78] J. T. Coyle, "Glutamate and schizophrenia: beyond the dopamine hypothesis," *Cellular and Molecular Neurobiology*, vol. 26, no. 4–6, pp. 365–384, 2006.

[79] S. Prabakaran, J. E. Swatton, M. M. Ryan et al., "Mitochondrial dysfunction in schizophrenia: evidence for compromised brain metabolism and oxidative stress," *Molecular Psychiatry*, vol. 9, no. 7, p. 643, 2004.

[80] E. Courchesne, H. J. Chisum, J. Townsend et al., "Normal brain development and aging: qantitative analysis at in vivo MR imaging in healthy volunteers," *Radiology*, vol. 216, no. 3, pp. 672–682, 2000.

[81] G. Bartzokis, M. Beckson, P. H. Lu, K. H. Nuechterlein, N. Edwards, and J. Mintz, "Age-related changes in frontal and temporal lobe volumes in men: a magnetic resonance imaging study," *Archives of General Psychiatry*, vol. 58, no. 5, pp. 461–465, 2001.

[82] T. L. Jernigan and C. Fennema-Notestine, "White matter mapping is needed," *Neurobiology of Aging*, vol. 25, no. 1, pp. 37–39, 2004.

[83] P. Katsel, K. L. Davis, C. Li et al., "Abnormal indices of cell cycle activity in schizophrenia and their potential association with oligodendrocytes," *Neuropsychopharmacology*, vol. 33, no. 12, pp. 2993–3009, 2008.

[84] K. Barley, S. Dracheva, and W. Byne, "Subcortical oligodendrocyte- and astrocyte-associated gene expression in subjects with schizophrenia, major depression and bipolar disorder," *Schizophrenia Research*, vol. 112, no. 1–3, pp. 54–64, 2009.

[85] R. S. Kern, J. M. Gold, D. Dickinson et al., "The MCCB impairment profile for schizophrenia outpatients: results from the MATRICS psychometric and standardization study," *Schizophrenia Research*, vol. 126, no. 1–3, pp. 124–131, 2011.

[86] G. T. Konopaske, K. A. Dorph-Petersen, R. A. Sweet et al., "Effect of chronic antipsychotic exposure on astrocyte and oligodendrocyte numbers in macaque monkeys," *Biological Psychiatry*, vol. 63, no. 8, pp. 759–765, 2008.

[87] B.-C. Ho, N. C. Andreasen, S. Ziebell, R. Pierson, and V. Magnotta, "Long-term antipsychotic treatment and brain volumes: a longitudinal study of first-episode schizophrenia," *Archives of General Psychiatry*, vol. 68, no. 2, pp. 128–137, 2011.

[88] J. Moncrieff and J. Leo, "A systematic review of the effects of antipsychotic drugs on brain volume," *Psychological Medicine*, pp. 1–14, 2010.

[89] J. Steiner, Z. Sarnyai, S. Westphal et al., "Protective effects of haloperidol and clozapine on energy-deprived OLN-93 oligodendrocytes," *European Archives of Psychiatry and Clinical Neuroscience*. In press.

[90] H. Wang, H. Xu, J. Niu et al., "Haloperidol activates quiescent oligodendroglia precursor cells in the adult mouse brain," *Schizophrenia Research*, vol. 119, no. 1–3, pp. 164–174, 2010.

[91] B. D. Butts, C. Houde, and H. Mehmet, "Maturation-dependent sensitivity of oligodendrocyte lineage cells to apoptosis: implications for normal development and disease," *Cell Death and Differentiation*, vol. 15, no. 7, pp. 1178–1186, 2008.

[92] A. Gritti, M. D. Molin, C. Foroni, and L. Bonfanti, "Effects of developmental age, brain region, and time in culture on long-term proliferation and multipotency of neural stem cell populations," *Journal of Comparative Neurology*, vol. 517, no. 3, pp. 333–349, 2009.

[93] Y. He, W. Cai, L. Wang, and P. Chen, "A developmental study on the expression of PDGFαR immunoreactive cells in the brain of postnatal rats," *Neuroscience Research*, vol. 65, no. 3, pp. 272–279, 2009.

[94] A. Reif, S. Fritzen, M. Finger et al., "Neural stem cell proliferation is decreased in schizophrenia, but not in depression," *Molecular Psychiatry*, vol. 11, no. 5, pp. 514–522, 2006.

[95] F. M. Benes, "The relationship between structural brain imaging and histopathologic findings in schizophrenia research," *Harvard Review of Psychiatry*, vol. 1, no. 2, pp. 100–109, 1993.

[96] S. Akbarian, J. J. Kim, S. G. Potkin, W. P. Hetrick, W. E. Bunney Jr., and E. G. Jones, "Maldistribution of interstitial neurons in prefrontal white matter of the brains of schizophrenic patients," *Archives of General Psychiatry*, vol. 53, no. 5, pp. 425–436, 1996.

[97] N. Mellios, H. S. Huang, S. P. Baker, M. Galdzicka, E. Ginns, and S. Akbarian, "Molecular determinants of dysregulated GABAergic gene expression in the prefrontal cortex of subjects with schizophrenia," *Biological Psychiatry*, vol. 65, no. 12, pp. 1006–1014, 2009.

2

Clinical Practice Associated with a Switch from and to Ziprasidone during Routine Inpatient Treatment of Patients with Schizophrenia

Matthias J. Müller

Clinic for Psychiatry and Psychotherapy Giessen and Marburg, Vitos Clinical Centre Giessen-Marburg, Academic Teaching Hospital, University of Giessen, Licher Strasse 106, 35392 Giessen, Germany

Correspondence should be addressed to Matthias J. Müller, mjmueller@gmx.de

Academic Editor: Luis San

Ziprasidone (ZIP) shows a low propensity for metabolic side effects but can prolong QTc time. It is unclear how these features translate into clinical reality. Charts of inpatients with schizophrenia and switched from (ZIP−, $n = 27$) or to ZIP (ZIP+, $n = 24$) were reviewed. Clinical data including documented switch reasons were anonymously analyzed. Comorbidity, body mass index (BMI) at admission, illness severity, side effects, illness duration, and length of stay were comparable in both groups. About 2/3 of ZIP+ were women (1/3 of ZIP−, $P = 0.035$); ZIP+ patients were younger ($P = 0.017$), had higher BMI values ($P = 0.042$), and received higher chlorpromazine equivalents before switch ($P = 0.004$) whereas ZIP doses were comparable (136 versus 141 mg/d). More patients in ZIP− versus ZIP+ were switched because of previous weight gain ($P = 0.006$) and depression ($P = 0.085$) whereas single reasons for ZIP− versus ZIP+ were mainly persisting positive symptoms ($P = 0.089$) and patients' choice ($P = 0.10$). The results of the naturalistic study corroborate controlled trials.

1. Introduction

Ziprasidone (ZIP) is one of the second-generation antipsychotics (SGA) with proven low propensity for unwanted metabolic changes (weight gain, hyperlipidemia, hyperglycemia, etc.) [1, 2]. Thus, together with aripiprazole, ZIP is an alternative to conventional, first-generation antipsychotics (FGA), particularly if metabolic syndrome has to be avoided or if metabolic changes have occurred under treatment with other SGAs or FGAs.

ZIP was approved in 2001 as the fifth SGA by the FDA for treatment of schizophrenia (approval in Germany 2002). The approval has been extended for acute treatment of mania and mixed states associated with bipolar disorder. ZIP has a highly selective affinity for 5-HT2A receptors relative to D2 and 5-HT2C receptors compared to other FGAs and SGAs and shows also high blocking affinity for alpha-adrenergic receptors and a moderate antagonistic affinity for histamine H1-receptors [3]. This pharmacodynamic profile of ZIP explains the antipsychotic effects and some of the side effects of ZIP such as sedation and orthostasis [4, 5]. A modest inhibition of synaptic serotonin and norepinephrine reuptake of ZIP has been suggested to be involved in some antidepressant properties, although clinical significance is questionable [6]. ZIP is hepatically metabolized by aldehyde oxidase and via cytochrome P450 3A4 (CYP3A4). Absorption and sufficient bioavailability are dependent on sufficient preceding food intake (>500 kcal) [7, 8]. ZIP can slightly increase the QTc interval and the risk of potentially fatal arrhythmias [9].

In recent meta-analyses [2, 10] the effects of ZIP were compared with other SGAs in patients with schizophrenia and related disorders. According to these data, the rate of premature study discontinuation with ZIP was very high (59.1%) and early discontinuation—due to any reason—was higher than with olanzapine and risperidone, but not higher than with other SGAs. Additionally, ZIP was found to be slightly less efficacious than amisulpride, olanzapine, and risperidone in a meta-analysis [2]. Due to limited data no significant differences in tolerability between ZIP and amisulpride or clozapine were found, but ZIP produced consistently less weight gain than olanzapine, quetiapine, or risperidone. ZIP was associated with less cholesterol increase than olanzapine, quetiapine and risperidone. ZIP produced slightly higher rates of extrapyramidal side effects than olanzapine, but lower than risperidone. Prolactin increase with ZIP was greater than with quetiapine, but lower than with risperidone. In summary, despite a slightly lower efficacy compared to amisulpride, olanzapine, and risperidone, the greatest advantage of ZIP is a low propensity to induce weight gain [1, 2, 10, 11] and associated adverse effects (metabolic syndrome).

Open studies reporting on the switch from other antipsychotics to ZIP have found beneficial effects of ZIP on metabolic changes and no worsening of psychopathology [5, 12–15]. These studies were partially extensions of randomized controlled studies or open studies designed to investigate clinical effects of ZIP. However, whereas these studies have reported effects of switching to ZIP (ZIP+) under more or less standardized conditions, little is known regarding the reasons for a switch from ZIP (ZIP−) to other antipsychotics and ZIP+ under real-life conditions. Therefore, the clinical database of a routine care psychiatric hospital was searched for patients with ZIP+ and ZIP− to explore the characteristics of both patients' groups and main reasons for switch.

2. Materials and Methods

We searched for all inpatients of the psychiatric state hospital (107 inpatient beds) in Marburg, Germany, hospitalized in the years 2007–2009 using the following criteria: diagnosis of schizophrenic disorder according to ICD-10 (F20), documented switch from other antipsychotics to ZIP (antipsychotic monotherapy; ZIP+), or documented switch from ZIP (antipsychotic monotherapy) to other antipsychotics (ZIP−) within the first two weeks of hospitalization.

The available guidelines for schizophrenia treatment, for rationale, individualized pharmacotherapy, and for informed consent are part of the quality management of the clinic and summarized in a clinical pathway. Nonetheless, switch of antipsychotic drugs is to a great extent still left up to the discretion of physicians and patients.

A total group of 1059 inpatients (1737 cases) with schizophrenia (ICD-10 F20) was found in the register. Out of this population, 27 patients (2.5%) were switched to ziprasidone (ZIP+), and 24 patients (2.3%) were switched from ziprasidone to other antipsychotics (ZIP−) during hospitalization and routine inpatient treatment and were eligible according to the above criteria. In total, eight psychiatrists and one attending were involved in the treatment of ZIP+ and ZIP− patients.

A chart analysis of these two groups was carried out by two independent experienced clinicians not involved in the treatment of the patients. Severity of global illness at admission and discharge were judged with 7-point global assessment ratings (clinical global impression, CGI; (1) normal, not at all ill; (2) borderline mentally ill; (3) mildly ill; (4) moderately ill; (5) markedly ill; (6) severely ill; (7) extremely ill) using all available information. Accordingly, global severity of side effects was judged on a pragmatic 4-point scale (0 = none; 1 = mild; 2 = moderate; 3 = severe). The severity rating of side effects comprised all documented aspects of possibly drug-related signs and symptoms, for example, extrapyramidal symptoms (EPS), sedation, agitation, and sexual dysfunction. Variation in reporting and documentation made it impossible to analyze specific side effects.

Only patients with documented switch were included in the present study. All documented reasons for ZIP+ or ZIP− were listed and categorized in two steps. The first categorization step comprised nine switch reasons (multiple entries were possible): persisting positive symptoms, severe and burdensome depression, severe and disabling negative symptoms, interfering sedation, intolerable weight gain, severe agitation, intolerable EPS, other side effects, and the patient's choice. The latter consisted of admitted discontinuation and noncompliance and of alleged specific desires to change the antipsychotic without further explanation. The second step of categorizing reasons led to three broad categories of one main switch reason per patient: lack of effectiveness, side effects, and patients' choice. As more than one reason for a switch was possible at the first categorization step, the assumed single main reason (second step) was finally judged using all available information.

Body weight and body mass indices were obtained from the charts at admission or within 1 week after admission. Further laboratory and metabolic parameters and changes could not be analyzed.

Psychotropic medication at discharge and antipsychotic medication directly before switching was assessed in both groups. Chlorpromazine equivalents (CPZE) were calculated on the basis of daily doses for antipsychotic medication according to the literature [16–18]. Clinical data were compared between both groups (ZIP−/ZIP+). For categorical data, χ^2 tests were used, for continuous data t-tests for independent groups were applied. The level of statistical significance was set at $\alpha = 0.05$; results with $P < 0.10$ were reported as statistical trend due to the exploratory nature of the study.

3. Results

In both groups switch of antipsychotics occurred in most cases at admission or by cross-tapering within 10 days (Table 1) due to acute exacerbation requiring hospitalization. Table 1 shows clinical data of the two groups with patients switched either from or to ZIP.

Significantly more female patients were switched to ZIP ($P < 0.05$); additionally, these patients were younger ($P < 0.05$) and had higher BMI values ($P < 0.05$) than patients switched from ZIP to other antipsychotics (ZIP+). At admission chlorpromazine equivalents (CPZE) were significantly higher in ZIP+, and after switching to ZIP+, CPZE were significantly lower at discharge ($P < 0.01$). ZIP daily doses were comparable in both groups (after or before switching, resp.). Comparably high proportions of patients in ZIP+ and

Table 1: Switch from or to ziprasidone: clinical data.

	ZIP+ switch to ziprasidone	ZIP− switch from ziprasidone	Difference
N	24	27	n.s.[b]
Diagnoses (ICD-10)			n.s.[b]
F20.0	18 (75.0%)	21 (77.8%)	
F20.1	2 (8.3%)	1 (3.7%)	
F20.3	4 (4.2%)	3 (11.1%)	
F20.4	0	2 (7.4%)	
Comorbidity (ICD-10)			
None	6 (25.0%)	16 (59.3%)	$P = 0.025$[b]
1	11 (45.8%)	9 (33.3%)	
2	7 (29.2%)	2 (7.4)%)	
F1 substance abuse[c]	12 (50.0%)	8 (29.6%)	n.s[b]
F43 adjustment disorder	6 (25.0%)	2 (7.4%)	$P = 0.085$[b]
F60 personality disorder	2 (8.3%)	1 (3.7%)	n.s.[b]
Women	16 (67%)	10 (37%)	$P = 0.035$[b]
Age	40.6 (8.9)	47.2 (10.3)	$P = 0.017$[a]
BMI at admission (kg/m^2)	26.9 (3.2)	25.1 (2.7)	$P = 0.042$[a]
Women	26.9 (3.8)	24.0 (2.4)	$P = 0.047$[a]
Men	26.8 (1.5)	25.7 (2.8)	n.s[a]
Switch modalities			
Start/stop (abrupt change)	16 (67%)	17 (63%)	n.s.[b]
Tapering time (days)	2.3 (3.5)	2.4 (3.6)	n.s.[a]
Illness duration (years)	14.3 (7.8)	16.4 (10.0)	n.s.[a]
Hospitalization (days)	40.0 (21.2)	46.1 (43.7)	n.s.[a]
Ziprasidone dose	140.8 (27.8)	136.3 (38.0)	n.s.[a]
Minimum	80	80	
Maximum	180	240	
CPZE before switch	889 (291)	681 (190)	$P = 0.004$[a]
CPZE after switch	704 (140)	831 (340)	$P = 0.094$[a]
Psychotropic comedication: none	5 (20.8%)	5 (18.5%)	n.s.[b]
Laboratory abnormalities[d]	3 (12.5%)	1 (3.7%)	n.s.[b]
ECG abnormalities[e]	4 (16.7%)	4 (14.8%)	n.s.[b]
QTc prolongation >460 msec	0	0	n.s.[b]
Severity at admission	5.3 (0.61)	5.2 (0.64)	n.s.[a]
Severity at discharge	3.2 (0.89)	3.0 (0.85)	n.s.[a]
Change severity	2.0 (0.95)	2.2 (1.08)	n.s.[a]
Side effects at admission	1.1 (0.88)	0.9 (0.70)	n.s.[a]
Side effects at discharge	0.5 (0.59)	0.6 (0.64)	n.s.[a]
Change side effects	0.5 (0.78)	0.3 (0.62)	n.s.[a]

[a]t-test (independent groups); [b]χ^2 test; [c]F1 including alcohol abuse/dependence, THC abuse/dependence, benzodiazepine dependence, opioid abuse, multiple substance abuse (excluded: nicotine dependence); [d]ZIP+: creatine kinase (2-fold), hyperglycemia, yGT (189 U/L); ZIP−: serum creatinine (1.4 mg/dL); [e]ZIP+: AVB I°, repolarisation disturbance, nonspecific conduction disturbance (2); ZIP−: AVB I° (2), nonspecific conduction disturbance, abnormal repolarisation; n.s.: not significant; severity of illness was judged by 7-point ratings (CGI), side effects by a global severity rating (0–3).

ZIP− received psychotropic comedication (ZIP+ 79% versus ZIP− 82%). Clinical severity and side-effect judgements were comparable in both groups. Table 2 shows the psychotropic medication before and after switching from or to ZIP.

The patterns of medication were similar in both groups, in the ZIP+ seven patients were switched from FGA to ZIP; in the ZIP+ group seven patients versus four in the ZIP− group received concomitant antidepressant treatment, one patient in ZIP+ received two antidepressants (sertraline + mirtazapine). In Table 3 clinical reasons for switching to or from ZIP are reported; in some cases more than one reason for switching was recorded.

Significantly more patients were switched to ZIP because of weight gain during pretreatment ($P < 0.05$), depression, and extrapyramidal symptoms were found as reasons for a switch with a statistical tendency in favor of ZIP+

Table 2: Switching from or to ZIP: psychotropic medication.

	ZIP+ switch to ziprasidone	ZIP− switch from ziprasidone
Antipsychotic medication before	Amisulpride (1)	Amisulpride (2)
switch/after switch[a]	Aripiprazole (2)	Aripiprazole (2)
		Clozapine (3)
	Flupenthixol (4)	
	Haloperidol (2)	
	Olanzapine (2)	Olanzapine (1)
		Paliperidone (4)
	Perazine (1)	Perazine (1)
	Quetiapine (5)	Quetiapine (7)
	Risperidone (7)	Risperidone (6)
		None (1)
Comedication at discharge[b]		
Low-potency neuroleptics	Chlorprothixene (1)	Chlorprothixene (4)
	Promethazine (1)	Promethazine (1)
	Melperone (6)	Melperone (4)
	Pipamperone (3)	Pipamperone (3)
Mood stabilizer	Valproic acid (3)	Valproic acid (1)
	Pregabalin (2)	Carbamazepine (1)
Antidepressants		Doxepin (1)
	Mirtazapine (2)	Mirtazapine (2)
	Citalopram (3)	
	Sertraline (1)	Sertraline (1)
	Trimipramine (1)	
	Moclobemide (1)	
Other	Benzodiazepine (8)	Benzodiazepine (10)
	Biperiden (1)	Biperiden (3)

[a]monotherapy; [b]combination treatment in 57% of patients (29/51).

Table 3: Switching to or from ziprasidone-reasons for switch of antipsychotics.

Reason for switch	ZIP+ switch to ziprasidone	ZIP− switch from ziprasidone	Difference χ^2 test
N	24	27	
Positive symptoms[a]	6 (25.0%)	13 (48.1%)	$P = 0.088$
Depression[a]	6 (25.0%)	2 (7.4%)	$P = 0.085$
Negative symptoms[a]	5 (20.8%)	7 (25.9%)	n.s.
Sedation[b]	1 (4.2%)	3 (11.1%)	n.s.
Weight gain[b]	8 (33.3%)	1 (3.7%)	$P = 0.006$
Agitation[b]	—	1 (3.7%)	n.s.
EPS[b]	5 (20.8%)	1 (3.7%)	$P = 0.058$
Other side effects[b]	2 (8.3%)	1 (3.7%)	n.s.
Patient's choice[c]	4 (16.7%)	10 (37.0%)	$P = 0.10$

More than one reason possible (multiple entries); [a]lack of effectiveness; [b]side effects; [c]patients' choice; EPS, extrapyramidal symptoms.

($P < 0.10$). Reasons for a switch from ZIP were persisting positive symptoms and patients' choice with a slightly higher frequency ($P \leq 0.10$) in ZIP− compared to ZIP+.

The categorized main reasons for switch (lack of effectiveness, side effects, and patients' choice; only one per patient) were not significantly different between ZIP+ and ZIP− (χ^2 test, $P = 0.39$). Figure 1 illustrates the distribution of categories in both groups.

The main reason for a switch from ZIP (ZIP−) was lack of effectiveness regarding positive, negative, or affective symptoms of schizophrenia (approximately 50%). Side effects and the subjective choice of patients possibly relating

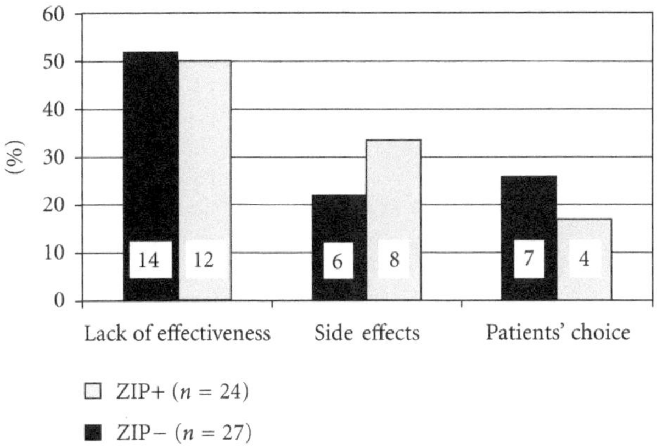

FIGURE 1: Main reasons for a switch from or to ziprasidone ZIP−, switch from ziprasidone; ZIP+, switch to ziprasidone.

to both psychopathology and unwanted effects of treatment were nearly equally distributed (both approximately 25%).

4. Discussion

The switch to or from ZIP during routine clinical treatment of schizophrenia was reviewed in a German psychiatric state hospital. Data were retrospectively analyzed to investigate whether the properties of ZIP found in controlled studies and meta-analyses are implicitly or explicitly considered in real-life situations. A proportion of patients <10% received ZIP indicating that ZIP is not a first-line treatment for schizophrenia in Germany. If the low propensity of ZIP for unwanted metabolic changes compared to other antipsychotic compounds is clinically relevant, reasons for a switch to ZIP (ZIP+) should reflect this aspect compared to ZIP−. The results of the present study corroborate this hypothesis as more patients with ZIP+ were switched because of previous weight gain than patients with ZIP−. Moreover, BMI values at baseline were significantly higher at least in women with schizophrenia switched to ZIP (ZIP+) in comparison to ZIP−.

Despite guidelines and clinical pathways the decision to change an antipsychotic drug and which substance is used remains often on a consensus between the patient and the physicians who are in charge. Thus, the results of the present analysis are not independent of subjective aspects of clinical decision making [19]. According to available guidelines and recommendations, ZIP and aripiprazole are considered superior in patients with schizophrenia and weight or metabolic problems [19, 20]. However, in large-scale analyses of US data the physicians' adherence to these recommendations seems to be low [21]. In larger trials [2, 22] ZIP treatment of schizophrenia was discontinued in a high proportion of >50% of patients within 12–18 months, probably more than under other SGAs. This question could not be evaluated with the present data, as only a single switch (from or to ZIP) was focused in the present study, the switch occurred in the first two weeks of treatment, and patients were not followedup. Nonetheless, the patients' choice to change ZIP was one reason among others to switch in 1/3 and the main reason to switch from ZIP in 1/4 of patients in the present study and may reflect the early discontinuation found in meta-analyses which was not caused by metabolic effects or weight gain but by a lack of efficacy [2, 10].

Patients switched to ZIP were younger and had tentatively more affective symptoms and psychiatric comorbidity, and more women were in the ZIP+ group whereas subtype of schizophrenia, severity and duration of illness, and global severity of side-effect were not different between ZIP+ and ZIP−. These findings are in line with previous reports [14, 15, 23, 24]. The mean daily doses of ZIP were approximately 140 mg in both groups according to recommended and widely used doses of ZIP [25, 26]. The results can thus not confirm findings that higher doses of ZIP are more effective in some patients with schizophrenia [27] although the proportion of patients switched from ZIP due to apparent ineffectiveness was rather high. Switching to ZIP resulted in lower daily chlorpromazine equivalents for patients. This finding is conforming with recent suggestions [28] but could also have resulted from still questionable equivalent doses [18].

The methodological limitations of a retrospective chart analysis based on semistandardized clinical data hamper the generalization of the present findings. First, the low proportion of patients switched to or from ZIP within three years seems to reflect the actual market share of ZIP in Germany for schizophrenia treatment but resulted in a rather low sample size. Selection bias due to specific implicit treatment strategies in this single-site study cannot be ruled out completely despite an implemented clinical pathway for the treatment of schizophrenia. Mult-center studies could avoid this source of bias in the future. The data concerning psychopathology and the decision to switch were derived from the original charts whereas medication at admission and discharge were taken from discharge letters. Both parts of information can be questioned regarding reliability. However, continuous reports during the course of treatment and widely standardized discharge letters support the applied method.

Furthermore, one could criticize that subjective "weight gain" and not objectively assessed body weight, body mass index, or laboratory measures of metabolic changes were reported as in controlled studies published in the literature. However, beside the fact that reliable data on weight before and after switch to or from ZIP were not obtainable objective weight gain during a rather short time period is of questionable value. From the clinical standpoint, the patients' view [22] seems to be much more important for treatment success and adherence. A recent study in first-episode patients showed that patients' attitudes beside positive symptoms and sexual dysfunction were the strongest predictors of treatment success [29]. In this perspective our data may offer some "ecological validity" in addition to controlled, but more artificial conditions in many randomized trials. Furthermore, the aspect of "shared decision making" contains the patients' view explicitly and is in the present study also reflected in the finding, that a great number of patients (14/51, 27%) were switched mainly due to their own choice. This was by tendency more frequently the case for a switch from ZIP.

5. Conclusions

In summary, the data reflect some findings from large randomized trials regarding the use of ZIP in the treatment of schizophrenia in a routine inpatient care setting but show also the limitations and restrictions of transferring such results into real life. Switching antipsychotics should be considered early in the course of treatment if effectiveness is lacking [30], and a switch due to side effects, particularly weight gain and metabolic changes, can be cost-effective [31] in the long run. In this regard, ZIP seems to be a reasonable option in clinical routine for the treatment of schizophrenia. However, medication decisions should always be made collaboratively between the patient and his treating clinician.

References

[1] C. Rummel-Kluge, K. Komossa, S. Schwarz et al., "Head-to-head comparisons of metabolic side effects of second generation antipsychotics in the treatment of schizophrenia: a systematic review and meta-analysis," *Schizophrenia Research*, vol. 123, no. 2-3, pp. 225–233, 2010.

[2] K. Komossa, C. Rummel-Kluge, H. Hunger et al., "Ziprasidone versus other atypical antipsychotics for schizophrenia," *Cochrane Database of Systematic Reviews*, no. 4, Article ID CD006627, 2009.

[3] T. F. Seeger, P. A. Seymour, A. W. Schmidt et al., "Ziprasidone (CP-88,059): a new antipsychotic with combined dopamine and serotonin receptor antagonist activity," *Journal of Pharmacology and Experimental Therapeutics*, vol. 275, no. 1, pp. 101–113, 1995.

[4] A. Schotte, P. F. M. Janssen, W. Gommeren et al., "Risperidone compared with new and reference antipsychotic drugs: in vitro and in vivo receptor binding," *Psychopharmacology*, vol. 124, no. 1-2, pp. 57–73, 1996.

[5] S. W. Kim, I. S. Shin, J. M. Kim, K. Y. Bae, S. J. Yang, and J. S. Yoon, "Effectiveness of switching from aripiprazole to ziprasidone in patients with schizophrenia," *Clinical Neuropharmacology*, vol. 33, no. 3, pp. 121–125, 2010.

[6] H. J. Möller, "Antipsychotic and antidepressive effects of second generation antipsychotics: two different pharmacological mechanisms?" *European Archives of Psychiatry and Clinical Neuroscience*, vol. 255, no. 3, pp. 190–201, 2005.

[7] J. J. Miceli, P. Glue, J. Alderman et al., "The effect of food on the absorption of oral ziprasidone," *Psychopharmacology Bulletin*, vol. 40, pp. 58–68, 2007.

[8] J. Lincoln, M. E. Stewart, and S. H. Preskorn, "How sequential studies inform drug development: evaluating the effect of Food intake on optimal bioavailability of ziprasidone," *Journal of Psychiatric Practice*, vol. 16, no. 2, pp. 103–114, 2010.

[9] P. A. Alvarez and J. Pahissa, "QT alterations in psychopharmacology: proven candidates and suspects," *Current Drug Safety*, vol. 5, no. 1, pp. 97–104, 2010.

[10] S. Leucht, D. Arbter, R. R. Engel, W. Kissling, and J. M. Davis, "How effective are second-generation antipsychotic drugs? A meta-analysis of placebo-controlled trials," *Molecular Psychiatry*, vol. 14, no. 4, pp. 429–447, 2009.

[11] B. Parsons, D. B. Allison, A. Loebel et al., "Weight effects associated with antipsychotics: a comprehensive database analysis," *Schizophrenia Research*, vol. 110, no. 1–3, pp. 103–110, 2009.

[12] P. F. Buckley, P. D. Harvey, C. R. Bowie, and A. Loebel, "The relationship between symptomatic remission and neuropsychological improvement in schizophrenia patients switched to treatment with ziprasidone," *Schizophrenia Research*, vol. 94, no. 1–3, pp. 99–106, 2007.

[13] G. M. Simpson, C. J. O'Gorman, A. Loebel, and R. Yang, "Long-term improvement in efficacy and safety after switching to ziprasidone in stable outpatients with schizophrenia," *CNS Spectrums*, vol. 13, no. 10, pp. 898–905, 2008.

[14] K. Alptekin, J. Hafez, S. Brook et al., "Efficacy and tolerability of switching to ziprasidone from olanzapine, risperidone or haloperidol: an international, multicenter study," *International Clinical Psychopharmacology*, vol. 24, no. 5, pp. 229–238, 2009.

[15] E. Stip, S. Zhornitsky, S. Potvin, and V. Tourjman, "Switching from conventional antipsychotics to ziprasidone: a randomized, open-label comparison of regimen strategies," *Progress in Neuro-Psychopharmacology and Biological Psychiatry*, vol. 34, no. 6, pp. 997–1000, 2010.

[16] S. W. Woods, "Chlorpromazine equivalent doses for the newer atypical antipsychotics," *Journal of Clinical Psychiatry*, vol. 64, no. 6, pp. 663–667, 2003.

[17] O. Benkert and H. Hippius, *Kompendium der Psychiatrischen Pharmakotherapie*, Springer, Berlin, Germany, 2010.

[18] N. C. Andreasen, M. Pressler, P. Nopoulos, D. Miller, and B. C. Ho, "Antipsychotic dose equivalents and dose-years: a standardized method for comparing exposure to different drugs," *Biological Psychiatry*, vol. 67, no. 3, pp. 255–262, 2010.

[19] P. J. Weiden, S. H. Preskorn, P. A. Fahnestock, D. Carpenter, R. Ross, and J. P. Docherty, "Translating the psychopharmacology of antipsychotics to individualized treatment for severe mental illness: a roadmap," *Journal of Clinical Psychiatry*, vol. 68, supplement 7, pp. 1–48, 2007.

[20] A. Mukundan, G. Faulkner, T. Cohn, and G. Remington, "Antipsychotic switching for people with schizophrenia who have neuroleptic-induced weight or metabolic problems," *Cochrane Database of Systematic Reviews*, vol. 12, Article ID CD006629, 2010.

[21] E. H. Morrato, B. Cuffel, J. W. Newcomer, I. Lombardo, S. Kamat, and J. Barron, "Metabolic risk status and second-generation antipsychotic drug selection: a retrospective study of commercially insured patients," *Journal of Clinical Psychopharmacology*, vol. 29, no. 1, pp. 26–32, 2009.

[22] D. Naber and M. Lambert, "The CATIE and CUtLASS studies in schizophrenia: results and implications for clinicians," *CNS Drugs*, vol. 23, no. 8, pp. 649–659, 2009.

[23] A. W. Nyhuis, D. E. Faries, H. Ascher-Svanum, V. L. Stauffer, and B. J. Kinon, "Predictors of switching antipsychotic medications in the treatment of schizophrenia," *BMC Psychiatry*, vol. 10, p. 75, 2010.

[24] S. M. Stahl, A. Malla, J. W. Newcomer et al., "A post hoc analysis of negative symptoms and psychosocial function in patients with schizophrenia: a 40-week randomized, double-blind study of ziprasidone versus haloperidol followed by a 3-year double-blind extension trial," *Journal of Clinical Psychopharmacology*, vol. 30, no. 4, pp. 425–430, 2010.

[25] P. J. Weiden, N. Iqbal, A. J. Mendelowitz et al., "Best clinical practice with ziprasidone: update after one year of experience," *Journal of Psychiatric Practice*, vol. 8, pp. 81–97, 2002.

[26] A. Fagiolini, F. Caas, B. Gallhofer et al., "Strategies for successful clinical management of schizophrenia with ziprasidone," *Expert Opinion on Pharmacotherapy*, vol. 11, no. 13, pp. 2199–2220, 2010.

[27] D. Kudla, M. Lambert, S. Domin, S. Kasper, and D. Naber, "Effectiveness, tolerability, and safety of ziprasidone in patients with schizophrenia or schizoaffective disorder: results of a multi-centre observational trial," *European Psychiatry*, vol. 22, no. 3, pp. 195–202, 2007.

[28] S. Yamin and K. Vaddadi, "Are we using excessive neuroleptics? an argument for systematic neuroleptic dose reduction in stable patients with schizophrenia with specific reference to clozapine," *International Review of Psychiatry*, vol. 22, no. 2, pp. 138–147, 2010.

[29] W. Gaebel, M. Riesbeck, M. von Wilmsdorff et al., "Drug attitude as predictor for effectiveness in first-episode schizophrenia: results of an open randomized trial (EUFEST)," *European Neuropsychopharmacology*, vol. 20, no. 5, pp. 310–316, 2010.

[30] E. M. Derks, W. W. Fleischhacker, H. Boter, J. Peuskens, and R. S. Kahn, "Antipsychotic drug treatment in first-episode psychosis should patients be switched to a different antipsychotic drug after 2, 4, or 6 weeks of nonresponse?" *Journal of Clinical Psychopharmacology*, vol. 30, no. 2, pp. 176–180, 2010.

[31] R. S. McIntyre, L. Cragin, S. Sorensen, H. Naci, T. Baker, and J. P. Roussy, "Comparison of the metabolic and economic consequences of long-term treatment of schizophrenia using ziprasidone, olanzapine, quetiapine and risperidone in Canada: a cost-effectiveness analysis," *Journal of Evaluation in Clinical Practice*, vol. 16, no. 4, pp. 744–755, 2010.

3

Cannabinoids for the Treatment of Schizophrenia? A Balanced Neurochemical Framework for Both Adverse and Therapeutic Effects of Cannabis Use

Carissa M. Coulston,[1,2] Michael Perdices,[1,3] Antony F. Henderson,[1] and Gin S. Malhi[1,2]

[1] *Discipline of Psychiatry, Sydney Medical School, University of Sydney, NSW 2006, Australia*
[2] *Department of Psychiatry, CADE Clinic, Royal North Shore Hospital, St. Leonards, Sydney, NSW 2065, Australia*
[3] *Department of Neurology, Royal North Shore Hospital, St. Leonards, Sydney, NSW 2065, Australia*

Correspondence should be addressed to Gin S. Malhi, gin.malhi@sydney.edu.au

Academic Editor: David C. Henderson

Recent studies have found that cannabinoids may improve neuropsychological performance, ameliorate negative symptoms, and have antipsychotic properties for a subgroup of the schizophrenia population. These findings are in contrast to the longstanding history of adverse consequences of cannabis use, predominantly on the positive symptoms, and a balanced neurochemical basis for these opposing views is lacking. This paper details a review of the neurobiological substrates of schizophrenia and the neurochemical effects of cannabis use in the normal population, in both cortical (in particular prefrontal) and subcortical brain regions. The aim of this paper is to provide a holistic neurochemical framework in which to understand how cannabinoids may impair, or indeed, serve to ameliorate the positive and negative symptoms as well as cognitive impairment. Directions in which future research can proceed to resolve the discrepancies are briefly discussed.

1. Introduction

A body of literature over the past three decades has established cannabis use to be a significant risk factor for the onset and development of schizophrenia [1–5], with early onset of use (by age 15) believed to confer greater risk than later onset of use [6]. In a comprehensive meta-analysis of prospective and population-based studies by Moore et al. [7], an increased risk of psychosis was found in individuals who had ever used cannabis, and a dose-response effect was yielded in which greater risk applied to people who used cannabis most frequently. The authors could not, however, draw a definitive causal link between cannabis use and psychosis on grounds that the studies were observational in nature, and no robust evidence supports the view that early-age onset of cannabis use might be more harmful than later-age onset of use. The increased risk of psychosis in people using cannabis from a younger age could indicate greater cumulative exposure to cannabis rather than a sensitive period of exposure.

The high prevalence of cannabis use in schizophrenia combined with observations that cannabis exacerbates the positive symptoms has driven research to investigate why cannabis is used so widely in this population. According to the self-medication hypothesis, there are beneficial effects of cannabis and cannabinoids on the symptoms of schizophrenia. Cross-sectional studies comparing users and nonusers have shown that cannabis use is associated with a reduction in negative symptoms [8–14]. Animal and human models have also suggested that cannabinoids possess antipsychotic properties [15–17]. One of these studies [15] involved a randomised, double-blind controlled trial in 42 patients with acute schizophrenia and found antipsychotic properties of cannabidiol (CBD) that were comparable to amisulpride. Other studies in which CBD has been administered to rats as well as healthy human volunteers have also demonstrated antipsychotic properties of CBD [16, 17].

These mixed findings on how cannabis or cannabinoids impact on the positive and negative symptoms of schizophrenia may in part be attributable to differences in methodology and research design. For example, studies have used different methods to measure cannabis exposure and assess outcome [7], and results are likely to be influenced by whether the studies were observational (prospective versus cross sectional) or experimental (direct drug administration by way of randomised controlled trials or other means). A range of other potential confounding factors are also likely to have contributed to the inconsistent results, particularly where observational designs were employed.

From a neuropsychological perspective, a paucity of research exists. Cannabis use, in some studies of schizophrenia, has been found to be associated with worse neuropsychological performance [18–20]. Conversely, cannabis has been suggested to improve neuropsychological functioning [21–25]. Only one of these studies [18] involved a randomised, double-blind, placebo-controlled trial, in which the effects of i.v. Δ^9-tetrahydrocannabinol (THC) on cognition were studied in 13 stabilised schizophrenia patients and 22 healthy controls, 30 minutes after drug administration. All participants administered THC relative to their placebo baseline performance demonstrated cognitive impairments in domains such as memory and attention, and the schizophrenia group performed more poorly than the control group. Five of the remaining studies [19, 21–25] were cross sectional in nature in which current or past cannabis users with schizophrenia were compared to non current users or those without a past history of use; and one study [20] performed a correlational analysis examining the relationship between level of cannabis use over the preceding year and cognition in persons with a psychotic illness.

Again, the inconsistencies in the findings between these neuropsychological studies are likely to be at least, in part, attributable to methodological variability between the studies, as well as methodological limitations within each study (for full review, see Coulston et al. [26]). For example, different methods were used to measure cannabis exposure, as per the studies detailed earlier which assessed the clinical symptoms. All seven neuropsychological studies used only a single index to classify cannabis use, which does not adequately reflect the variable and fluctuating level of cannabis use that may occur over time in the schizophrenia population. In three instances [19, 22, 23], cannabis use was defined solely with respect to abuse/dependence according to the Diagnostic and Statistical Manual of Mental Disorders, Fourth Edition (DSM-IV) [27]. In one study [18], only the acute effects of cannabis were examined, whilst in another study [21], only the residual, longer-term effects of cannabis were examined in participants who had been abstinent for at least 28 days. Such indices of cannabis use fail to consider factors such as recency and frequency of use (beyond the acute intoxication phase), which have been found to impact on cognition in the normal population [28].

Other limitations in several of these neuropsychological studies, some of which are also relevant to those studies mentioned earlier that focused on the associations between cannabis use and the positive/negative symptoms, include absence of drug screening procedures prior to assessment, restricted range of cognitive functions assessed, minimal or no control of important confounding variables such as current and past history of other substance use (including caffeine and nicotine), and a range of demographic and medical/psychiatric variables (e.g., gender, level of education, premorbid IQ, early-age onset of psychosis, duration of mental illness, medications). Furthermore, several of these studies did not include a control group which limits interpretation of their findings, because it cannot be determined if the cognitive performance of the cannabis users was frankly impaired (i.e., fell below the normal range of performance) or, was in fact within the normal range of performance.

One of the most comprehensive cross-sectional neuropsychological studies to date [29] was conducted by considering all the limitations and range of potential confounds detailed above. The investigators found that cannabis use was associated with enhanced cognitive functioning, predominantly in the areas of attention, processing speed, and executive functioning, domains which rely heavily on prefrontal cortical networks.

Additional reasons for the discrepancies across the literature on the effects of cannabis use on symptomatology and cognition may pertain to the fact that separate and specialised groups of people with schizophrenia react differently to cannabis and other substances. Empirical literature indicates that systematic research on schizophrenia is difficult due to the disorder's heterogeneity and different diagnostic conceptualisations [30], which would imply that the neurochemical imbalances in different brain regions are not equal in all persons. As such, the schizophrenia population is deemed pharmacologically heterogenous [31], in which case the interaction between cannabinoids, neurotransmitters, and antipsychotic treatments is likely to vary between individuals. Subsequently, a balanced neurochemical framework to conceptualise *both* the adverse and potential therapeutic use of cannabinoids for respective groups of the population would be useful for two reasons; first, in light of the new emerging literature supporting a therapeutic benefit for all symptoms, and second, in the context of relatively minimal research that has been conducted in the field of neuropsychology. Further, positing a more balanced neurochemical framework that perhaps underpins an aspect of the core pathophysiology of schizophrenia allows a reconceptualisation of aetiology and treatment of this complex disorder. In particular, a balanced framework promotes awareness that there may not be a unidirectional method of treatment for all subgroups of the population, thereby providing a foundation for novel approaches to investigating the basis of this neuropsychiatric condition.

This paper briefly outlines the neurochemical processes associated with schizophrenia and cannabis use in the normal population, with implications for the effects of cannabinoids on the positive and negative symptoms, as well as cognitive impairment.

2. Symptomatology in Schizophrenia and Neurotransmitter Systems

The effectiveness of conventional antipsychotic medications in alleviating positive symptoms is largely attributed to the blockade of dopamine transmission, especially in the mesolimbic system [32, 33]. Atypical antipsychotics are also believed to exert their therapeutic benefits on psychotic symptoms (in the same cerebral regions) via their antagonistic actions on serotonin, acetylcholine, and noradrenaline receptors [34–37], and via agonistic actions on GABA [35] and glutamate transmission [38]. This suggests that in the unmedicated state, the positive symptoms of schizophrenia are, at least in part, attributable to hyperactivation of dopamine, serotonin, acetylcholine, and noradrenaline, and hypoactivity of GABA and glutamate in the mesolimbic and other subcortical regions.

Moreover, reduced prefrontal dopamine activity is associated with exaggerated striatal dopaminergic activity [39], which is thought to account for the negative symptoms and cognitive impairment. Negative symptoms and cognitive impairments have also been associated with decreased prefrontal acetylcholine, serotonin, noradrenaline, and glutamate [39–47]. The therapeutic action of atypical antipsychotics involves facilitating prefrontal neurotransmission across all of these neurotransmitter systems, except GABA [48–53]. This suggests that in the unmedicated state, the negative symptoms and cognitive impairments of schizophrenia are, at least in part, attributable to hypoactivity of dopamine, serotonin, acetylcholine, noradrenaline, and glutamate in the prefrontal region.

With respect to GABA, although direct enhancement of prefrontal activity would be a potential treatment for schizophrenia [54], atypical antipsychotics tend to exert their effect in the prefrontal cortex by inhibiting release of GABA from interneurons [55]. This subsequently enhances prefrontal neurotransmitter activity. Dopamine and serotonin signalling, associated with antipsychotics, may therefore be responsible for the inhibition of GABAergic currents, and subsequent increase in prefrontal activity [56, 57].

3. The Endocannabinoid System

Cannabinoids exert their effect by binding to specific *endogenous cannabinoid receptors* [58] known as CB1 and CB2, which are located in the CNS and peripherally in the spleen and immune cells [59, 60]. The CB1 receptors are widely distributed in the brain including the cerebral cortex (especially the frontal and medial temporal lobes), limbic areas, basal ganglia, ventral tegmental area, thalamus, hypothalamus, cerebellum, and brainstem [58, 61–65].

CB1 receptors reside within the lipid membrane of the presynaptic neuron terminals, are modulated by the postsynaptic release of endocannabinoids (namely anandamide and 2-arachidonoyl glycerol), and are also influenced by exogenously consumed cannabinoids. CB1 receptors act as neuromodulators through coupling with intracellular G-proteins controlling cyclic adenosine monophosphate (c-AMP) formation and Ca2+ and K+ transport. In this respect, the cannabinoid system has important interactions with several neurotransmitter systems.

Cannabinoids augment potassium stimulated striatal dopamine efflux and subsequently dopamine release in the mesolimbic system (especially the nucleus accumbens), medial prefrontal cortex, midbrain regions, and substantia nigra [58, 66–74]. THC has been shown to facilitate stimulation of dopamine release in the medial forebrain bundle of the mesolimbic system at dose ranges pharmacologically relevant to human recreational use [68]. As the positive symptoms of schizophrenia are related to elevated dopamine release, particularly in the mesolimbic system, cannabinoids have long been implicated in worsening the positive symptoms of schizophrenia [73, 75, 76].

In contrast to the effect of cannabinoids on dopamine release in the mesolimbic system, significant evidence exists for the CB1 receptor mechanism to play an important role in "dampening" neuroexcitability [59, 60, 77]. It has been demonstrated that in the cerebral cortex, serotonin activity is inhibited by cannabinoid receptor agonists (e.g., WIN 55,212 and CP-55,940) [78]. Conversely, studies employing CB1 receptor antagonists (e.g., SR 141716A) have demonstrated increases in serotonin in various brain regions including the medial prefrontal cortex and nucleus accumbens [79].

Cannabinoids have been demonstrated to decrease acetylcholine release in the medial prefrontal cortex, hippocampus, and striatum [80–82]. Likewise, the CB1 receptor antagonist (SR 141716A) has resulted in an increase in acetylcholine in the medial prefrontal cortex and hippocampus [79, 83].

Noradrenaline activity in various areas of the brain including the hippocampus, cerebellum, hypothalamus, and cerebral cortex, has been inhibited by the cannabinoid receptor agonist (WIN 55,212) [84]. This inhibition was subsequently attenuated by the cannabinoid receptor antagonist (SR 141716). Cannabinoid-inhibited release of noradrenaline has also been demonstrated in the hypothalamus and striatum [60, 85–87].

The CB1 receptor has been demonstrated to be present in high concentration at presynaptic terminals of glutaminergic synapses in the hippocampus and other areas of the brain [88]. In general, activation of the CB1 receptor has been shown to inhibit glutamate release in the cerebellum, hippocampus, prefrontal cortex, and substantia nigra [77, 78, 89–91].

CB1 receptor mediated decreases in GABA has also been demonstrated in brain regions including the prefrontal cortex [78, 88, 92, 93], hippocampus [90, 94, 95], and subcortical regions including the basal ganglia [96–100].

4. Cannabinoids and Prefrontal Neurotransmission

Despite the general consensus that cannabinoids inhibit all major neurotransmitters (except dopamine) in various brain regions including the prefrontal cortex, a number of studies have supported the converse notion that cannabinoids in fact stimulate neurotransmission release in the prefrontal cortex [88, 92, 93].

An example of how neurotransmission of dopamine could be theoretically enhanced by cannabinoids in the prefrontal cortex is related to CB1 receptors being preferentially located on GABAergic interneurons in areas including the cerebral cortex, ventral tegmental area, and hippocampus

Table 1: Directions of neurotransmitter release in the prefrontal cortex and subcortical regions.

	Prefrontal cortex			Subcortical regions		
	Schizophrenia (unmedicated)	Atypical antipsychotic treatment	Cannabis use	Schizophrenia (unmedicated)	Atypical antipsychotic treatment	Cannabis use
Dopamine	↓ (grey)	↑ (black)	↑ (black)	↑ (grey)	↓ (black)	↑ (grey)
Serotonin	↓ (grey)	↑ (black)	↑ (black) ↓ (grey)	↑ (grey)	↓ (black)	↓ (black)
Acetylcholine	↓ (grey)	↑ (black)	↑ (black) ↓ (grey)	↑ (grey)	↓ (black)	↓ (black)
Noradrenaline	↓ (grey)	↑ (black)	↑ (black) ↓ (grey)	↑ (grey)	↓ (black)	↓ (black)
Glutamate	↓ (grey)	↑ (black)	↑ (black) ↓ (grey)	↓ (grey)	↑ (black)	↓ (grey)
GABA	↓ (grey)	↓ (grey)	↑ (black) ↓ (grey)	↓ (grey)	↑ (black)	↓ (grey)

[92]. Cannabinoids such as THC decrease the excitability of GABA-ergic interneurons, and therefore, given GABA is the major inhibitory neurotransmitter in the CNS, disinhibition of dopamine and glutamate follows. Consequently, increases in the outflow of neurotransmission parallel the decrease in extracellular GABA.

As another example of how neurotransmission is theoretically enhanced by cannabinoids in the prefrontal cortex, studies have demonstrated that increased dopamine neurotransmission in the mesolimbic projections from the nucleus accumbens triggers an inhibition of GABA-ergic efferents to the basal forebrain. The process of inhibiting the release of GABA, in turn, decreases the inhibition of other neurotransmitters such as dopamine, acetylcholine, noradrenaline, and glutamate. A specific example of this process has been postulated where dopamine's direct inhibitory effect on both glutamate and GABA-ergic activity leads to an increased excitability of cholinergic flow [46, 101].

Proceeding from these lines of reasoning, studies have demonstrated that in the prefrontal region, cannabinoids mediate increases in noradrenaline [102], acetylcholine [103, 104], and glutamate [92, 105]. With respect to serotonin and GABA, studies have demonstrated that cannabinoids mediate the inhibition of *reuptake* in cortical areas, which leads to their increase [106].

5. The Effects of Cannabis on Cognition and the Positive/Negative Symptoms of Schizophrenia

Table 1 presents a summary of the information discussed thus far. The grey arrows in the "Schizophrenia" columns represent the directions of neurotransmitter release in the unmedicated state of the disorder in both the prefrontal cortex and subcortical regions. As discussed above, the negative symptoms and cognitive impairments are generally conceptualised in terms of decreased neurotransmission of all six major systems in the prefrontal cortex, whilst the positive symptoms are generally thought to arise because of increased neurotransmission of dopamine, serotonin, acetylcholine and noradrenaline systems, and decreased neurotransmission of glutamate and GABA systems in subcortical regions.

The black arrows in the "Atypical antipsychotic treatment" columns represent how these medications are purported to ameliorate the symptoms and cognitive impairments of schizophrenia. Specifically, atypical antipsychotics are postulated to ameliorate the negative symptoms and cognitive impairment by stimulating neurotransmission in the prefrontal cortex (of all neurotransmitters except GABA), and are thought to ameliorate the positive symptoms by inhibiting dopamine, serotonin, acetylcholine, and noradrenaline, and by increasing glutamate and GABA in subcortical regions.

Of pertinent interest to this review is the theoretical amelioration and/or exacerbation of the symptoms and cognitive impairments of schizophrenia that cannabis use may produce. As Table 1 shows, cannabis in the normal population leads to excitation of dopamine in the prefrontal cortex. However, what remains relatively less certain is whether cannabis leads to excitation or inhibition of the other five major neurotransmitters in the prefrontal cortex (i.e., serotonin, acetylcholine, noradrenaline, glutamate, and GABA), given that evidence for both modes of action have been presented. Hence, the postulated effect of cannabis on these five systems is indicated by both grey and black arrows.

Consequently, looking at the "Schizophrenia (unmedicated)" and "Cannabis use" columns in conjunction, Table 1 shows that although cannabis has the potential to exacerbate the negative symptoms and cognitive impairments of schizophrenia via contributing further to the "hypofrontal" nature of the disorder, cannabis also has a therapeutic potential by facilitating neurotransmission (at least in the dopaminergic system) in the prefrontal cortex. In line with the latter perspective, research has demonstrated enhanced cognitive performance in schizophrenia with comorbid cannabis use [21–25, 29], which may be attributable to stimulation of prefrontal neurotransmission.

In subcortical regions, Table 1 shows that cannabis use is associated with excitation of dopamine and inhibition of all the other five major neurotransmitters (i.e., serotonin, noradrenaline, acetylcholine, glutamate, and GABA). Hence, cannabis has the potential to counteract increased levels of serotonin, acetylcholine, and noradrenaline that occur in subcortical regions in untreated schizophrenia and thus, provide an antipsychotic therapeutic effect. However, excitation of dopamine and inhibition of glutamate and GABA in subcortical regions produced by cannabis use may augment the dysregulation that occurs in these three systems in untreated schizophrenia, and possibly exacerbate the positive symptoms.

6. Summary and Conclusion

Cannabis use in the schizophrenia population has been shown to worsen the prognosis and increase the burden of the disorder. However, evidence exists for a subgroup of the population to suggest that cannabinoids have therapeutic effects on the negative and positive symptoms, as well as cognitive impairments. Although this evidence is not conclusive and requires further research and replication, a more comprehensive and broad-based neurochemical framework has been presented in this paper, offering an explanation for the potentially therapeutic effects of cannabinoids in addition to its adverse effects.

Whilst the neurochemical effects of cannabinoids are complex, cannabinoids appear to have at least in part, a "restorative" effect on neurotransmitter dysfunctions in schizophrenia, which may underpin the biological substrate of the therapeutic effects cannabis has been demonstrated to have in recent studies.

In the context of recent research by Coulston et al. [29], future studies need to establish which subgroups of schizophrenia most benefit from cannabinoids as a putative "treatment"; which subgroups demonstrate nil or minimal exacerbation of positive symptoms in the context of cannabis use, or indeed, which subgroups may experience antipsychotic effects of cannabis; how such a treatment may complement or interact with standard antipsychotics and other psychiatric treatments; what constitutes an effective quantity or dose of cannabinoids to exert a beneficial impact on cognition; what precise frequency of administration would be required; how long the effects of cannabinoids last on cognition following a recent dose; how such a treatment may generalise to other domains of real-life functioning such as employment and social settings (and in particular, cognitive processes required to function well in these settings); and whether such a treatment can be generalised to older age groups. Methods by which future research could proceed to address these questions include randomised, double-blind, controlled drug trials.

Clearly there are many questions that need to be addressed and the use of further randomised, double-blind studies is necessary to establish the effects of cannabis across the domains of cognition, mood, and mentation. However, given the prevalence of cannabis use and its integral role in the clinical manifestation of psychosis, this is an area for future research, and reconceptualising our neurochemical understanding is perhaps a useful first step. In this context, the consideration, appraisal, and rigorous testing of novel models are necessary, and are likely to advance our understanding.

References

[1] S. Andréasson, P. Allebeck, A. Engström, and U. Rydberg, "Cannabis and schizophrenia. A longitudinal study of Swedish conscripts," *Lancet*, vol. 2, no. 8574, pp. 1483–1486, 1987.

[2] D. M. Fergusson, L. J. Horwood, and N. R. Swain-Campbell, "Cannabis dependence and psychotic symptoms in young people," *Psychological Medicine*, vol. 33, no. 1, pp. 15–21, 2003.

[3] P. A. Silva and W. R. Stanton, *From Child to Adult: The Dunedin Multidisciplinary Health and Development Study*, Oxford University Press, Auckland, UK, 1996.

[4] J. Van Os, M. Bak, M. Hanssen, R. V. Bijl, R. De Graaf, and H. Verdoux, "Cannabis use and psychosis: a longitudinal population-based study," *American Journal of Epidemiology*, vol. 156, no. 4, pp. 319–327, 2002.

[5] S. Zammit, P. Allebeck, S. Andréasson, I. Lundberg, and G. Lewis, "Self reported cannabis use as a risk factor for schizophrenia in Swedish conscripts of 1969: historical cohort study," *British Medical Journal*, vol. 325, no. 7374, pp. 1199–1201, 2002.

[6] L. Arseneault, M. Cannon, R. Poulton, R. Murray, A. Caspi, and T. E. Moffitt, "Cannabis use in adolescence and risk for adult psychosis: longitudinal prospective study," *British Medical Journal*, vol. 325, no. 7374, pp. 1212–1213, 2002.

[7] T. H. Moore, S. Zammit, A. Lingford-Hughes et al., "Cannabis use and risk of psychotic or affective mental health outcomes: a systematic review," *Lancet*, vol. 370, no. 9584, pp. 319–328, 2007.

[8] G. Bersani, V. Orlandi, S. Gherardelli, and P. Pancheri, "Cannabis and neurological soft signs in schizophrenia: absence of relationship and influence on psychopathology," *Psychopathology*, vol. 35, no. 5, pp. 289–295, 2002.

[9] G. Bersani, V. Orlandi, G. D. Kotzalidis, and P. Pancheri, "Cannabis and schizophrenia: impact on onset, course, psychopathology and outcomes," *European Archives of Psychiatry and Clinical Neuroscience*, vol. 252, no. 2, pp. 86–92, 2002.

[10] M. T. Compton, A. C. Furman, and N. J. Kaslow, "Lower negative symptom scores among cannabis-dependent patients with schizophrenia-spectrum disorders: preliminary evidence from an African American first-episode sample," *Schizophrenia Research*, vol. 71, no. 1, pp. 61–64, 2004.

[11] M. T. Compton, N. E. Whicker, and K. M. Hochman, "Alcohol and cannabis use in urban, African American, first-episode schizophrenia-spectrum patients: associations with positive and negative symptoms," *Journal of Clinical Psychiatry*, vol. 68, no. 12, pp. 1939–1945, 2007.

[12] C. Dubertret, I. Bidard, J. Adès, and P. Gorwood, "Lifetime positive symptoms in patients with schizophrenia and cannabis abuse are partially explained by co-morbid addiction," *Schizophrenia Research*, vol. 86, no. 1–3, pp. 284–290, 2006.

[13] V. Peralta and M. J. Cuesta, "Influence of cannabis abuse on schizophrenic psychopathology," *Acta Psychiatrica Scandinavica*, vol. 85, no. 2, pp. 127–130, 1992.

[14] P. D. Skosnik, S. Park, L. Dobbs, and W. L. Gardner, "Affect processing and positive syndrome schizotypy in cannabis users," *Psychiatry Research*, vol. 157, no. 1–3, pp. 279–282, 2008.

[15] F. M. Leweke, D. Koethe, C. W. Gerth, et al., "Cannabidiol as an antipsychotic agent," *European Psychiatry*, vol. 22, supplement 1, p. S21, 2007.

[16] A. W. Zuardi, J. A. S. Crippa, J. E. C. Hallak, F. A. Moreira, and F. S. Guimarães, "Cannabidiol, a Cannabis sativa constituent, as an antipsychotic drug," *Brazilian Journal of Medical and Biological Research*, vol. 39, no. 4, pp. 421–429, 2006.

[17] A. W. Zuardi, J. A. Rodrigues, and J. M. Cunha, "Effects of cannabidiol in animal models predictive of antipsychotic activity," *Psychopharmacology*, vol. 104, no. 2, pp. 260–264, 1991.

[18] D. C. D'Souza, W. M. Abi-Saab, S. Madonick et al., "Delta-9-tetrahydrocannabinol effects in schizophrenia: implications for cognition, psychosis, and addiction," *Biological Psychiatry*, vol. 57, no. 6, pp. 594–608, 2005.

[19] F. Liraud and H. Verdoux, "Effect of comorbid substance use on neuropsychological performance in subjects with psychotic or mood disorders," *Encephale*, vol. 28, no. 2, pp. 160–168, 2002.

[20] A. Pencer and J. Addington, "Substance use and cognition in early psychosis," *Journal of Psychiatry and Neuroscience*, vol. 28, no. 1, pp. 48–54, 2003.

[21] M. C. Jockers-Scherübl, T. Wolf, N. Radzei et al., "Cannabis induces different cognitive changes in schizophrenic patients and in healthy controls," *Progress in Neuro-Psychopharmacology and Biological Psychiatry*, vol. 31, no. 5, pp. 1054–1063, 2007.

[22] S. Kumra, E. Thaden, C. DeThomas, and H. Kranzler, "Correlates of substance abuse in adolescents with treatment-refractory schizophrenia and schizoaffective disorder," *Schizophrenia Research*, vol. 73, no. 2-3, pp. 369–371, 2005.

[23] S. Sevy, K. E. Burdick, H. Visweswaraiah et al., "Iowa Gambling Task in schizophrenia: a review and new data in patients with schizophrenia and co-occurring cannabis use disorders," *Schizophrenia Research*, vol. 92, no. 1–3, pp. 74–84, 2007.

[24] J. Stirling, C. White, S. Lewis et al., "Neurocognitive function and outcome in first-episode schizophrenia: a 10-year follow-up of an epidemiological cohort," *Schizophrenia Research*, vol. 65, no. 2-3, pp. 75–86, 2003.

[25] J. Stirling, S. Lewis, R. Hopkins, and C. White, "Cannabis use prior to first onset psychosis predicts spared neurocognition at 10-year follow-up," *Schizophrenia Research*, vol. 75, no. 1, pp. 135–137, 2005.

[26] C. M. Coulston, M. Perdices, and C. T. Tennant, "The Neuropsychology of cannabis and other substance use in schizophrenia: review of the literature and critical evaluation of methodological issues," *Australian and New Zealand Journal of Psychiatry*, vol. 41, no. 11, pp. 869–884, 2007.

[27] American Psychiatric Association, *Diagnostic and Statistical Manual of Mental Disorders*, APA, Washington, DC, USA, 4th edition, 1994.

[28] H. G. Pope Jr., A. J. Gruber, J. I. Hudson, M. A. Huestis, and D. Yurgelun-Todd, "Neuropsychological performance in long-term cannabis users," *Archives of General Psychiatry*, vol. 58, no. 10, pp. 909–915, 2001.

[29] C. M. Coulston, M. Perdices, and C. C. Tennant, "The neuropsychological correlates of cannabis use in schizophrenia: lifetime abuse/dependence, frequency of use, and recency of use," *Schizophrenia Research*, vol. 96, no. 1–3, pp. 169–184, 2007.

[30] M. Keyes, "Assessing schizophrenia with the MMPI-2," *Dissertation Abstracts International. Section B*, vol. 64, p. 5788, 2004.

[31] T. A. Ban, "Neuropsychopharmacology and the genetics of schizophrenia: a history of the diagnosis of schizophrenia," *Progress in Neuro-Psychopharmacology and Biological Psychiatry*, vol. 28, no. 5, pp. 753–762, 2004.

[32] E. B. Binder, B. Kinkead, M. J. Owens, and C. B. Nemeroff, "The role of neurotensin in the pathophysiology of schizophrenia and the mechanism of action of antipsychotic drugs," *Biological Psychiatry*, vol. 50, no. 11, pp. 856–872, 2001.

[33] L. Farde, "Brain imaging of schizophrenia—the dopamine hypothesis," *Schizophrenia Research*, vol. 28, no. 2-3, pp. 157–162, 1997.

[34] F. P. Bymaster, D. L. Nelson, N. W. DeLapp et al., "Antagonism by olanzapine of dopamine D1, serotonin2, muscarinic, histamine H1 and α1-adrenergic receptors in vitro," *Schizophrenia Research*, vol. 37, no. 1, pp. 107–122, 1999.

[35] J. Ma, N. Ye, N. Lange, and B. M. Cohen, "Dynorphinergic GABA neurons are a target of both typical and atypical antipsychotic drugs in the nucleus accumbens shell, central amygdaloid nucleus and thalamic central medial nucleus," *Neuroscience*, vol. 121, no. 4, pp. 991–998, 2003.

[36] D. Tarsy, R. J. Baldessarini, and F. I. Tarazi, "Effects of newer antipsychotics on extrapyramidal function," *CNS Drugs*, vol. 16, no. 1, pp. 23–45, 2002.

[37] J. L. Waddington, P. J. Scully, and E. O'Callaghan, "The new antipsychotics, and their potential for early intervention in schizophrenia," *Schizophrenia Research*, vol. 28, no. 2-3, pp. 207–222, 1997.

[38] D. C. Goff and J. T. Coyle, "The emerging role of glutamate in the pathophysiology and treatment of schizophrenia," *American Journal of Psychiatry*, vol. 158, no. 9, pp. 1367–1377, 2001.

[39] A. Meyer-Lindenberg, R. S. Miletich, P. D. Kohn et al., "Reduced prefrontal activity predicts exaggerated striatal dopaminergic function in schizophrenia," *Nature Neuroscience*, vol. 5, no. 3, pp. 267–271, 2002.

[40] F. M. Benes, S. L. Vincent, A. Marie, and Y. Khan, "Up-regulation of GABA(A) receptor binding on neurons of the prefrontal cortex in schizophrenic subjects," *Neuroscience*, vol. 75, no. 4, pp. 1021–1031, 1996.

[41] H. F. Clarke, J. W. Dalley, H. S. Crofts, T. W. Robbins, and A. C. Roberts, "Cognitive inflexibility after prefrontal serotonin depletion," *Science*, vol. 304, no. 5672, pp. 878–880, 2004.

[42] J. T. Coyle, "The GABA-glutamate connection in schizophrenia: which is the proximate cause?" *Biochemical Pharmacology*, vol. 68, no. 8, pp. 1507–1514, 2004.

[43] J. W. Dalley, D. E. Theobald, E. A. C. Pereira, P. M. M. C. Li, and T. W. Robbins, "Specific abnormalities in serotonin release in the prefrontal cortex of isolation-reared rats measured during behavioural performance of a task assessing visuospatial attention and impulsivity," *Psychopharmacology*, vol. 164, no. 3, pp. 329–340, 2002.

[44] J. I. Friedman, H. Temporini, and K. L. Davis, "Pharmacologic strategies for augmenting cognitive performance in schizophrenia," *Biological Psychiatry*, vol. 45, no. 1, pp. 1–16, 1999.

[45] J. Ichikawa, J. Dai, I. A. O'Laughlin, W. L. Fowler, and H. Y. Meltzer, "Atypical, but not typical, antipsychotic drugs increase cortical acetylcholine release without an effect in the nucleus accumbens or striatum," *Neuropsychopharmacology*, vol. 26, no. 3, pp. 325–339, 2002.

[46] M. Sarter and J. P. Bruno, "Abnormal regulation of corticopetal cholinergic neurons and impaired information processing in neuropsychiatric disorders," *Trends in Neurosciences*, vol. 22, no. 2, pp. 67–74, 1999.

[47] K. Zavitsanou, P. B. Wards, and X.-F. Huang, "Selective alterations in inotropic glutamate receptors in the anterior cingulated cortex in schizophrenia," *Neuropsychopharmacology*, vol. 27, pp. 826–833, 2002.

[48] P. Hertel, G. G. Nomikos, B. Schilström, L. Arborelius, and T. H. Svensson, "Risperidone dose-dependently increases extracellular concentrations of serotonin in the rat frontal cortex: role of α2-adrenoceptor antagonism," *Neuropsychopharmacology*, vol. 17, no. 1, pp. 44–55, 1997.

[49] J. Ichikawa, T. Kuroki, J. Dai, and H. Y. Meltzer, "Effect of antipsychotic drugs on extracellular serotonin levels in rat medial prefrontal cortex and nucleus accumbens," *European Journal of Pharmacology*, vol. 351, no. 2, pp. 163–171, 1998.

[50] K. E. Jardemark, I. Ninan, X. Liang, and R. Y. Wang, "Protein kinase C is involved in clozapine's facilitation of N-methyl-D-aspartate- and electrically evoked responses in pyramidal cells of the medial prefrontal cortex," *Neuroscience*, vol. 118, no. 2, pp. 501–512, 2003.

[51] L. P. Lacroix, M. E. Hows, A. J. Shah, J. J. Hagan, and C. A. Heidbreder, "Selective antagonism at dopamine D3 receptors enhances monoaminergic and cholinergic neurotransmission in the rat anterior cingulate cortex," *Neuropsychopharmacology*, vol. 28, no. 5, pp. 839–849, 2003.

[52] S. Potvin, E. Stip, and J.-Y. Roy, "Clozapine, quetiapine and olanzapine among addicted schizophrenic patients: towards testable hypotheses," *International Clinical Psychopharmacology*, vol. 18, no. 3, pp. 121–132, 2003.

[53] W. Zhang, K. W. Perry, D. T. Wong et al., "Synergistic effects of olanzapine and other antipsychotic agents in combination with fluoxetine on norepinephrine and dopamine release in rat prefrontal cortex," *Neuropsychopharmacology*, vol. 23, no. 3, pp. 250–262, 2000.

[54] E. Costa, J. M. Davis, E. Dong et al., "A GABAergic cortical deficit dominates schizophrenia pathophysiology," *Critical Reviews in Neurobiology*, vol. 16, no. 1-2, pp. 1–23, 2004.

[55] A. J. Bourdelais and A. Y. Deutch, "The effects of haloperidol and clozapine on extracellular GABA levels in the prefrontal cortex of the rat: an in vivo microdialysis study," *Cerebral Cortex*, vol. 4, no. 1, pp. 69–77, 1994.

[56] X. Wang, P. Zhong, and Z. Yan, "Dopamine D4 receptors modulate GABAergic signaling in pyramidal neurons of prefrontal cortex," *Journal of Neuroscience*, vol. 22, no. 21, pp. 9185–9193, 2002.

[57] Z. Yan, "Regulation of GABAergic inhibition by serotonin signaling in prefrontal cortex: molecular mechanisms and functional implications," *Molecular Neurobiology*, vol. 26, no. 2-3, pp. 203–216, 2002.

[58] C. H. Ashton, "Pharmacology and effects of cannabis: a brief review," *British Journal of Psychiatry*, vol. 178, pp. 101–106, 2001.

[59] I. Grant, R. Gonzalez, C. L. Carey, L. Natarajan, and T. Wolfson, "Non-acute (residual) neurocognitive effects of cannabis use: a meta-analytic study," *Journal of the International Neuropsychological Society*, vol. 9, no. 5, pp. 679–689, 2003.

[60] M. Kathmann, U. Bauer, E. Schlicker, and M. Göthert, "Cannabinoid CB1 receptor-mediated inhibition of NMDA- and kainate- stimulated noradrenaline and dopamine release in the brain," *Naunyn-Schmiedeberg's Archives of Pharmacology*, vol. 359, no. 6, pp. 466–470, 1999.

[61] C. S. Breivogel and S. R. Childers, "The functional neuroanatomy of brain cannabinoid receptors," *Neurobiology of Disease*, vol. 5, no. 6, pp. 417–431, 1998.

[62] A. N. Gifford, A. Makriyannis, N. D. Volkow, and S. J. Gatley, "In vivo imaging of the brain cannabinoid receptor," *Chemistry and Physics of Lipids*, vol. 121, no. 1-2, pp. 65–72, 2002.

[63] A. B. Ilan, M. E. Smith, and A. Gevins, "Effects of marijuana on neurophysiological signals of working and episodic memory," *Psychopharmacology*, vol. 176, no. 2, pp. 214–222, 2004.

[64] Y. B. Shah, M. J. W. Prior, A. L. Dixon, P. G. Morris, and C. A. Marsden, "Detection of cannabinoid agonist evoked increase in BOLD contrast in rats using functional magnetic resonance imaging," *Neuropharmacology*, vol. 46, no. 3, pp. 379–387, 2004.

[65] P. W. Vik, T. Cellucci, A. Jarchow, and J. Hedt, "Cognitive impairment in substance abuse," *Psychiatric Clinics of North America*, vol. 27, no. 1, pp. 97–109, 2004.

[66] M. Diana, M. Melis, A. L. Muntoni, and G. L. Gessa, "Mesolimbic dopaminergic decline after cannabinoid withdrawal," *Proceedings of the National Academy of Sciences of the United States of America*, vol. 95, no. 17, pp. 10269–10273, 1998.

[67] E. D. French, K. Dillon, and X. Wu, "Cannabinoids excite dopamine neurons in the ventral tegmentum and substantia nigra," *NeuroReport*, vol. 8, no. 3, pp. 649–652, 1997.

[68] G. Gessa, M. Melis, A. Muntoni, and M. Diana, "Cannabinoids activate mesolimbic dopamine neurons by an action on cannabinoid CB1 receptors," *European Journal of Pharmacology*, vol. 341, no. 1, pp. 39–44, 1998.

[69] N. Hiroi, "Dependence, tolerance, and alteration in gene expression," in *Marihuana and Medicine*, G. G. Nahas, K. M. Sutin, and D. Harvey, Eds., pp. 207–211, Humana Press, Totowa, NJ, USA, 1999.

[70] V. Patel, M. Borysenko, and M. S. A. Kumar, "Effect of Δ9-THC on brain and plasma catecholamine levels as measured by HPLC," *Brain Research Bulletin*, vol. 14, no. 1, pp. 85–90, 1985.

[71] S. M. Stahl, "Getting stoned without inhaling: anandamide is the brain's natural marijuana," *Journal of Clinical Psychiatry*, vol. 59, no. 11, pp. 566–567, 1998.

[72] E. Valjent, C. Pagès, M. Rogard, M.-J. Besson, R. Maldonado, and J. Caboche, "δ9-tetrahydrocannabinol-induced MAPK/ERK and Elk-1 activation in vivo depends on dopaminergic transmission," *European Journal of Neuroscience*, vol. 14, no. 2, pp. 342–352, 2001.

[73] L. N. P. Voruganti, P. Slomka, P. Zabel, A. Mattar, and A. G. Awad, "Cannabis induced dopamine release: an in-vivo SPECT study," *Psychiatry Research: Neuroimaging*, vol. 107, no. 3, pp. 173–177, 2001.

[74] X. Wu and E. D. French, "Effects of chronic Δ9-tetrahydrocannabinol on rat midbrain dopamine neurons: an electrophysiological assessment," *Neuropharmacology*, vol. 39, no. 3, pp. 391–398, 2000.

[75] L. Degenhardt, W. Hall, and M. Lynskey, "Testing hypotheses about the relationship between cannabis use and psychosis," *Drug and Alcohol Dependence*, vol. 71, no. 1, pp. 37–48, 2003.

[76] W. Hall, "Reducing the harms caused by cannabis use: the policy debate in Australia," *Drug and Alcohol Dependence*, vol. 62, no. 3, pp. 163–174, 2001.

[77] B. E. Akinshola, R. E. Taylor, A. B. Ogunseitan, and E. S. Onaivi, "Anandamide inhibition of recombinant AMPA receptor subunits in Xenopus oocytes is increased by forskolin and 8-bromo-cyclic AMP," *Naunyn-Schmiedeberg's Archives of Pharmacology*, vol. 360, no. 3, pp. 242–248, 1999.

[78] M. Nakazi, U. Bauer, T. Nickel, M. Kathmann, and E. Schlicker, "Inhibition of serotonin release in the mouse brain via presynaptic cannabinoid CB1 receptors," *Naunyn-Schmiedeberg's Archives of Pharmacology*, vol. 361, no. 1, pp. 19–24, 2000.

[79] E. T. Tzavara, R. J. Davis, K. W. Perry et al., "The CB1 receptor antagonist SR141716A selectively increases monoaminergic neurotransmission in the medial prefrontal cortex: implications for therapeutic actions," *British Journal of Pharmacology*, vol. 138, no. 4, pp. 544–553, 2003.

[80] G. Carta, F. Nava, and G. L. Gessa, "Inhibition of hippocampal acetylcholine release after acute and repeated delta-9-tetrahydrocannabinoid administration in rats," *Brain Research*, vol. 809, pp. 1–4, 1998.

[81] E. F. Domino, "Cannabinoids and the cholinergic system," *Journal of Clinical Pharmacology*, vol. 21, supplement 8-9, pp. 2495–2555, 1981.

[82] G. L. Gessa, M. S. Mascia, M. A. Casu, and G. Carta, "Inhibition of hippocampal acetylcholine release by cannabinoids: reversal by SR 141716A," *European Journal of Pharmacology*, vol. 327, no. 1, pp. R1–R2, 1997.

[83] G. L. Gessa, M. A. Casu, G. Carta, and M. S. Mascia, "Cannabinoids decrease acetylcholine release in the medial-prefrontal cortex and hippocampus, reversal by SR 141716A," *European Journal of Pharmacology*, vol. 355, no. 2-3, pp. 119–124, 1998.

[84] E. Schlicker, J. Timm, J. Zentner, and M. Göthert, "Cannabinoid CB1 receptor-mediated inhibition of noradrenaline release in the human and guinea-pig hippocampus," *Naunyn-Schmiedeberg's Archives of Pharmacology*, vol. 356, no. 5, pp. 583–589, 1997.

[85] I. Göbel, A. U. Trendelenburg, S. L. Cox, A. Meyer, and K. Starke, "Electrically evoked release of [3H]noradrenaline from mouse cultured sympathetic neurons: release-modulating heteroreceptors," *Journal of Neurochemistry*, vol. 75, no. 5, pp. 2087–2094, 2000.

[86] E. T. Tzavara, K. W. Perry, D. E. Rodriguez, F. P. Bymaster, and G. G. Nomikos, "The cannabinoid CB1 receptor antagonist SR141716A increases norepinephrine outflow in the rat anterior hypothalamus," *European Journal of Pharmacology*, vol. 426, no. 3, pp. R3–R4, 2001.

[87] E. S. Vizi, I. Katona, and T. F. Freund, "Evidence for presynaptic cannabinoid CB1 receptor-mediated inhibition of noradrenaline release in the guinea pig lung," *European Journal of Pharmacology*, vol. 431, no. 2, pp. 237–244, 2001.

[88] L. Ferraro, M. C. Tomasini, T. Cassano et al., "Cannabinoid receptor agonist WIN 55,212-2 inhibits rat cortical dialysate γ-aminobutyric acid levels," *Journal of Neuroscience Research*, vol. 66, no. 2, pp. 298–302, 2001.

[89] N. Auclair, S. Otani, P. Soubrie, and F. Crepel, "Cannabinoids modulate synaptic strength and plasticity at glutamatergic synapses of rat prefrontal cortex pyramidal neurons," *Journal of Neurophysiology*, vol. 83, no. 6, pp. 3287–3293, 2000.

[90] A. F. Hoffman and C. R. Lupica, "Mechanisms of cannabinoid inhibition of GABA(A) synaptic transmission in the hippocampus," *Journal of Neuroscience*, vol. 20, no. 7, pp. 2470–2479, 2000.

[91] J. M. Sullivan, "Mechanisms of cannabinoid-receptor-mediated inhibition of synaptic transmission in cultured hippocampal pyramidal neurons," *Journal of Neurophysiology*, vol. 82, no. 3, pp. 1286–1294, 1999.

[92] M. Pistis, L. Ferraro, L. Pira et al., "Δ9-tetrahydrocannabinol decreases extracellular GABA and increases extracellular glutamate and dopamine levels in the rat prefrontal cortex: an in vivo microdialysis study," *Brain Research*, vol. 948, no. 1-2, pp. 155–158, 2002.

[93] J. Trettel and E. S. Levine, "Cannabinoids depress inhibitory synaptic inputs received by layer 2/3 pyramidal neurons of the neocortex," *Journal of Neurophysiology*, vol. 88, no. 1, pp. 534–539, 2002.

[94] N. Hájos, I. Katona, S. S. Naiem et al., "Cannabinoids inhibit hippocampal GABAergic transmission and network oscillations," *European Journal of Neuroscience*, vol. 12, no. 9, pp. 3239–3249, 2000.

[95] R. E. Hampson and S. A. Deadwyler, "Cannabinoids, hippocampal function and memory," *Life Sciences*, vol. 65, no. 6-7, pp. 715–723, 1999.

[96] P. K. Chan, S. C. Chan, and W. H. Yung, "Presynaptic inhibition of GABAergic inputs into rat substantia nigra pars reticulate neurons by cannabinoid agonists," *Neuroreport*, vol. 9, pp. 671–675, 1998.

[97] A. F. Hoffman and C. R. Lupica, "Direct actions of cannabinoids on synaptic transmission in the nucleus accumbens: a comparison with opioids," *Journal of Neurophysiology*, vol. 85, no. 1, pp. 72–83, 2001.

[98] O. J. Manzoni and J. Bockaert, "Cannabinoids inhibit GABAergic synaptic transmission in mice nucleus accumbens," *European Journal of Pharmacology*, vol. 412, no. 2, pp. R3–R5, 2001.

[99] B. Szabo, S. Siemes, and I. Wallmichrath, "Inhibition of GABAergic neurotransmission in the ventral tegmental area by cannabinoids," *European Journal of Neuroscience*, vol. 15, no. 12, pp. 2057–2061, 2002.

[100] I. Wallmichrath and B. Szabo, "Cannabinoids inhibit striatonigral GABAergic neurotransmission in the mouse," *Neuroscience*, vol. 113, no. 3, pp. 671–682, 2002.

[101] J. M. Crook, E. Tomaskovic-Crook, D. L. Copolov, and B. Dean, "Low muscarinic receptor binding in prefrontal cortex from subjects with schizophrenia: a study of brodmann's areas 8, 9, 10, and 46 and the effects of neuroleptic drug treatment," *American Journal of Psychiatry*, vol. 158, no. 6, pp. 918–925, 2001.

[102] J. D. Jentsch, E. Andrusiak, A. Tran, M. B. Bowers Jr., and R. H. Roth, "δ9-tetrahydrocannabinol increases prefrontal cortical catecholaminergic utilization and impairs spatial working memory in the rat: blockade of dopaminergic effects with HA966," *Neuropsychopharmacology*, vol. 16, no. 6, pp. 426–432, 1997.

[103] E. Acquas, A. Pisanu, P. Marrocu, S. R. Goldberg, and G. Di Chiara, "Δ9-tetrahydrocannabinol enhances cortical and hippocampal acetylcholine release in vivo: a microdialysis study," *European Journal of Pharmacology*, vol. 419, no. 2-3, pp. 155–161, 2001.

[104] C. D. Verrico, J. D. Jentsch, L. Dazzi, and R. H. Roth, "Systemic, but not local, administration of cannabinoid CB1 receptor agonists modulate prefrontal cortical acetylcholine efflux in the rat," *Synapse*, vol. 48, no. 4, pp. 178–183, 2003.

[105] L. Ferraro, M. C. Tomasini, G. L. Gessa, B. W. Bebe, S. Tanganelli, and T. Antonelli, "The cannabinoid receptor agonist WIN 55,212-2 regulates glutamate transmission in rat cerebral cortex: an in vivo and in vitro study," *Cerebral Cortex*, vol. 11, no. 8, pp. 728–733, 2001.

[106] M. Steffens and T. J. Feuerstein, "Receptor-independent depression of DA and 5-HT uptake by cannabinoids in rat neocortex—involvement of Na^+/K^+-ATPase," *Neurochemistry International*, vol. 44, no. 7, pp. 529–538, 2004.

4

Health-Related Quality of Life and Overall Life Satisfaction in People with Serious Mental Illness

Amy L. Barnes, Meghan E. Murphy, Christopher A. Fowler, and Melisa V. Rempfer

Department of Psychology, University of Missouri-Kansas City, 5030 Cherry Hall, Kansas City, MO 64110, USA

Correspondence should be addressed to Melisa V. Rempfer, rempferm@umkc.edu

Academic Editor: Robin Emsley

Quality of life (QoL) in people with schizophrenia and other serious mental illnesses (SMI) is an important outcome goal, yet there is no consistent definition of the construct. We examined three aspects of QoL in persons with SMI: overall life satisfaction, physical health-related QoL (HRQoL), and mental HRQoL. This study had two primary aims: first, to examine whether there are differences in physical and mental HRQoL in persons with SMI, and, second, to investigate the cognitive, clinical, and functional correlates of the three QoL indicators. Participants were 48 persons with SMI who completed assessments of QoL, cognition, functional capacity, psychiatric symptomatology, and medical comorbidity. Results indicate that participants experience similar levels of physical and mental HRQoL, and these two constructs are not related to one another. Physical HRQoL is associated with less medical comorbidity, while mental HRQoL is associated with negative and depressive symptoms. Overall life satisfaction was associated with fewer psychiatric symptoms and less medical comorbidity. This study adds to the important literature defining distinct domains of QoL and supports the necessity of addressing both physical and mental health factors as they relate to recovery and well-being among persons with SMI.

1. Introduction

Quality of life (QoL) among persons with schizophrenia and other serious mental illnesses (SMI) has become an important outcome assessment for both research and treatment in recent years [1–4]. However, it remains unclear what factors best predict QoL in this population [3, 5, 6] and a significant challenge for researchers has been the varied methods used to define and measure the broad concept. In an attempt to reduce some of this heterogeneity, research in this area has begun to distinguish between objective and subjective assessments of QoL, as these appear to represent distinct constructs [6]. For instance, objective QoL has been operationalized by examining factors such as the frequency of social interactions, number of hours worked per week, or housing status [5]. However, subjective QoL measurement, which addresses perceived life satisfaction, may be a particularly meaningful treatment goal in this population [4] and is consistent with the recovery model, which emphasizes the lived experience of individuals with SMI [7, 8].

To date, much of the research on life satisfaction in SMI has focused on its relationship with cognitive and clinical symptoms. In terms of cognition, some studies have reported significant correlations between life satisfaction and cognition [9], while others, including a meta-analysis by Tolman and Kurtz [6], have reported either no correlations or inverse correlations between life satisfaction and cognitive functioning. With regard to psychiatric symptomatology, current research has revealed variable relationships. For example, life satisfaction has been associated with psychiatric symptoms, such as depressive and negative symptomatology [8, 10, 11]. However, Narvaez et al. [3] reported that symptom reduction alone did not translate into improved life satisfaction.

Another proposed approach of operationally defining overall life satisfaction in schizophrenia has included examining the impact of disease-related or health-related factors on an individual's perceived QoL, which is referred to as health-related quality of life (HRQoL). HRQoL is a particularly relevant outcome indicator for this population, given that individuals with schizophrenia and other SMIs experience significantly elevated rates of medical comorbidity and early mortality compared to the general population [12]. Thus, the assessment of HRQoL has the benefit of incorporating a broader definition of physical/mental health and its impact on life satisfaction than other general life satisfaction measures, which often have limited coverage of physical health [4, 13, 14]. Previous studies have demonstrated that individuals with schizophrenia and other SMIs report poorer HRQoL than people without SMI [4, 15, 16]. HRQoL in this population has been consistently associated with psychiatric symptomatology, such as depression and general psychopathology [5, 11].

The most widely used measure of HRQoL is the Short Form Health Survey (SF-36), which distinguishes between mental HRQoL (Mental Health Component Summary Scale (MHC)) and physical HRQoL (Physical Health Component Summary Scale (PHC)) [17]. However, few researchers in SMI have begun to examine the distinctions between physical and mental HRQoL [5]. Notably, Meijer et al. [18] reported recently that mental HRQoL, compared to physical HRQoL, was a stronger predictor of overall life satisfaction. In general, little is known about the distinction between mental and physical HRQoL or the relative determinants of each. Given that there are multiple methods for assessing QoL, which have been demonstrated to be distinct from one another [5, 19], further research is needed to understand the unique determinants of the various QoL indicators [5].

The current study simultaneously examined three important aspects of life satisfaction for persons with schizophrenia and other SMIs: overall life satisfaction, mental HRQoL, and physical HRQoL. Specifically, the current study has two aims: (1) to evaluate the subjective concern with physical HRQoL relative to the concern with mental HRQoL and (2) to investigate the cognitive, clinical, and functional correlates of the three QoL indicators.

2. Methods

2.1. Participants. Forty-eight participants with SMI were recruited from an outpatient treatment program at an urban community mental health center. The Structured Clinical Interview for DSM-IV Disorders (SCID) [20] was used to confirm the diagnosis. Of this sample, 46.9% (n = 23) had a SCID-confirmed diagnosis of schizophrenia, 10.2% (n = 5) with schizoaffective disorder, 28.6% (n = 14) with major depressive disorder, and 12.2% (n = 6) with bipolar disorder. One person did not complete the SCID, but diagnosis was confirmed through the chart review and consultation with the treating staff. Exclusionary criteria for the study included known neurological disease, developmental disability, significant sensory/physical impairment that would affect task performance (e.g., blindness), or substance abuse/dependence in the prior 30 days. Additional descriptive information is presented in Table 1.

2.2. Procedures. All participants provided an informed consent and all study procedures were approved by the Institutional Review Board at the University of Missouri-Kansas City. Assessments were conducted in a quiet room at the university-affiliated mental health center where participants were enrolled in outpatient psychosocial treatment.

2.3. Measures

2.3.1. Health-Related QoL Assessment. The SF-36 [17] is a 36-item measure of subjective health. Widely used in many populations as an HRQoL assessment, the SF-36 contains two primary components, physical health (PHC) and mental health (MHC) [17, 21]. The MHC and PHC share a common standardized metric that utilizes a t-distribution ranging from 0 to 100 (M = 50, SD = 10). The SF-36 has an extensive evidence supporting its reliability and validity in various populations, including persons with SMI [13, 21–23].

2.3.2. Overall Life Satisfaction. As a measure of overall life satisfaction, we utilized participant scores from item number 23 on the Quality of Life Enjoyment and Satisfaction Questionnaire (Q-LES-Q-23 [24, 25]). This item asks participants to rate their "overall life satisfaction and contentment" in the past week on a 5-point Likert-type scale. This item was selected as the variable of interest, because there are several health-related items on the overall Q-LES-Q measure and we wished to avoid construct overlap with the health-related SF-36 indices. Indeed, this rating of overall life satisfaction and contentment has been found to be distinct from the health domain factor on the Q-LES-Q [25].

2.3.3. Clinical Assessment. The Brief Psychiatric Rating Scale (Expanded) (BPRS-E, [26]) was used to assess the severity of total symptoms, positive symptoms, and negative symptoms. The Hamilton Rating Scale for Depression (HAM-D, [27]) was used to assess the severity of depressive symptoms.

2.3.4. Neurocognitive Assessment. A composite neurocognitive measure was formed using z-scores from a battery of 7 measures that are known to be of functional significance in people with SMI [28], including measures of *executive functions* (the Wisconsin Card Sorting Test (WCST-64, [29]), the Trail Making Test, part B (TMT, [30]), and The Controlled Oral Word Association Test (FAS, [31])), *attention/concentration* (the D2 Test of Attention [32]), *processing speed* (the Trail Making Test, part A (TMT A, [30])), *working memory* (Letter-Number Sequencing (LNS, [33])), and *secondary verbal memory* (the California Verbal Learning Test (CVLT-II, [34])).

2.3.5. Functional Capacity. The Brief UCSD Performance-Based Skill Assessment (UPSA-Brief, [35]) was administered as a measure of functional skill capacity. This instrument consists of the finance and communication subscales of the original UCSD Performance-Based Skill Assessment (UPSA, [36]). Validity evidence for the UPSA-Brief has been reported in terms of significant relationships with real-world outcomes [37].

TABLE 1: Descriptive characteristics of the sample.

Total $N = 48$	N (%)
Gender	
Male	25 (52%)
Female	23 (48%)
Race/ethnicity	
African American	30 (62.5%)
Caucasian	13 (27.1%)
Multiracial	5 (10.4%)
Marital status	
Never married	23 (47.9%)
Divorced/widowed/separated	18 (37.5%)
Married/living together	7 (14.6%)
Education	
Less than high school	17 (35.4%)
High school/GED	13 (27.1%)
Posthigh school/no college	1 (2.1%)
Some college	16 (33.3%)
College beyond 4 year degree	1 (2.1%)
Living situation	
Lives independently	31 (64.6%)
Lives with relatives	7 (14.6%)
Supervised care housing	6 (12.5%)
Long-term care facility	1 (2.1%)
Homeless	3 (6.3%)

2.3.6. Medical Comorbidity. Participants completed a health checklist indicating if they had ever been diagnosed with any of the 25 listed health problems. Similar to the methods of Dixon et al. [38], an index of the total number of health problems reported by participants was created.

2.4. Statistical Analyses. Diagnostic subgroups were combined for all analyses; there were no significant differences among SMI diagnostic groups in terms of age, education, nor any of the study variables. To address our first aim of directly comparing physical HRQoL and mental HRQoL, a paired-sample t-test was conducted to examine mean differences in PHC and MHC scores. In addition, we used one sample t-test to compare observed PHC and MHC scores in our sample to established population norms for these indices. For our second aim to investigate the cognitive, clinical, and functional correlates of the three QoL indicators, Pearson correlation coefficients were computed to examine the relevant interrelationships.

3. Results

Demographic characteristics of the sample are presented in Table 1, while means and standard deviations for the study variables are presented in Table 2.

The first aim of the study was to directly compare physical HRQoL and mental HRQoL. A paired-sample t-test revealed no significant difference between mean scores on the PHC ($M = 43.49$) and MHC ($M = 39.59$), $t(46) = 1.63$.

TABLE 2: Means and standard deviations.

Total $N = 48$	Mean (SD)
PHC	43.49 (9.97)
MHC	39.59 (12.20)
Life satisfaction	3.50 (1.05)
BPRS-E (total score)	45.67 (10.77)
Positive symptoms	1.68 (0.63/range 1–4)
Negative symptoms	2.32 (0.79/range 1–4)
HAM-D	20.02 (10.87)
UPSA-B	70.43 (14.65)
Medical comorbidity	5.27 (3.43)

Note: PHC: physical health component of the SF-36, MHC: mental health component of the SF-36, BPRS-E: brief psychiatric rating scale (expanded), HAM-D: hamilton depression rating scale, and UPSA-B: University of California San Diego performance-based skills assessment (brief).

The second aim of this study was to examine the respective correlates of three QoL indicators, physical HRQoL, mental HRQoL, and overall life satisfaction. With regard to correlates of physical HRQoL, the PHC and MHC were not related to one another ($r(48) = -0.087$, $P > .05$), suggesting the participant's subjective concerns with physical health may be independent of their subjective concerns with mental health. As expected, higher physical HRQoL was associated with less medical comorbidity ($r(48) = -0.518$, $P < .01$). Physical HRQoL was not associated with any of the psychiatric, cognitive, or functional measures. See Table 3.

Mental HRQoL was significantly associated with overall life satisfaction ($r(48) = 0.621$, $P < .01$), as well as total symptoms on the BPRS-E ($r(48) = -0.370$, $P < .05$) and depressive symptomatology ($r(48) = -.662$, $P < .01$). This association between mental HRQoL and the BPRS-E appears to be driven by the significant relationship between mental HRQoL and negative symptoms ($r(48) = -.607$, $P < .01$); positive symptoms were not significantly associated with mental HRQoL. In addition, mental HRQoL was not significantly associated with cognitive or functional capacity measures. Better overall life satisfaction was associated with fewer negative ($r(48) = -.379$, $P < .01$) and depressive ($r(48) = -.427$, $P < .01$) psychiatric symptoms, as well as less medical comorbidity ($r(48) = -.339$, $P < .05$). Correlations between overall life satisfaction and cognition and functional capacity did not reach significance ($P < .10$). See Table 3.

4. Discussion

The overall purpose of this study was to examine three aspects of subjective QoL in persons with SMI: overall life satisfaction, physical HRQoL, and mental HRQoL. This study differs from the previous QoL research in that it directly compared self-reported physical HRQoL with self-reported mental HRQoL (aim 1). We found no significant difference between physical and mental HRQoL, indicating that participants in this sample were as concerned with their physical health status as they were with mental health status. HRQoL reports in this sample were consistent with those

Table 3: Summary of bivariate correlations among quality of life indicators and psychiatric symptoms, cognition, functional capacity, and medical comorbidity.

	PHC	MHC	Life satisfaction
PHC		−0.087	0.159
MHC			0.621**
BPRS-E (total score)	−0.079	−0.370*	−0.306*
Positive symptoms	0.070	−0.016	−0.058
Negative symptoms	−0.038	−0.607**	−0.379**
HAM-D	0.071	−0.662**	−0.427**
Cognitive composite	0.014	0.094	−0.281+
UPSA-B	0.044	−0.024	−0.243+
Medical comorbidity	−0.518**	−0.262+	−0.339*

Note: PHC: physical health component of the SF-36, MHC: mental health component of the SF-36, BPRS-E: brief psychiatric rating scale (expanded), HAM-D: Hamilton depression rating scale, and UPSA-B: University of California San Diego performance-based skills assessment (brief). *P is significant at the 0.05 level (two tailed), **P is significant at the 0.01 level (two tailed), and $^{+}P < 0.10$.

from previous research, which are significantly lower than the general population [4, 39, 40].

Given the significant and well-documented physical health concerns in persons with SMI [12, 38, 41], it is noteworthy that persons with SMI report statistically similar rates of role limitations due to physical and mental health factors. Further, it was interesting to note that although persons are similarly concerned about mental HRQoL and physical HRQoL, there is evidence that these are nonetheless distinct constructs. We found that physical HRQoL and mental HRQoL were not significantly correlated, and with regard to aim 2 each showed distinct patterns of associations with other variables, as described below.

The second aim of this study was to examine patterns of associations between the three distinct QoL indices and measures of clinical, functional, and cognitive status. Physical HRQoL was strongly associated with less medical comorbidity experienced by participants, but not with other variables. This pattern supports the face validity of physical HRQoL and suggests that it is a very specific construct, at least as perceived by respondents with SMI. Similarly, mental HRQoL was associated with psychiatric symptomatology but not with other measures. On the other hand, general life satisfaction showed a broader pattern of correlations and was significantly associated with psychiatric symptoms (total and negative symptoms, and depression), mental HRQoL, and medical comorbidity. Further, there were trend associations for overall life satisfaction with cognitive functioning and functional capacity. These findings are generally consistent with other literature on life satisfaction in this population. Recently, for instance, Meijer et al. [18] reported that depression and anxiety predicted general QoL and that HRQoL (particularly mental HRQoL) was a mediator in this relationship.

Interestingly, however, in our study physical HRQoL was not associated with overall life satisfaction. This finding is in need of further examination in the literature, but one explanation may be that persons with SMI, although concerned about their medical status, do not perceive these health-related limitations as related to other, more general, aspects of their well-being. Given the significant health comorbidities in this population, and the fact that persons with SMI are concerned about their physical HRQoL, further research on this issue is warranted.

Further, our findings highlight the potentially limited influence of positive psychiatric symptoms on life satisfaction. In this vein, Lysaker and LaRocco [42] note the importance of not assuming that reductions in QoL are directly related to symptoms of the SMI itself. Perhaps it should come as no surprise that some psychiatric symptoms may have limited influence on overall life satisfaction given that researchers have debated the relative contributions of psychiatric symptoms on other domains of functional outcomes, such as social and community functioning [43].

Our findings should be viewed in light of the associated methodological limitations. Most notably, our study included a relatively small sample size, which may limit the generalizability of our findings to the larger, broad population of persons with SMI. Further, we examined only a subset of the factors that are surely associated with overall life satisfaction. Future studies, with larger samples, are needed that allow for the simultaneous examination of additional social-environmental predictors of QoL, such as trauma history, relationship status, or vocational factors.

An additional limitation is that our findings may be limited to those persons who are actively involved in treatment. Participation within a mental health system may influence some individuals to become more aware of and/or knowledgeable about the influence of factors such as symptoms or medical comorbidities on their functioning. Certainly, as mental health service systems increasingly address physical health issues, one would expect that service consumers would become more attuned to their physical functioning. Thus, our findings may not be consistent with the experiences of those individuals with SMI who are not actively participating in mental health services, or receiving health care in general. Thus, further work is needed to replicate and extend the current findings in other SMI populations, such as younger (and older) participants and those not involved in the formal mental health system.

5. Conclusion

This study adds to the important line of research on overall life satisfaction, which ultimately may have important policy and clinical implications in this population. A growing body of outcomes research has revealed that improvements in cognition, reduction of psychiatric symptoms, and access to social services may be necessary, but not sufficient methods of improving life satisfaction in people with SMI [6, 44]. Our findings that persons with SMI are concerned with both mental and physical HRQoL and that various aspects of QoL have distinct patterns of association indicate that recovery and improvements in well-being require attention to multiple levels of factors, including medical, psychiatric, and psychosocial ones. These findings therefore support the growing emphasis on more integrated mental and physical health services, particularly for populations such as persons with SMI who have significant health comorbidities. The appreciation of the physical health care needs of individuals within the mental health system is consistent with emerging state and national trends, which advocate for addressing both mental health and physical health as a part of a whole-body approach to well-being [45].

Acknowledgments

This study was supported in part by a Grant from the University of Missouri Research Board to M. Rempfer. All authors declare that they have no conflict of interests relevant to this research project. They thank Dr. Kym Bennett for her helpful feedback on this project and paper.

References

[1] S. Evans, S. Banerjee, M. Leese, and P. Huxley, "The impact of mental illness on quality of life: a comparison of severe mental illness, common mental disorder and healthy population samples," *Quality of Life Research*, vol. 16, no. 1, pp. 17–29, 2007.

[2] F. Dickerson, C. H. Brown, L. Fang et al., "Quality of life in individuals with serious mental illness and type 2 diabetes," *Psychosomatics*, vol. 49, no. 2, pp. 109–114, 2008.

[3] J. M. Narvaez, E. W. Twamley, C. L. McKibbin, R. K. Heaton, and T. L. Patterson, "Subjective and objective quality of life in schizophrenia," *Schizophrenia Research*, vol. 98, no. 1–3, pp. 201–208, 2008.

[4] D. P. Folsom, C. Depp, B. W. Palmer et al., "Physical and mental health-related quality of life among older people with schizophrenia," *Schizophrenia Research*, vol. 108, no. 1–3, pp. 207–213, 2009.

[5] S. M. Eack and C. E. Newhill, "Psychiatric symptoms and quality of life in schizophrenia: a meta-analysis," *Schizophrenia Bulletin*, vol. 33, no. 5, pp. 1225–1237, 2007.

[6] A. W. Tolman and M. M. Kurtz, "Neurocognitive predictors of objective and subjective quality of life in individuals with schizophrenia: a meta-analytic investigation," *Schizophrenia Bulletin*, vol. 38, no. 2, pp. 304–315, 2012.

[7] C. Brown, M. Rempfer, and E. Hamera, "Correlates of insider and outsider conceptualizations of recovery," *Psychiatric Rehabilitation Journal*, vol. 32, no. 1, pp. 23–31, 2008.

[8] M. Lambert, B. G. Schimmelmann, A. Schacht et al., "Long-term patterns of subjective wellbeing in schizophrenia: cluster, predictors of cluster affiliation, and their relation to recovery criteria in 2842 patients followed over 3 years," *Schizophrenia Research*, vol. 107, no. 2-3, pp. 165–172, 2009.

[9] S. Wegener, M. A. Redoblado-Hodge, S. Lucas, D. Fitzgerald, A. Harris, and J. Brennan, "Relative contributions of psychiatric symptoms and neuropsychological functioning to quality of life in first-episode psychosis," *Australian and New Zealand Journal of Psychiatry*, vol. 39, no. 6, pp. 487–492, 2005.

[10] M. Ritsner, A. Gibel, and Y. Ratner, "Determinants of changes in perceived quality of life in the course of schizophrenia," *Quality of Life Research*, vol. 15, no. 3, pp. 515–526, 2006.

[11] M. S. Ritsner, A. Lisker, and M. Arbitman, "Ten-year quality of life outcomes among patients with schizophrenia and schizoaffective disorders: I. Predictive value of disorder-related factors," *Quality of Life Research*, vol. 21, no. 5, pp. 837–847, 2012.

[12] D. L. Kelly, D. L. Boggs, and R. R. Conley, "Reaching for Wellness in Schizophrenia," *Psychiatric Clinics of North America*, vol. 30, no. 3, pp. 453–479, 2007.

[13] P. Auquier, M. C. Simeoni, C. Sapin et al., "Development and validation of a patient-based health-related quality of life questionnaire in schizophrenia: the S-QoL," *Schizophrenia Research*, vol. 63, no. 1-2, pp. 137–149, 2003.

[14] F. Porzsolt, C. P. Wolpl, C. E. Rist, R. Kosa, G. Buchele, and W. Gaus, "Comparison of three instruments (QLQ-C30, SF-36, QWB-7) measuring health-related quality of life/quality of well-being," *Psycho-Oncology*, vol. 5, pp. 103–117, 1996.

[15] L. M. Arnold, K. A. Witzeman, M. L. Swank, S. L. McElroy, and P. E. Keck, "Health-related quality of life using the SF-36 in patients with bipolar disorder compared with patients with chronic back pain and the general population," *Journal of Affective Disorders*, vol. 57, no. 1–3, pp. 235–239, 2000.

[16] D. Vancampfort, M. Probst, T. Scheewe et al., "Lack of physical activity during leisure time contributes to an impaired health related quality of life in patients with schizophrenia," *Schizophrenia Research*, vol. 129, no. 2-3, pp. 122–127, 2011.

[17] J. E. Ware, K. K. Snow, M. Kosinski, and B. Gandek, *The SF-36 Health Survey Manual and Interpretation Guide*, The Health Institute, New England Medical Centre, Boston, Mass, USA, 1993.

[18] C. J. Meijer, M. W. J. Koeter, M. A. G. Sprangers, and A. H. Schene, "Predictors of general quality of life and the mediating role of health related quality of life in patients with schizophrenia," *Social Psychiatry and Psychiatric Epidemiology*, vol. 44, no. 5, pp. 361–368, 2009.

[19] C. J. Meijer, A. H. Schene, and M. W. J. Koeter, "Quality of life in schizophrenia measured by the MOS SF-36 and the Lancashire Quality of Life Profile: a comparison," *Acta Psychiatrica Scandinavica*, vol. 105, no. 4, pp. 293–300, 2002.

[20] M. B. First, R. L. Spitzer, M. Gibbon, and J. B. W. Williams, *Structured Clinical Interview for DSM-IV Axis I Disorders, Clinician Version (SCID-CV)*, American Psychiatric Press, Washington, DC, USA, 1996.

[21] J. Hewitt, "Critical evaluation of the use of research tools in evaluating quality of life for people with schizophrenia," *International Journal of Mental Health Nursing*, vol. 16, no. 1, pp. 2–14, 2007.

[22] J. D. Burke, K. C. Burke, J. H. Baker, and A. Hillis, "Test-retest reliability in psychiatric patients of the sf-36 health survey," *International Journal of Methods in Psychiatric Research*, vol. 5, no. 3, pp. 189–194, 1996.

[23] R. Pukrop, V. Schlaak, A. M. Möller-Leimkühler et al., "Reliability and validity of Quality of Life assessed by the Short-Form 36 and the Modular System for Quality of Life in patients with schizophrenia and patients with depression," *Psychiatry Research*, vol. 119, no. 1-2, pp. 63–79, 2003.

[24] J. Endicott, J. Nee, W. Harrison, and R. Blumenthal, "Quality of life enjoyment and satisfaction questionnaire: a new measure," *Psychopharmacology Bulletin*, vol. 29, no. 2, pp. 321–326, 1993.

[25] M. Ritsner, R. Kurs, A. Gibel, Y. Ratner, and J. Endicott, "Validity of an abbreviated Quality of Life Enjoyment and Satisfaction Questionnaire (Q-LES-Q-18) for schizophrenia, schizoaffective,and mood disorder patients," *Quality of Life Research*, vol. 14, no. 7, pp. 1693–1703, 2005.

[26] D. Lukoff, K. H. Nuechterlein, and J. Ventura, "Manual for the expanded BPRS," *Schizophrenia Bulletin*, vol. 12, pp. 594–602, 1986.

[27] M. Hamilton, "Development of a rating scale for primary depressive illness.," *The British Journal of Social Clinical Psychology*, vol. 6, no. 4, pp. 278–296, 1967.

[28] M. F. Green, R. S. Kern, D. L. Braff, and J. Mintz, "Neurocognitive deficits and functional outcome in schizophrenia: are we measuring the "right stuff"?" *Schizophrenia Bulletin*, vol. 26, no. 1, pp. 119–136, 2000.

[29] S. K. Kongs, L. L. Thompson, G. L. Iverson, and R. K. Heaton, *Wisconsin Card Sorting Test-64 Card Version: Professional Manual*, Psychological Assessment Resources, Odessa, Fla, USA, 2000.

[30] R. M. Reitan, *Trail Making Test*, Reitan Neuropsychology Laboratory, Tucson, Ariz, USA, 1992.

[31] A. L. Benton and K. S. Hamsher, *Multilingual Aphasia Examination Manual*, University of Iowa, Iowa City, Iowa, USA, 1976.

[32] R. Brickenkamp and E. Zillmer, *D2 Test of Attention*, Hogrefe and Huber Publishers, Seattle, Wash, USA, 1998.

[33] D. Wechsler, *Wechsler Adult Intelligence Scale: Administration and Scoring Manual*, The Psychological Corporation, San Antonio, Tex, USA, 3rd edition, 1997.

[34] D. C. Delis, J. H. Kramer, E. Kaplan, and B. A. Ober, *California Verbal Learning Test—Second Edition: Adult Version Manual*, The Psychological Corporation, San Antonio, Tex, USA, 2000.

[35] B. T. Mausbach, P. D. Harvey, S. R. Goldman, D. V. Jeste, and T. L. Patterson, "Development of a brief scale of everyday functioning in persons with serious mental illness," *Schizophrenia Bulletin*, vol. 33, no. 6, pp. 1364–1372, 2007.

[36] T. L. Patterson, S. Goldman, C. L. McKibbin, T. Hughs, and D. V. Jeste, "UCSD Performance-Based Skills Assessment: development of a new measure of everyday functioning for severly mentally ill adults," *Schizophrenia Bulletin*, vol. 27, no. 2, pp. 235–245, 2001.

[37] B. T. Mausbach, R. Moore, C. Bowie, V. Cardenas, and T. L. Patterson, "A Review of instruments for measuring functional recovery in those diagnosed with psychosis," *Schizophrenia Bulletin*, vol. 35, no. 2, pp. 307–318, 2009.

[38] L. Dixon, L. Postrado, J. Delahanty, P. J. Fischer, and A. Lehman, "The association of medical comorbidity in schizophrenia with poor physical and mental health," *Journal of Nervous and Mental Disease*, vol. 187, no. 8, pp. 496–502, 1999.

[39] M. Ritsner, R. Kurs, H. Kostizky, A. Ponizovsky, and I. Modai, "Subjective quality of life in severely mentally ill patients: a comparison of two instruments," *Quality of Life Research*, vol. 11, no. 6, pp. 553–561, 2002.

[40] D. Schechter, J. Endicott, and J. Nee, "Quality of life of "normal" controls: association with lifetime history of mental illness," *Psychiatry Research*, vol. 152, no. 1, pp. 45–54, 2007.

[41] A. L. Hackman, R. W. Goldberg, C. H. Brown et al., "Use of emergency department services for somatic reasons by people with serious mental illness," *Psychiatric Services*, vol. 57, no. 4, pp. 563–566, 2006.

[42] P. H. Lysaker and V. A. LaRocco, "Health-related quality of life and trauma history in adults with schizophrenia spectrum disorders," *Journal of Nervous and Mental Disease*, vol. 197, no. 5, pp. 311–315, 2009.

[43] J. Ventura, G. S. Hellemann, A. D. Thames, V. Koellner, and K. H. Nuechterlein, "Symptoms as mediators of the relationship between neurocognition and functional outcome in schizophrenia: a meta-analysis," *Schizophrenia Research*, vol. 113, no. 2-3, pp. 189–199, 2009.

[44] M. A. Test, J. S. Greenberg, J. D. Long, J. S. Brekke, and S. S. Burke, "Construct validity of a measure of subjective satisfaction with life of adults with serious mental illness," *Psychiatric Services*, vol. 56, no. 3, pp. 292–300, 2005.

[45] A. Q. Radke, J. Parks, and T. J. Ruter, "A call for improved prevention and reduction of obesity among persons with serious mental illness," *Psychiatric Services*, vol. 61, no. 6, pp. 617–619, 2010.

5

Role of Long-Acting Injectable Second-Generation Antipsychotics in the Treatment of First-Episode Schizophrenia: A Clinical Perspective

Radovan Přikryl,[1,2] Hana Přikrylová Kučerová,[1,2] Michaela Vrzalová,[2] and Eva Češková[1,2]

[1] *Central European Institute of Technology, Masaryk University (CEITEC-MU), Kamenice 753/5, 62500 Brno, Czech Republic*
[2] *Department of Psychiatry, Faculty of Medicine Masaryk University, University Hospital Brno, Jihlavska 20, 62500 Brno, Czech Republic*

Correspondence should be addressed to Radovan Přikryl, radovan.prikryl@post.cz

Academic Editor: Dawn I. Velligan

Approximately 80% of patients with the first-episode schizophrenia reach symptomatic remission after antipsychotic therapy. However, within two years most of them relapse, mainly due to low levels of insight into the illness and nonadherence to their oral medication. Therefore, although the formal data available is limited, many experts recommend prescribing long-acting injectable second-generation antipsychotics (mostly risperidone or alternatively paliperidone) in the early stages of schizophrenia, particularly in patients who have benefited from the original oral molecule in the past and agree to receive long-term injectable treatment. Early application of long-acting injectable second-generation antipsychotics can significantly reduce the risk of relapse in the future and thus improve not only the social and working potential of patients with schizophrenia but also their quality of life.

1. Depot Antipsychotics for the Treatment of Schizophrenia

First-generation long-acting injectable (depot) antipsychotics (AP1G) emerged in clinical practice in the 1960s. For the treatment of schizophrenia, their use resulted in a significant decrease in the number of patients relapses, including length and frequency of hospitalizations [1]. However, when oral second-generation antipsychotics (AP2G) were introduced thirty years later, the position (in clinical practice) of depot AP1G dramatically changed. Despite the benefits of AP1G, psychiatrists prescribed them for long-term therapy of schizophrenia much less often and started to switch to oral AP2G as they were seen as more efficient and better tolerated [2]. This trend persisted for many years, despite evidence to suggest from meta-analyses and naturalistic studies that depot AP1G were more effective in reducing schizophrenic relapses than oral AP2G [3]. The same finding was later logically replicated also for long-acting injectable (LAI) AP2G [4–7]. Although patients with schizophrenia are often willing to use depot or LAI antipsychotics, these preparations are today prescribed only for approximately 20% of them [8–10]. In a survey [11] psychiatrists answered that they only offer long-acting injectable antipsychotics to one in every three patients with schizophrenia.

2. Specifics for First-Episode Schizophrenia Therapy

Therapy for the first episode of schizophrenia has certain specific features. Patients respond to low doses of antipsychotics relatively well; yet they are more sensitive to the adverse effects, particularly extrapyramidal ones [12, 13]. Patients with first-episode schizophrenia, however, typically show low willingness to use antipsychotics in the long-term treatment, likely due to their high unawareness of the disease severity. Recommended duration of antipsychotic administration after the first episode of schizophrenia usually ranges from 1 to 2 years [12–14]. A five-year observation study of first-episode patients showed that the risk of relapse is five times higher after discontinuation of therapy compared to continuous medication [15]. Despite the recommendations from their psychiatrists, patients with schizophrenia discontinue their therapy often. Results of the clinical antipsychotic trials of intervention effectiveness (CATIE) study indicate that up to 74% of patients with schizophrenia discontinued their therapy after 18 months; the European First Episode Schizophrenia Trial (EUFEST) shows that up to 42% of patients terminated their treatment within one year after the disease onset [16, 17]. When considering the length of subsequent prophylactic treatment after the first episode of schizophrenia; not only its efficacy but also the profile or severity of adverse events of the given antipsychotic must be taken into account. Moreover, it should be taken into consideration that approximately 20% of first-episode patients will never experience a subsequent exacerbation of schizophrenia, irrespective of whether they receive or the type of therapy they receive [14, 18].

3. Problems Associated with Nonadherence to Pharmacological Treatment of Schizophrenia

Schizophrenia is a chronic mental disease characterized among other things by a high degree of nonadherence to prescribed medication [19]. It has been reported that patients take on average only 58% of their prescribed drugs, 41.2% of patients do not use their medication according to prescription, and one- to two-thirds of patients take their pills irregularly [20–22]. These are the results of questionnaire surveys, and therefore they reflect only the situation of patients that agreed to take part in the research; in reality, therefore the rates of nonadherence may be much higher. In general, the current guidelines on schizophrenia treatment consider depot or long-acting injectable antipsychotics as drugs of choice for long-term therapy in patients who are nonadherent with antipsychotic medication [12–14]. Systematic surveys of specific studies indicate that patients treated with depot antipsychotics show only a 24% non-adherence rate while they are sufficiently covered by medication for 91% of the total therapy time [23–25].

4. Long-Acting Injectable versus Oral Antipsychotics in the Treatment of Schizophrenia

Since available studies differ in methodology and primary observation goals [26], it is difficult to generalize on the effects of oral or long-acting injectable administration of antipsychotics on the course of schizophrenia. In a meta-analysis, Adams et al. [27] did not prove dominance of depot AP1G over oral antipsychotics in terms of reduction of the number of relapses. Nevertheless, overall improvement was seen more often in patients treated with depot antipsychotics [27]. On the other hand, a recent meta-analysis [7] found lower levels of relapse in patients with schizophrenia treated with depot AP1G or LAI AP2G, compared with those treated with oral antipsychotics. Still, the two therapeutic strategies did not differ in the number of rehospitalizations, terminations of therapy, or cases of non-adherence. Inconsistency of results might be explained by the nature of double-blind randomized studies that, of course, do not typically enroll non-adherent patients who are likely to benefit most from the depot/LAI formulation of antipsychotic therapy. Conditions of real clinical practice are therefore better simulated by observation studies where depot and oral antipsychotics are often compared with a mirror design. These studies describe almost consistently lower number of days of hospitalization during depot or LAI antipsychotic therapy, as compared with the same period of oral medication [1, 28]. The main methodological problem of these studies lies in the fact that, when the initial oral antipsychotic medication fails, a new oral treatment is prescribed, whilst the injectable medication remains the same. This can significantly affect the comparison of the therapy efficacy in identical time periods [26].

5. Long-Acting Injectable Antipsychotics in First-Episode Schizophrenia

Depot AP1Gs, let alone LAI AP2G, are rarely prescribed for patients with first-episode schizophrenia, although their levels of non-adherence and hence the risk of subsequent relapse are in reality very high [29, 30]. Importantly, adverse course of early schizophrenia has a profound negative influence on psychosocial integration of patients, not to mention a patients ability to remain in education and/or employment. Economic consequences of schizophrenia therefore represent a burden not only for health system but also for the social system of public health insurance. Psychiatrists usually explain the low prescription rate of LAI antipsychotics in the initial/early stage of schizophrenia treatment as an unwillingness of patient to receive injections on an outpatient basis or generally by negative attitudes to depot/LAI antipsychotics [31, 32].

6. Long-Acting Injectable Antipsychotics in First-Episode Schizophrenia: Attitudes of Psychiatrists

Heres et al. [33] used a questionnaire to ask almost 200 German psychiatrists at the national congress in 2008 about their attitudes towards the use of LAI antipsychotics in patients with first-episode schizophrenia. They found that long-term injectable therapy was only offered to 26.7% of patients with first-episode schizophrenia; it was actually prescribed to 13.3% of those offered (i.e., one of every two). Respondents also reported that up to 60.4% patients taking antipsychotics irregularly will relapse within one year after the first episode [33]. The main outcome of this questionnaire was that it identified the three principal reasons for *not* using LAI antipsychotics in patients with first-episode schizophrenia. German psychiatrists stated that they find it difficult to present the benefits of a long-term injectable antipsychotic therapy to patients who do not have any personal experience with schizophrenia relapse, as they are still at the very beginning of their illness. Poor availability of LAI AP2G was identified as another reason, particularly when AP2G are strongly preferred over AP1G, especially in patients with first-episode schizophrenia. The last reason was mainly personal reservations of the psychiatrists associated associated with difficult control of adverse effects of depot antipsychotics, negative impact on patient-psychiatrist relationship, or higher amount of psychiatrist's time needed to manage depot medication administration [33]. The survey indicates that the only barrier to more frequent use of LAI AP2G in patients with first-episode schizophrenia, which is not influenced by perceptions of patients and psychiatrists, is the issue with market availability, price, and method of reimbursement. At present, only LAI risperidone, olanzapine pamoate, and paliperidone palmitate are available in most countries. For many reasons, limited availability of these drugs is today considered as the main barrier of their more common use in the therapy of schizophrenia [2, 11, 32]. This is problem mainly in first-episode patients in whom AP2G are strongly preferred as drugs of first choice [13, 34, 35]. Hopefully, better availability of LAI AP2G, simpler prescription rules, and better reimbursement from public health insurance will result in more common use of these products in clinical practice. However, this logical sequence of thoughts is in conflict with the real situation in the UK where better availability of LAI risperidone did not increase the use of LAI antipsychotics for treatment of schizophrenia despite previous belief of British psychiatrists that availability of these products was highly desirable and would significantly change their prescription habits in favor of LAI antipsychotics [2, 32]. Keeping this in mind, the latter assumption that better availability of LAI AP2G would make psychiatrists prescribe LAI preparations more often sounds ironic [32]. Other reasons for not prescribing LAIs reflect subjective attitudes of psychiatrists and patients towards injectable therapy in general. The questionnaire by Heres et al. clearly highlighted that only one in four patients with first-episode schizophrenia was offered the possibility of treatment with LAI AP2G and half of those that were, agreed. That means that three out of four patients were not offered this type of therapy from their psychiatrist. Actually, the fact that psychiatrists, driven by their own personal negative attitudes/perceptions, offer LAI AP2G less frequently is a true barrier to using these products more commonly in patients with first-episode schizophrenia. Psychiatrists often say that first-episode patients reject LAI AP2G because they have not yet experienced a schizophrenic relapse. In this sense, higher efficacy of a LAI AP2G in prevention of relapses may not be a feasible argument [1, 5, 36]. Alternatively, low prescription rates can be explained by the fact that psychiatrists suppose beforehand (without discussing the issue with patients) that first-episode patients will not be interested in LAI AP2G therapy for the above-mentioned reasons. Interestingly, high self-confidence of psychiatrists to foreknow attitudes of their patients is considered to be one of the key factors of less frequent use of LAI AP2G in clinical practice [2, 32].

7. Long-Acting Injectable Antipsychotics in First-Episode Schizophrenia: Current Knowledge

Recent studies show that long-term injectable AP2G therapy is effective and also acceptable for first-episode patients, which is in opposition to the above-mentioned "conservative" attitudes [30, 37]. Unfortunately, studies comparing long-term injection or depot therapy with oral antipsychotic treatment after the first episode of schizophrenia are rare [38]. From this perspective, unique data can be drawn from a nation wide cohort study aimed at identification of the risk of rehospitalization and therapy discontinuation in more than 2,500 patients first hospitalized for schizophrenia between 2000 and 2007 in Finland [26]. The results show that in Finland, where antipsychotics are fully reimbursed from general health insurance systems, only 45.7% patients pick up prescribed drugs within one month and continue their therapy. Data are highly representative, since the study used the national registry and incorporated every single patient in Finland who was hospitalized for schizophrenia for the first time. Although information about medication during hospitalization was not available, almost all patients were recommended to start subsequent antipsychotic therapy. As compared with studies such as CATIE [16] or EUFEST [17], the Finnish study indicated higher rate of therapy discontinuation. This could be explained by the nature of the study which made it possible to capture real everyday behavior of patients, irrespective of their motivations or willingness to cooperate. As Finland, just as the majority of other countries, has not established any compulsory outpatient psychiatric screening, comparison of efficiency of individual antipsychotics can be generalized only for persons who were willing to visit their psychiatrist on an outpatient basis. It turned out that administration of depot AP1G and LAI risperidone resulted in reduction of the risk of rehospitalization by 50% or 65%, respectively, compared with oral formulations of the same antipsychotics. Depot AP1G or LAI risperidone were the first-choice drug in 8% of patients, and, in total, they comprised 10% of treated patient-years [26]. This is relatively low, especially when compared with patients with chronic schizophrenia. So far, these antipsychotic formulations have been earmarked mainly for patients with low insight into the illness and poor adherence to the therapy. However, if the target population for LAI AP2G would be extended to include also patients with better insight and apparent adherence, rehospitalization rate should decrease. Of course, this would apply only to patients who are willing to use these products on an outpatient basis.

Table 1: Survey of studies on LAI risperidone in first-episode schizophrenia patients.

Author, year	Study design	Duration of schizophrenia	N	Comparator	Result
Parellada et al., 2005 [39]	Six-month open study	Median one year, no more than 3 years	382	0	73% patients completed the study, statistically significant decrease of PANSS; 40% patients achieved at least 20% reduction of total PANSS score.
Malla et al., 2006 [44]	Two-year open study	Up to 3 years	15	Oral AP2G	More significant reduction of total PANSS score versus oral risperidone.
Emsley et al. 2009 [30]	Two-year open study	First episode	50	0	72% patients completed the study; 78% of them reached at least 50% reduction of symptoms; remission persisted for two years in 62% patients [42].

8. Long-Acting Injectable Second-Generation Antipsychotics in First-Episode Schizophrenia

As far as LAI AP2G products are concerned, researchers have clinical experience with LAI risperidone, olanzapine pamoate, and paliperidone palmitate. Although many studies in schizophrenia with these products have been performed, relatively limited data on their use specifically in first-episode patients is available. Only LAI risperidone has been specifically studied for the use in early stage of schizophrenia (see Table 1) in addition specific post-hoc analyses have been performed in patients classified as having recent onset schizophrenia. Parellada et al. [39] designed a six-month open-label study with LAI risperidone to analyze a subgroup of 382 patients with recent schizophrenia or schizoaffective disorder (diagnosed $\leq$ 3 years ago) [40]. Schizophrenia was diagnosed in 84% of patients, with median of one year after the diagnosis was established. Previous medication included mainly AP2G (70%) and depot AP1G (24%). Non-adherence (42%) and poor efficacy (31%) of previous medication were the main reasons for changing the therapy. The study was completed by 73% patients who showed significant decrease of severity of schizophrenic symptomatology, reflected by statistically significant reduction of not only total PANSS score (positive and negative syndrom scale) [41] but also all PANSS subscales. In 40% of patients, total PANSS score decreased by at least 20%. At the same time, patients showed an improvement of overall functioning, quality of life, and satisfaction [39]. In other study, Emsley et al. [30] administered LAI risperidone monotherapy to fifty patients with the first episode of schizophrenia: this two-year observation study was completed by 36 patients (72%), 39 patients (78%) showed reduction of symptoms by at least 50%; 4 of them relapsed, 32 patients (64%) reached remission according to the proposed criteria for the remission in schizophrenia [42], and 31 patients (62%) reached remission that persisted throughout the two years of the study [30]. After two years, 33 patients decided to terminate the therapy. Seventy-nine percent (79%) of those then subsequently relapsed (median to relapse: 163 days). Based on these results, Emsley et al. [43] assert that first-episode patients who reached remission are prone to relapse after discontinuation of continuous long-acting injectable risperidone therapy. Antipsychotic treatment in such patients should therefore be continuous and maintained for at least two years [43]. Malla et al. [44] published data from their two-year prospective open multicentric study that was performed with young patients (aged 18 to 30 years) suffering from schizophreniform disorder, schizophrenia, or schizoaffective disorder (for no longer than 3 years). Patients were randomized to treatment with oral AP2G or LAI risperidone. Although it is difficult to generalize the results due to low number of subjects enrolled in the study ($n = 15$), patients treated with LAI risperidone showed more significant reduction of total PANSS score (by 16.1), as compared with oral AP2G (by 5.0) [44]. Weiden et al. [37] published preliminary data about early adherence from their randomized controlled study that compared LAI risperidone with oral AP2G in first-episode patients [37]. Nineteen (19, 73%) of 26 patients who were asked to participate in the study agreed to be treated with LAI risperidone; the other group consisted of 11 patients. Adherence rate in the twelfth week of observation was comparable in both groups. However, adherence questionnaires indicated that patients accepting LAI risperidone therapy showed higher probability of adherence, as compared with patients treated with oral antipsychotics [37]. Bartzokis et al. [45] examined the impact of antipsychotic formulation on the myelination trajectory during a randomized six-month trial of LAI risperidone versus oral risperidone in first-episode schizophrenia subjects. Two groups (11 patients treated with LAI risperidone and 13 patients treated with oral risperidone) that were matched in prerandomization oral medication exposure and 14 healthy controls were prospectively examined. Frontal lobe white matter volume was estimated using inversion recovery MRI (magnetic resonance imaging) images. A brief neuropsychological battery that focused on reaction times was performed at the end of the study. White matter volume remained stable in the LAI risperidone group and decreased significantly in the oral risperidone group resulting in a significant differential treatment effect, while the healthy controls had a white matter change intermediate and not significantly different from the two schizophrenia groups. White matter increase was associated with faster reaction times in tests involving frontal lobe function. The results suggest that LAI risperidone may improve the trajectory of myelination in first-episode patients and has a beneficial impact on cognitive performance. Better adherence provided by LAI AP2G may underlie the modified trajectory of myelin development [45].

9. Benefits of Long-Acting Injectable Antipsychotics in First-Episode Patients with Schizophrenia: Clinical Perspective and Summary

LAI AP2G have been used in clinical practice for several years. Nowadays, LAI AP2G are reserved mainly for patients with long-term course of schizophrenia who show low adherence to oral medication. The studies performed especially with LAI risperidone in patients with first episode or early stage of schizophrenia clearly indicated that this form of therapy could be effective and well tolerated also in this subgroup of patients with schizophrenia. Thanks to the familiar mother molecule (paliperidone is 9-OH risperidone, which is the active metabolite of risperidone) data concerning efficacy and tolerability of LAI risperidone in first-episode schizophrenia, patients could be applicable for paliperidone palmitate as well. Combined benefits of AP2G characteristics with an assured route of administration raise a question whether LAI AP2G should be recommended also in first-episode patients [46, 47]. Instead of foreknowing/guessing whether patients will accept LAI therapy or not, psychiatrists should offer this form of treatment as a routine choice to all appropriate patients with schizophrenia, including first-episode subjects. Selection between long-term injectable therapy and oral medication should be based on educational and therapeutic dialogue of the psychiatrist and the patient who can then in turn discuss the potential benefits and disadvantages of the proposed therapeutic strategy [48, 49].

Approximately 80% of patients with a first episode of schizophrenia reach symptomatic remission after antipsychotic therapy. However, within two years most of them relapse mainly due to low insight into the illness and non-adherence to oral medication. Therefore, although the formal data available are limited many experts recommend prescribing long-acting second-generation antipsychotics (especially LAI risperidone or alternatively paliperidone palmitate) in the early stages of schizophrenia, particularly in patients who benefited from the original oral molecule in the past and agree to receive long-term injection treatment. Early application of long-acting injectable second-generation antipsychotics can significantly reduce the risk of relapses in future and thus improve not only social and working potential of patients with schizophrenia but also their quality of life.

Acknowledgment

This work was supported by the Research Plan MSM0021622404 of the Ministry of Education, Youth and Sports of the Czech Republic.

References

[1] J. M. Davis, L. Metalon, M. D. Watanabe, and L. Blake, "Depot antipsychotic drugs. Place in therapy," *Drugs*, vol. 47, no. 5, pp. 741–773, 1994.

[2] M. X. Patel, V. Nikolaou, and A. S. David, "Psychiatrists' attitudes to maintenance medication for patients with schizophrenia," *Psychological Medicine*, vol. 33, no. 1, pp. 83–89, 2003.

[3] J. Tiihonen, K. Wahlbeck, J. Lönnqvist et al., "Effectiveness of antipsychotic treatments in a nationwide cohort of patients in community care after first hospitalisation due to schizophrenia and schizoaffective disorder: observational follow-up study," *British Medical Journal*, vol. 333, no. 7561, pp. 224–227, 2006.

[4] P. Chue, P. M. Llorca, I. Duchesne, A. Leal, D. Rosillon, and A. Mehnert, "Hospitalization rates in patients during long-term treatment with long-acting risperidone injection," *Journal of Applied Research*, vol. 5, no. 2, pp. 266–274, 2005.

[5] R. Medori, R. Wapenaar, A. de Rosario et al., "Relapse prevention and effectiveness in schizophrenia with risperidone long-acting injectable (RLAI) versus quetiapine," in *Proceedings of the 116th Annual Convention of the APA*, Boston, Mass, USA, 2008.

[6] G. M. Simpson, R. A. Mahmoud, R. A. Lasser et al., "A 1-year double-blind study of 2 doses of long-acting risperidone in stable patients with schizophrenia or schizoaffective disorder," *Journal of Clinical Psychiatry*, vol. 67, no. 8, pp. 1194–1203, 2006.

[7] C. Leucht, S. Heres, J. M. Kane, W. Kissling, J. M. Davis, and S. Leucht, "Oral versus depot antipsychotic drugs for schizophrenia—a critical systematic review and meta-analysis of randomised long-term trials," *Schizophrenia Research*, vol. 127, no. 1-3, pp. 83–92, 2011.

[8] K. Sim, A. Su, G. S. Ungvari et al., "Depot antipsychotic use in schizophrenia: an East Asian perspective," *Human Psychopharmacology*, vol. 19, no. 2, pp. 103–109, 2004.

[9] H. A. Nasrallah, "The case for long-acting antipsychotic agents in the post-CATIE era," *Acta Psychiatrica Scandinavica*, vol. 115, no. 4, pp. 260–267, 2007.

[10] J. Ahn, J. S. McCombs, C. Jung et al., "Classifying patients by antipsychotic adherence patterns using latent class analysis: characteristics of nonadherent groups in the California Medicaid (Medi-Cal) program," *Value in Health*, vol. 11, no. 1, pp. 48–56, 2008.

[11] S. Heres, J. Hamann, W. Kissling, and S. Leucht, "Attitudes of psychiatrists toward antipsychotic depot medication," *Journal of Clinical Psychiatry*, vol. 67, no. 12, pp. 1948–1953, 2006.

[12] R. W. Buchanan, J. Kreyenbuhl, D. L. Kelly et al., "The 2009 schizophrenia PORT psychopharmacological treatment recommendations and summary statements," *Schizophrenia Bulletin*, vol. 36, no. 1, pp. 71–93, 2010.

[13] J. Raboch, M. Anders, P. Hellerová, and P. Uhlíková, "Psychiatrie: doporučené postupy psychiatrické péče III," *Tribun EU*, pp. 118–126, 2010.

[14] National Institute for Health and Clinical Excellence (NICE), "Schizophrenia: Core Interventions in the Treatment and Management of Schizophrenia in Adults in Primary and Secondary Care (Update), Final Version (NICE Clinical Guideline 82). NICE, London, UK," 2009, http://www.nice.org.uk/nicemedia/pdf/CG82NICEGuideline.pdf.

[15] D. Robinson, M. G. Woerner, J. M. J. Alvir et al., "Predictors of relapse following response from a first episode of schizophrenia or schizoaffective disorder," *Archives of General Psychiatry*, vol. 56, no. 3, pp. 241–247, 1999.

[16] J. A. Lieberman, T. Scott Stroup, J. P. McEvoy et al., "Effectiveness of antipsychotic drugs in patients with chronic schizophrenia," *New England Journal of Medicine*, vol. 353, no. 12, pp. 1209–1223, 2005.

[17] R. S. Kahn, W. W. Fleischhacker, H. Boter et al., "Effectiveness of antipsychotic drugs in first-episode schizophrenia and schizophreniform disorder: an open randomised clinical trial," *The Lancet*, vol. 371, no. 9618, pp. 1085–1097, 2008.

[18] P. M. Haddad and S. G. Sharma, "Adverse effects of atypical antipsychotics: differential risk and clinical implications," *CNS Drugs*, vol. 21, no. 11, pp. 911–936, 2007.

[19] J. Kreyenbuhl, E. P. Slade, D. R. Medoff et al., "Time to discontinuation of first- and second-generation antipsychotic medications in the treatment of schizophrenia," *Schizophrenia Research*, vol. 131, no. 1–3, pp. 127–132, 2011.

[20] J. A. Cramer and R. Rosenheck, "Compliance with medication regimens for mental and physical disorders," *Psychiatric Services*, vol. 49, no. 2, pp. 196–201, 1998.

[21] J. P. Lacro, L. B. Dunn, C. R. Dolder, S. G. Leckband, and D. V. Jeste, "Prevalence of and risk factors for medication nonadherence in patients with schizophrenia: a comprehensive review of recent literature," *Journal of Clinical Psychiatry*, vol. 63, no. 10, pp. 892–909, 2002.

[22] P. Thieda, S. Beard, A. Richter, and J. Kane, "An economic review of compliance with medication therapy in the treatment of schizophrenia," *Psychiatric Services*, vol. 54, no. 4, pp. 508–516, 2003.

[23] J. L. Young, H. V. Zonana, and L. Shepler, "Medication noncompliance in schizophrenia: codification and update," *Bulletin of the American Academy of Psychiatry and the Law*, vol. 14, no. 2, pp. 105–122, 1986.

[24] J. L. Young, R. T. Spitz, M. Hillbrand, and G. Daneri, "Medication adherence failure in schizophrenia: a forensic review of rates, reasons, treatments, and prospects," *Journal of the American Academy of Psychiatry and the Law*, vol. 27, no. 3, pp. 426–444, 1999.

[25] L. Shi, H. Ascher-Svanum, B. Zhu, D. Faries, W. Montgomery, and S. R. Marder, "Characteristics and use patterns of patients taking first-generation depot antipsychotics or oral antipsychotics for schizophrenia," *Psychiatric Services*, vol. 58, no. 4, pp. 482–488, 2007.

[26] J. Tiihonen, J. Haukka, M. Taylor, P. M. Haddad, M. X. Patel, and P. Korhonen, "A nationwide cohort study of oral and depot antipsychotics after first hospitalization for schizophrenia," *American Journal of Psychiatry*, vol. 168, no. 6, pp. 603–609, 2011.

[27] C. E. Adams, M. K. P. Fenton, S. Quraishi, and A. S. David, "Systematic meta-review of depot antipsychotic drugs for people with schizophrenia," *British Journal of Psychiatry*, vol. 179, pp. 290–299, 2001.

[28] P. M. Haddad, M. Taylor, and O. S. Niaz, "First-generation antipsychotic long-acting injections v. oral antipsychotics in schizophrenia: systematic review of randomised controlled trials and observational studies," *British Journal of Psychiatry*, vol. 195, no. 52, supplement, pp. s20–s28, 2009.

[29] E. L. Coldham, J. Addington, and D. Addington, "Medication adherence of individuals with a first episode of psychosis," *Acta Psychiatrica Scandinavica*, vol. 106, no. 4, pp. 286–290, 2002.

[30] R. Emsley, P. Oosthuizen, L. Koen et al., "A study of the clinical outcome following treatment discontinuation after remission in first-episode schizophrenia," *European Neuropsychopharmacology*, vol. 19, no. 3, supplement, pp. 486–487, 2009.

[31] L. Waddell and M. Taylor, "Attitudes of patients and mental health staff to antipsychotic long-acting injections: systematic review," *British Journal of Psychiatry*, vol. 195, no. 52, pp. s43–s50, 2009.

[32] M. X. Patel, P. M. Haddad, I. B. Chaudhry, S. McLoughlin, and A. S. David, "Psychiatrists' use, knowledge and attitudes to first- and second-generation antipsychotic long-acting injections: comparisons over 5 years," *Journal of Psychopharmacology*, vol. 24, no. 10, pp. 1473–1482, 2010.

[33] S. Heres, T. Reichhart, J. Hamann, R. Mendel, S. Leucht, and W. Kissling, "Psychiatrists' attitude to antipsychotic depot treatment in patients with first-episode schizophrenia," *European Psychiatry*, vol. 26, pp. 297–301, 2011.

[34] A. F. Lehman, J. A. Lieberman, L. B. Dixon et al., "Practice guideline for the treatment of partients with schizophrenia, 2nd Edition," *American Journal of Psychiatry*, vol. 161, no. 2, pp. 1–56, 2004.

[35] P. Falkai, T. Wobrock, J. Lieberman et al., "World Federation of Societies of Biological Psychiatry (WFSBP) guidelines for biological treatment of schizophrenia—part 2: long-term treatment of schizophrenia," *World Journal of Biological Psychiatry*, vol. 7, no. 1, pp. 5–40, 2006.

[36] C. Mentschel, "Depot-drugs may reduce relapse rates in schizophrenic outpatients: a meta-analysis," in *Proceedings of the 156th meeting of the American Psychiatric Association*, p. 71, San Francisco, Calif, USA, 2003.

[37] P. J. Weiden, N. R. Schooler, J. C. Weedon, A. Elmouchtari, A. Sunakawa, and S. M. Goldfinger, "A randomized controlled trial of long-acting injectable risperidone vs continuation on oral atypical antipsychotics for first-episode schizophrenia patients: initial adherence outcome," *Journal of Clinical Psychiatry*, vol. 70, no. 10, pp. 1397–1406, 2009.

[38] M. X. Patel, M. Taylor, and A. S. David, "Antipsychotic long-acting injections: mind the gap," *British Journal of Psychiatry*, vol. 195, no. 52, supplement, pp. s1–s4, 2009.

[39] E. Parellada, R. Andrezina, V. Milanova et al., "Patients in the early phases of schizophrenia and schizoaffective disorders effectively treated with risperidone long-acting injectable," *Journal of Psychopharmacology*, vol. 19, no. 5, pp. 5–14, 2005.

[40] H. J. Möller, P. M. Llorca, E. Sacchetti, S. D. Martin, R. Medori, and E. Parellada, "Efficacy and safety of direct transition to risperidone long-acting injectable in patients treated with various antipsychotic therapies," *International Clinical Psychopharmacology*, vol. 20, no. 3, pp. 121–130, 2005.

[41] S. R. Kay, A. Fiszbein, and L. A. Opler, "The positive and negative syndrome scale (PANSS) for schizophrenia," *Schizophrenia Bulletin*, vol. 13, no. 2, pp. 261–276, 1987.

[42] N. C. Andreasen, W. T. Carpenter, J. M. Kane, R. A. Lasser, S. R. Marder, and D. R. Weinberger, "Remission in schizophrenia: proposed criteria and rationale for consensus," *American Journal of Psychiatry*, vol. 162, no. 3, pp. 441–449, 2005.

[43] R. Emsley, P. Oosthuizen, L. Koen, D. J. H. Niehaus, R. Medori, and J. Rabinowitz, "Remission in patients with first-episode schizophrenia receiving assured antipsychotic medication: a study with risperidone long-acting injection," *International Clinical Psychopharmacology*, vol. 23, no. 6, pp. 325–331, 2008.

[44] A. Malla, C. Binder, and P. Chue, "Comparison of long-acting injectable risperidone and oral novel antipsychotic drugs for treatment in early phase of schizophrenia spectrum psychosis," in *Proceedings of the 61st Annual Convention Society of Biological Psychiatry*, Toronto, Canada, 2006.

[45] G. Bartzokis, P. H. Lu, C. P. Amar et al., "Long acting injection versus oral risperidone in first-episode schizophrenia: differential impact on white matter myelination trajectory," *Schizophrenia Research*, vol. 132, no. 1, pp. 35–41, 2011.

[46] P. Chue and R. Emsley, "Long-acting formulations of atypical antipsychotics: time to reconsider when to introduce depot antipsychotics," *CNS Drugs*, vol. 21, no. 6, pp. 441–448, 2007.

[47] M. X. Patel and A. S. David, "Why aren't depot antipsychotics prescribed more often and what can be done about it?" *Advances in Psychiatric Treatment*, vol. 11, no. 3, pp. 203–213, 2005.

[48] T. Lambert, "Selecting patients for long-acting novel antipsychotic therapy," *Australasian Psychiatry*, vol. 14, no. 1, pp. 38–42, 2006.

[49] R. Fraser, G. Berger, E. Killackey, and P. McGorry, "Emerging psychosis in young people—part 3— key issues for prolonged recovery," *Australian Family Physician*, vol. 35, no. 5, pp. 329–333, 2006.

6

Dissecting the Syndrome of Schizophrenia: Progress toward Clinically Useful Biomarkers

Brian Dean[1, 2]

[1] *The Rebecca L. Cooper Research Laboratories, The Mental Health Research Institute, Locked bag 11, Parkville, VIC 3052, Australia*
[2] *The Department of Psychiatry, The University of Melbourne, Parkville, VIC 3052, Australia*

Correspondence should be addressed to Brian Dean, anddali@unimelb.edu.au

Academic Editor: Vaibhav A. Diwadkar

The search for clinically useful biomarkers has been one of the holy grails of schizophrenia research. This paper will outline the evolving notion of biomarkers and then outline outcomes from a variety of biomarkers discovery strategies. In particular, the impact of high-throughput screening technologies on biomarker discovery will be highlighted and how new or improved technologies may allow the discovery of either diagnostic biomarkers for schizophrenia or biomarkers that will be useful in determining appropriate treatments for people with the disorder. History tells those involved in biomarker research that the discovery and validation of useful biomarkers is a long process and current progress must always be viewed in that light. However, the approval of the first biomarker screen with some value in predicting responsiveness to antipsychotic drugs suggests that biomarkers can be identified and that these biomarkers that will be useful in diagnosing and treating people with schizophrenia.

1. Introduction

There is a growing recognition that the development of drugs with an increasing efficacy for reducing the psychotic symptoms of schizophrenia (Sz) is slowing and there has been little progress in developing treatments for the negative symptoms and cognitive deficits associated with the disorder [1]. In addition, it is now acknowledged that the current symptom-based diagnoses of Sz defines a syndrome of disorders which are likely to have diverse pathophysiologies [2]. This hypothesis is supported by the existence of treatment resistant Sz [3] which does not appear to be primarily associated with the dopaminergic systems of the human CNS because they are the primary targets of antipsychotic drugs [4]. The limitation of having to study the syndrome of Sz is now recognised as hampering progress toward a better understanding of the pathophysiologies of its component disorders [2] whilst having to provide treatments at the level of the syndrome is a major factor preventing the development of personalised medicine [5]. As with other forms of medicine, the solution to both of these problems would be to divide subjects with Sz into more biologically homogenous subgroups using well validated biomarkers as diagnostic tests [6] which in some cases may result in separating groups into endophenotypes [7]. To fulfil the requirement of an endophenotype, subjects clustered by the use of a specific biomarker must have a disorder which is heritable, be primarily state independent and, within families, the endophenotype and illness cosegregate [8]. The differences between dissecting a syndrome using a diagnostic test or into endophenotypes is discussed extensively elsewhere [9]. Briefly, both a biomarker that can be used as a diagnostic test and the characteristics or tests used to define an endophenotype must be detectably different in the large majority, if not all, the subjects within the category defined by the biomarker or an endophenotype.

This paper will focus on the evolving notion of biomarkers and on the progress toward developing biomarkers that will allow subjects with Sz to be divided into more homogeneous subpopulations as a foundation to better understanding their pathophysiologies and responsiveness to treatments.

2. The Evolving Concept of a Biomarker

The initial definition of a biomarker was not focussed on purely medical requirements but defined a measurable event occurring in a biological system that could inform on the

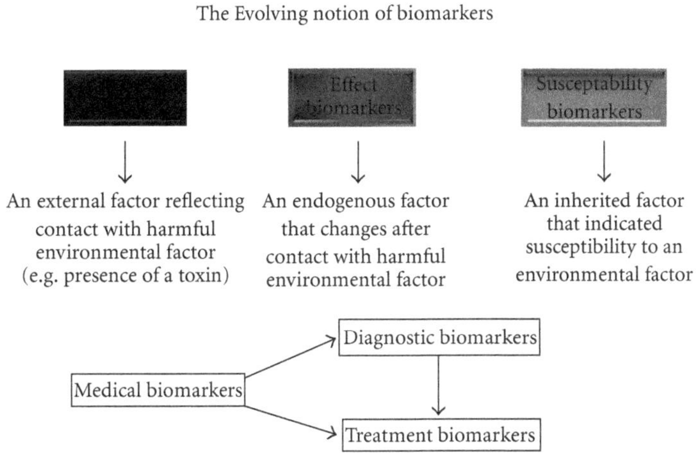

FIGURE 1: A schematic showing the evolving notion of biomarker utility from the inception of the concept of biomarkers to their use in medical research. This schema acknowledges that the discovery of diagnostic biomarkers is likely to also allow the separation of the different-component disorders in the syndrome of schizophrenia and that more tailored treatment of these component disorder will be possible. Hence diagnostic biomarkers, to a greater or lesser extent, are also likely to be treatment biomarkers.

general state of an organism, its life expectancy, or the well being of its environment (Figure 1) [10]. These concepts saw biomarkers divided into three categories: exposure biomarkers, effect biomarkers, and susceptibility biomarkers [11]. An exposure biomarker might be a xenobiotic or metabolites that reflect contact with a harmful environmental factor (e.g., toxin), an effective biomarker was an endogenous component of an organism that would change after exposure to an environmental factor whilst a susceptibility marker would be an inherited factor that provided a measure of susceptibility or sensitivity to an environmental factor. It was proposed that the major advantages of identifying biomarkers for these three categories were to elucidate pathogenic mechanisms, to improve etiologic classification of environmentally related disease and to allow an early recognition of contact with disadvantageous environmental factors [12].

More recently, in the medical arena, biomarkers are viewed as measurable factors that can enable diagnoses [13], inform on disease pathophysiology [13], or enable decisions to be made on the optimal treatment of an individual (personalised medicine) [14]. The value of well-validated biomarkers now has strong face validity as drug regulatory bodies have, for example, acknowledged that certain biomarkers do have predictive validity for treatment responsiveness in some forms of cancers [14]. It is also well recognised that well-validated biomarkers can differentiate component disorders within diagnostic syndromes and that the separation of the component disorders within a syndrome leads to rapid advances in understanding the underlying pathophysiologies of those disorders [13, 15, 16]. Existing experience in biomarker validation has shown this process to be a far from trivial undertaking. For example, perhaps the earliest biomarker was the sweet taste of urine first used by Thomas Willis to identify subjects with diabetes in 1674 [17]. However, it was not until 1949 that Himsworth proposed two disorders within the syndrome that could be delineated based on the presence or absence of insulin resistance [18]. Over time, the form of diabetes that was not associated with insulin resistance became known as insulin-dependent diabetes mellitus and is now recognised as an autoimmune disease [19] that can be treated with immunotherapy [20]. By contrast, the form of diabetes associated with noninsulin-dependent diabetes mellitus is now primarily defined by the presence of insulin resistance [21] and initial treatments usually involve lifestyle changes and drugs that can lessen tissue insulin resistance [22]. Research is still ongoing to better understand and develop better treatments for both forms of diabetes.

Given lessons learned in other discipline, those in the psychiatry arena must acknowledge that biomarker discovery and validation will be difficult and time consuming. However, the rewards following the discovery of reliable biomarkers will be significant advances in understanding the causes and treatment of the component disorders within diagnostic syndrome such as Sz.

3. Biomarker in Psychiatry

The identification of biomarkers has been one of the holy grails for psychiatric research for many years [23]. Given that biomarkers are not widely used for either diagnoses or treatment monitoring of psychiatric disorders, the challenge of identifying clinically useful biomarkers must remain a high research priority. Recently, biomarker discovery has seen a significant boost with the availability of "omic" technologies that permit the large-scale rapid screening of DNA sequence (genome) [24], levels of gene expression (transcriptome) [25], levels of gene translation (proteome) [26], and levels of metabolic activity (metabolome) [27]. These technologies are now producing large data sets that could well be the foundation for identifying biomarkers that will be useful in diagnosis and directing treatment for serous psychiatric disorders such as Sz. Hence it would seem appropriate to review the progress that has been made towards identifying biomarkers that can be used to assist in the diagnoses and treatment of Sz.

4. Peripheral Biomarkers for Sz: Biochemical, Genetic, and Pharmacogenomic Approaches

The initial search for biomarkers focussed on peripheral tissue. This was partly a pragmatic approach but also reflected the reality that a peripheral biomarker would have immediate clinical utility. One suggested diagnostic biomarker for Sz was the presence of 3,4-dimethoxyphenylethylamine in the urine of subjects with the disorder [28]. Importantly, when first reporting evidence to support this hypothesis, the authors stated that experiments would be required to validate the use of urinary 3,4-dimethoxyphenylethylamine as a biomarker for Sz. These subsequent experiments proved that urinary 3,4-dimethoxyphenylethylamine was not a biomarker for Sz and that there was doubt as to whether the "pink spot", by which the presence of 3,4-dimethoxyphenylethylamine was measured, was a measure of that chemical entity [29]. Thus, the outcome from the initial experiments that suggested a diagnostic biomarker for Sz had been identified was disappointing but the ensuing debate led to the realisation that "perhaps the time has now finally come to stop investigating "schizophrenics" en masse, and to concentrate on individuals" [29]. Importantly, it is still acknowledged that the study of the syndrome of Sz is a major impediment to identifying the causes of the symptoms associated with the disorder [2]. It is also now clear that it is unlikely that a single biomarker will be identified for any particular symptom such as psychoses [30]. These two hypotheses acknowledge that Sz is a complex syndrome, however it was hoped that an extensive study of the human genome in subjects with Sz would reveal DNA sequence variation that were associated with an increased risk of developing the symptoms experience by people with the disorder [31] and hence lead to biomarkers with which to diagnose the disorder.

The notion that changes in DNA sequence could be associated with an increased susceptibility to Sz came from the recognition that the disorder was highly heritable [32]. The hypotheses that changes in the genome could be used to diagnose Sz gained significant support from the identification of susceptibility locus for Sz in chromosome 5 [33]. More extensive studies showed that there was not a susceptibility marker for Sz on chromosome 5 [34] but other studies have generated a large body of data that may lead to the identification of genetic biomarkers that could be used for either the diagnosis of Sz [35] or as an indicator of the best treatment for an individual with Sz with a particular genetic background (pharmacogenomics) [36]. Unfortunately, the failure of large-scale genomewide associations studies (GWAS) to identify strong genetic markers that can predict altered risk for Sz [37] suggests that no one genetic marker is associated with a major susceptibility risk for the disorder at the level of the syndrome. This has led to two proposals, one is that genetic associations with an altered risk for Sz can be discovered if larger cohorts are used to compensate for the search for low-effect size genetic associations [24] or that Sz does not result from genetic changes at the level of single nucleotide polymorphisms [37]. The failure to identify genetic markers that show an increased susceptibility for Sz may also support the argument that genetic testing may be more effective in identifying the risk of symptom severity level. This idea is supported by the reports of genetic markers associated with the severity of psychotic symptoms [38], cognitive deficits [39] and decline in IQ [40] in subjects with Sz. However, these findings need replication in large cohorts before they can be judged to be of clinical value.

Although many genetic studies have focussed on identifying diagnostic biomarker, other studies have used pharmacogenomics approaches to identify changes in DNA sequence that may provide indicators of treatment responsiveness based on genetic background [41]. Pharmacogenomic studies have shown that genetic polymorphisms in the cytochrome P450 gene can influence antipsychotic drug treatment responsiveness [41]. The cytochrome P450 gene is critical in antipsychotic drug metabolism and hence can be an indicator of antipsychotic drug clearance which is often inversely related to drug responsiveness [42]. It has also been suggested that polymorphism in the dopamine D2 receptor [43, 44], dopamine D3 receptors [43], the serotonin 2A receptors [44], and catechol-O-methyl transferase [44] genes may be predictors of responsiveness to antipsychotic drugs and that polymorphisms in dopamine receptor genes and the serotonin 2C receptor gene may predict susceptibility for side-effects such as tardive dyskinesia and weight gain, respectively [43]. These findings have inherent face value as the proteins encoded by these genes are targeted by many antipsychotic drugs [45]. However, large-scale studies will be required to establish the clinical usefulness of these pharmacogenomics markers.

5. Biomarker for Sz: Blood Based Studies

Complimentary to studies using genetic material, predominantly obtained from white blood cells, there has been a long history of research trying to identify other blood-based markers for Sz. A lot of this research has focussed on the study of the human platelet which has some biochemical processes that are similar to those present in neurons [46, 47]. Many of the more recent studies have suggested that the functioning of the platelet may provide some indication as to likely antipsychotic drug responsiveness. For example, it has been suggested that low platelet serotonin 2A receptor levels prior to treatment may predict responsiveness to olanzapine [48] and that changes in dopamine uptake by platelets may provide a more generic indication of responsiveness to antipsychotic drug treatment [49]. Changes in basic platelet function, such as a blunted serotonin responsive aggregation [50] and neurotransmitter uptake [51], have also been suggested to be potential biomarkers for Sz. Finally, it has been reported that platelet functions such as dopamine uptake [52] and monoamine oxidase activity [53] may correlated with the severity symptoms such as delusions and auditory hallucinations, respectively. Unfortunately, many platelet-based findings need to be replicated in well-controlled studies involving large cohorts before their value as potential biomarkers can be fully assessed [54].

6. Biomarker for Sz: High Throughput Screening of Blood and Brain Gene Expression

Biomarker discovery research has been accelerated by the development of high-throughput screening techniques, such as microarrays, which allow levels of the expression of multiple genes in a tissue to be measured effectively in short-time frame [55]. The initial study using such technology to probe the transcriptome in human postmortem CNS suggested that Sz was a disorder of dysregulated synaptic-related gene expression [56]. This finding was interesting given the hypothesis that Sz is a disorder that only occurs in humans [57] and that one of the major differences between humans and other species, at the level of gene expression, are changes in synaptic-related gene expression [58]. In addition, other studies examining changes in the transcriptome in the CNS of subjects with Sz suggest that changes in gene expression in Sz vary with duration of illness [59, 60]. These findings raise the intriguing possibility that some biomarkers could be a measure of disease progression and may be useful in predicting changes in drug responsiveness that are known to occur with the progression of the disorder [61].

High-throughput screening presents the opportunity to bring together different findings relating to the pathophysiology of Sz that may prove seminal to biomarker discovery. Thus, microarray gene-expression studies using postmortem CNS tissue added to genetic studies using peripheral DNA (association studies) suggest a role of regulator of G protein signaling 4 in the pathophysiology of Sz [62]. This is an important finding in its own right but also serves to illustrate how a holistic approach using multiple technologies can serve to identify potential biomarkers for the disorder. In addition, combining results from studies using CNS and peripheral tissue is beginning to suggest that changes in CNS gene expression may, at least in part, be detected using peripheral tissue such as white blood cells. This hypothesis is supported by studies showing similar changes in gene expression levels for some genes in blood and brain tissue (e.g., B-cell translocation gene 1, glycogen synthase kinase 3α, major histocompatibility complex, class II, DR β1, heterogeneous nuclear ribonucleoprotein A3, selenium binding protein 1, and splicing factor, arginine/serine-rich 1 [63]) from subjects with Sz. These findings are particularly important as they indicate it is possible to translate biomarkers identified using postmortem CNS into clinically useful tools because they can be measured in peripheral tissue and that, conversely, some changes in peripheral gene expression may provide insight into changes in brain gene expression in the CNS of subjects with Sz. Such conclusions must still be tempered by acknowledging other findings from microarray studies suggesting that changes in gene expression in peripheral blood cells are not present in the CNS from subjects with Sz [64, 65].

There are now intriguing data that could support the use of peripheral changes in gene expression as biomarkers for Sz. For example, changes in levels of selenium binding protein 1 expression have been found in peripheral tissue [63] and in the CNS from subjects with Sz [66]. However, the study of selenium-binding protein 1 expression in blood has shown that levels of gene expression correlate with levels of psychotic symptoms independent of whether the blood donor had Sz of bipolar disorder (BD) [63]. These latter data suggest that changes in gene expression may be associated with symptom severity and be associated with phenotypes rather than diagnoses [67]. If that is the case, gene expression biomarkers may be confirming the suggestion that the time has finally come to stop investigating schizophrenia in isolation as suggested over four decades ago [29]. Rather, it may be time for a more holistic approach testing potential biomarkers on a gene by gene basis carefully assessing their diagnostic potential but also whether they are pointing to commonalities in genetic susceptibility to multiple psychiatric disorders.

7. Biomarker for Sz: High Throughput Screening of the Blood and Brain Proteome

Whilst changes in levels of gene transcription at the level of mRNA may be a biomarker for Sz it is now recognised that not all changes in the transcriptome translate into changes in levels of the encoded protein [59] and hence the physiological significance of altered gene transcription is not readily apparent. Given one goal of biomarker discovery is to improve knowledge of disease pathophysiology, high-throughput methodologies that allow the study of the human blood and brain proteome have been used to identify potential biomarkers for Sz. This approach has been validated by a recent report that 25% of subjects with Sz can be separated into a separate population based on the loss of the majority (~75%) of their cortical muscarinic M1 receptors [68] which shows that levels of proteins can be used to identify subgroups of subjects within the syndrome of Sz. Moreover, the subjects with Sz with a marked loss in muscarinic M1 receptors have been shown to have altered muscarinic M1 receptor signalling [69] and increased levels of a microRNA that targets muscarinic M1 receptor mRNA to reduce protein translation [70] that are not present in people with Sz that do not have changes in muscarinic M1 receptors. These data support the hypothesis that (i) it should be possible to discover biomarkers for the identification of subgroups of subjects within the syndrome of Sz and (ii) once these subgroups of subjects have been identified it should be possible to understand their specific pathophysiologies. The findings on cortical muscarinic M1 receptors also argues against the position that the use of high-throughput technologies are essential for biomarker discovery in Sz [71].

A number of studies of the human proteome have claimed to identify biomarkers for Sz. One study using surface-enhanced laser desorption/ionization time of flight mass spectrometry and postmortem brain tissue suggests that there are at least 21 potential biomarkers (Table 1)

TABLE 1: Proteins suggested as potential biomarkers for Sz or BPD due to diagnostic-specific changes detected using surface-enhanced laser desorption/ionization time of flight mass spectrometry in postmortem CNS.

Diagnoses	Proposed biomarker
Sz	CD58 molecule Calmodulin 1 (phosphorylase kinase, delta) Mago-nashi homolog, proliferation-associated (Drosophila) MYC associated factor X Regulator of G-protein signaling 11 Ubiquitin carboxyl-terminal hydroxylase isozyme L1 Cyclophilin A CEBPZ CCAAT/enhancer binding protein (C/EBP), zeta LOC153154 similar to short heat shock protein 60 Hsp60s2 Phosphoglycerate mutase 1 Tyrosine 3-monooxygenase/tryptophan 5-monooxygenase activation protein, eta polypeptide NK2 homeobox 4, 2,4-dienoyl CoA reductase 2 Peroxisomal, methylthioadenosine phosphorylase Purine nucleoside phosphorylase Bystin-like Ankyrin repeat domain 12 Proteasome (prosome, macropain) subunit, alpha type, 7 Aldolase C, fructose-bisphosphate Sphingomyelin phosphodiesterase 1, acid lysosomal Glutamate-ammonia ligase and enolase 2 (gamma, neuronal)
BPD	Myelin basic protein Dickkopf homolog 2 (Xenopus laevis) CEBPZ CCAAT/enhancer binding protein (C/EBP), zeta; 2,4-dienoyl CoA reductase 2, peroxisomal Bystin-like Ankyrin repeat domain 12 Aldolase C, fructose-bisphosphate

that can be used to separate Sz and/or BD from controls [72]. Again these data suggest that not all biomarkers will always show diagnostic specificity but some may be useful in assessing common factors that cross psychiatric diagnostic boundaries. A study using postmortem brain tissue and the same technology to measure protein levels found that no single protein could be used as a diagnostic-specific biomarker for Sz [73] but that a cluster analysis of the intensities of several proteins were required to separate subjects with Sz with an accuracy of 70%. Thus, whilst initial outcomes from the use of surface-enhanced laser desorption/ionization time of flight mass spectrometry are encouraging, there is now a need for follow-up data to support the proposed proteins, or groups of proteins, as biomarkers for Sz; of course these studies should also advance understanding of the pathophysiology of the disorder.

Using a liquid chromatography/mass spectrometry approach 10 proteins (CD5 molecule-like (CD5L), IGHM immunoglobulin heavy constant mu (IGHM), coagulation factor XIII, B polypeptide (F13B), transferring (TF), apolipoprotein D (APOD), apolipoprotein A-1 (APOA1), apolipoprotein A-IV (APOA4), apolipoprotein A-II (APOA2), apolipoprotein C-I (APOC1), and alpha-2-HS-glycoprotein (AHSG)) have been identified as altered in serum from drug naïve subjects with Sz compared to controls [74]. Clearly the identification of changes in the blood proteome in drug naive subjects is significant as the effects of antipsychotic drug treatment would not be a confound. Significantly, APOD [75, 76], APOA1 [77–79], and TF [80, 81] have previously been identified as being altered in blood from subjects with Sz. In addition, APOA4 has been reported as altered in the CSF from subjects with Sz [82]. These findings obtained in protein-specific studies add to the hypotheses that blood proteins can be used as biomarkers in Sz.

Another recent approach to identify biomarkers for psychiatric disorders is a large study comparing proteins levels in plasma from subjects with Sz, major depressive disorders (MDD), and control subjects [83]. In this study biomarker identification relied on a technology that examined levels of multiple chemokines, cytokines, hormones, growth factors, and antigens. Significantly, the study showed a greater separation of samples from subjects with Sz from controls than was achieved for MDD and controls using cluster analysis. The proteins that most strongly allowed the separation of Sz from controls and MDD were chemokine (C-C motif) ligand 4 (CCL4), chemokine (C-C motif) ligand 5 (CCL5), chemokine (C-C motif) ligand 22 (CCL22), chemokine (C-X-C motif) ligand 5 (CXCL5), TIMP metallopeptidase inhibitor 1 (TIMP1), epidermal growth factor (EGF), serpin peptidase inhibitor, clade A (alpha-1 antiproteinase, antitrypsin), member 7 (SERPINA7), and KIT ligand (KITLG). Conversely, changes in blood levels of insulin (INS), alpha-2-macroglobulin (A2M), matrix metallopeptidase 9 (gelatinase B, 92 kDa gelatinase, and 92 kDa type IV collagenase) (MMP3) and tumour necrosis factor receptor superfamily, member 1B (TNFRSF1B) allowed the separation of MDD from controls and subjects with Sz. Finally, brain-derived neurotrophic factor (BDNF), serpin peptidase inhibitor, clade E (nexin, plasminogen activator inhibitor type 1), member 1 (SERPINA1), and APODA1 allowed the separation of Sz and MDD from controls but did not show diagnostic specificity.

Reviewing results from blood-based biomarker studies critically, it is notable that there is no agreement on potential biomarkers across two studies. This could be due to many uncontrolled variables across the studies as blood proteins levels are known to vary with multiple factors including time of day [84], menstrual cycle [85], and food intake status [86]. Hence, at some point those involved in blood biomarker discovery for Sz should attempt to come to a consensus with regard to standardisation blood collecting with regards to fasting status, time of bleed, and other critical factors which can add variability to blood protein levels, as has been advocated for biomarker discovery for other diseases [87].

Another approach to identifying potential biomarkers at the level of the protein has been to study the CNS proteome in subjects with psychiatric disorders [88]. Whilst the study of the human CNS proteome in Sz has been ongoing for over a decade [89, 90] only 16 gray matter proteins (aldolase C, fructose-bisulphate, creatine kinase (brain), dynamin 1, dihydropyrimidinase-like 2, enolase 1 α, enolase 2 (γ neuronal), glial fibrillary acidic protein, glutamate-ammonia ligase, guanine nucleotide binding protein β polypeptide 1, internexin neuronal intermediate filament protein α, and N-ethylmaleimide-sensitive factor) and 8 white matter proteins (dihydropyrimidinase-like 2, inositol-monophosphatase 1, neurofilament, light polypeptide, Parkinson Disease 7, 14-3-3 zeta, l-lactate dehydrogenase Chain B, and stathmin 1) have been reported as altered in the same direction in more than one study of the human proteome [91]. Of equal concern is that some of these proteins, such as dynamin 1 [92], N-ethylmaleimide-sensitive factor [93], glial fibrillary acidic protein [94], and 14-3-3 zeta [95], have been reported to be unaltered in the CNS of subjects with Sz when measured using Western blotting. However, it has to be acknowledged that current studies on the human CNS proteome have been completed using relatively small number of cases and this is an issue given the need for the adequately powered cohort sizes needed when attempting to identify clinically valid biomarkers in any form of disease [96].

8. Towards Clinically Useful Biomarkers for Sz

There is a high expectation that the discovery of biomarkers will greatly accelerate our understanding of the pathophysiology of syndromes such as Sz [2]. This high expectation brings the danger that "apparent" failures to identify useful biomarkers may lead to the perception that biomarker discovery is an impossible goal. However, biomarker discovery in Sz is still in its infancy and the likelihood of identifying biomarkers is dependent on a number of factors, not the least is the ongoing development of the high-throughput technologies that allow the probing of the human genome, transcriptome, proteome, and metabolome.

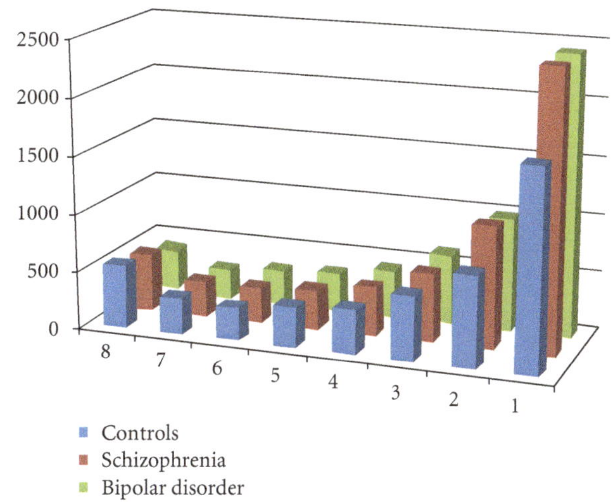

Figure 2: The number of protein spots visualised in Brodmann's area 46 from subjects with Sz, bipolar disorder, and schizophrenia after differential detergent solubilisation and separation across 5 two dimensional gels.

In this respect, deep sequencing is a new technology that will allow a much more comprehensive analysis of the human genome in much larger cohorts of subjects with disorders such as Sz [97] and this technology may be able to identify genetic biomarkers even in a complex syndrome such as Sz [31]. At the level of transcriptomics, an increasing knowledge of the complexities of gene expression is producing technologies that can probe mRNA at ever increasing levels of complexity [98]. In addition, there are efforts to refine existing technologies [99] and utilise new technologies [100, 101] to increase the proportion of the human proteome that can be effectively measured in blood, CNS, or other tissues.

The capacity to significantly increase the reach of proteomics technologies in psychiatric disease is illustrated by the application of a differential-detergent solubility, multi-gel approach to analysis of the human CNS proteome in tissue from subjects with Sz, BD, and control subjects [99]. This approach has led to the visualisation of approximately 3,800 protein spots in the acidic protein fraction from cortex and caudate-putamen, this is close to triple the number of protein spots visualised using crude homogenates as reported in most studies from subjects with Sz [99].

This methodology has now been applied to studying the acidic and basic proteins in Brodmann's area 46 (BA 46) from subjects with Sz, BD, and controls with 8 subjects in each cohort. Using this methodology, a total of 8152 protein spots were visualised across all of the cases studied, of which 5590 (69%) were present in two or more cases. Significantly, as is the case in some studies, if data analyses was limited to the study of protein spots visualised in every case then only 245 protein spots (3%) would be included for analyses. This would exclude the analyses of spots that seemed to have a significant variation with diagnoses (e.g., present in >75% of controls and <25% of cases with Sz). At the level of disease cohorts, the highest number of protein spots were visualised in tissue from subjects with Sz ($n = 5917$), followed by tissue

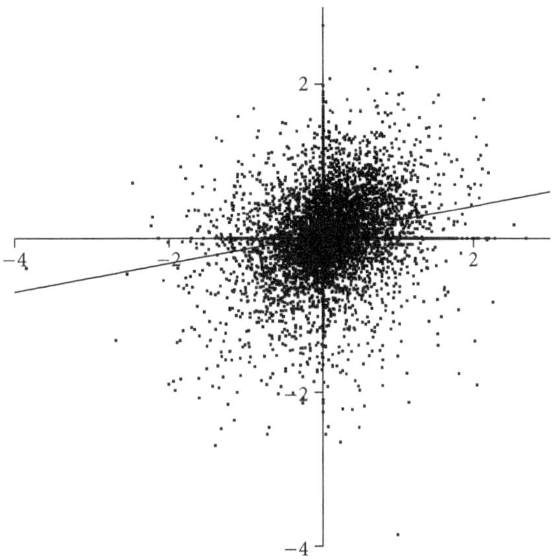

FIGURE 3: A comparison of the intensity of protein spots, normalised to the intensity of the corresponding protein spot in control CNS, in Brodmann's area 46 from subjects with Sz (Y-axis) and bipolar disorder (X-axis). Spots in the upper left quadrant show increased levels in Sz compared to bipolar disorder whereas those in the lower right quadrant show increased levels of proteins in bipolar disorder with lower levels in Sz.

from subjects with BD ($n = 5746$) and the fewest spots were detected in tissue from control subjects ($n = 4946$). These data are interesting as they suggest that subjects with Sz and BD expressed more CNS proteins or have overall higher levels of lower abundance CNS proteins, than do control subjects. Importantly, 3503 (59%) protein spots were detected in two or more subjects with Sz, 3322 (58%) in two or more subjects with BD and 3211 (65%) in two or more of the control subjects (Figure 2).

The data from a simple modification of an established methodology serve to show how existing technologies can still have value in the study of the human CNS proteome. The increased utility of such modifications can be illustrated by comparing the intensity of each protein spot, for protein present in at least two cases, from subjects with Sz and BD normalised to the intensity of the same spot in the proteome of control subjects (Figure 3). These data show that differential changes in many relative protein intensities are occurring in the CNS of subjects of Sz and BD and the challenge is to mine this rich data set to identify candidate proteins that may prove valuable as biomarkers to separate the two disorders.

9. Conclusions

There are clear and urgent needs to develop biomarkers to aid in the diagnoses and monitoring of treatment in subjects with psychiatric disorders such as Sz [5]. It will be important not to grow impatient and prematurely discard the hypothesis that biomarkers can be identified to aid in the diagnoses and treatment of the disorder. For example, in diabetes, the development of clinically useful biomarkers has spanned several centuries from the discovery of sweet urine to immunological diagnostic tests for certain forms of diabetes [13]. Moreover, the recognition of the Federal Drug Authority that at least one pharmacogenomics test (based on genetic variation in cytochrome P450) is of value in assessing likely treatment responsiveness in people with Sz [102] suggest that progress is being made toward biomarker discovery, validation and eventually widespread clinical use. This being said, those in the biomarker research space need to be considering some form of standardisation of blood collection to attempt to minimise blood protein level variation due to factors other than disease pathophysiology or treatment response. In addition, those involved in biomarker research using postmortem CNS or neuroimaging need to develop networks that will facilitate a rapid validation of potential biomarkers across brain collections and between imaging centres. Both these strategies may be essential for the rigorous testing of potential biomarkers to occur rapidly as a prelude to moving such validated biomarkers into the clinic.

Acknowledgments

The author would like to acknowledge Geoffrey Pavey, Simone Boer, and Alison Digney for assisting in running and analysing 2D gels to visualise proteins in Brodmann's area 46 from subjects with schizophrenia, bipolar disorder, and controls. The work described in the manuscript was supported in part by NHMRC Grant no. APP1002240, NHMRC Grant no. 192339, R01 MH069696-01 and grants-in aid from the Rebecca L. Cooper Medical Research Foundation. The study was supported by Operational Infrastructure Support (OIS) from the Victorian State Government.

References

[1] T. R. Insel, "Disruptive insights in psychiatry: transforming a clinical discipline," *Journal of Clinical Investigation*, vol. 119, no. 4, pp. 700–705, 2009.

[2] C. A. Tamminga, "Accelerating new knowledge in schizophrenia," *American Journal of Psychiatry*, vol. 165, no. 8, pp. 949–951, 2008.

[3] H. Elkis, "Treatment-Resistant Schizophrenia," *Psychiatric Clinics of North America*, vol. 30, no. 3, pp. 511–533, 2007.

[4] S. Miyamoto, G. E. Duncan, C. E. Marx, and J. A. Lieberman, "Treatments for schizophrenia: a critical review of pharmacology and mechanisms of action of antipsychotic drugs," *Molecular Psychiatry*, vol. 10, no. 1, pp. 79–104, 2005.

[5] L. J. Lesko, "Personalized medicine: elusive dream or imminent reality?" *Clinical Pharmacology and Therapeutics*, vol. 81, no. 6, pp. 807–816, 2007.

[6] E. Schwarz and S. Bahn, "The utility of biomarker discovery approaches for the detection of disease mechanisms in psychiatric disorders," *British Journal of Pharmacology*, vol. 153, supplement 1, pp. S133–S136, 2008.

[7] T. R. Insel and B. N. Cuthbert, "Endophenotypes: bridging Genomic Complexity and Disorder Heterogeneity," *Biological Psychiatry*, vol. 66, no. 11, pp. 988–989, 2009.

[8] I. I. Gottesman and T. D. Gould, "The endophenotype concept in psychiatry: etymology and strategic intentions,"

American Journal of Psychiatry, vol. 160, no. 4, pp. 636–645, 2003.

[9] C. L. Arfken, S. Carney, and N. N. Boutros, "Translating biological parameters into clinically useful diagnostic tests," *Current Psychiatry Reports*, vol. 11, no. 4, pp. 320–323, 2009.

[10] Committee on Biological Markers of the National Research Council, "Biological markers in environmental health research," *Environmental Health Perspectives*, vol. 74, pp. 1–191, 1987.

[11] P. Grandjean, "Biomarkers in epidemiology," *Clinical Chemistry*, vol. 41, no. 12, pp. 1800–1803, 1995.

[12] B. S. Hulka and T. Wilcosky, "Biological markers in epidemiologic research," *Archives of Environmental Health*, vol. 43, no. 2, pp. 83–89, 1988.

[13] E. A. M. Gale, "Perspectives in diabetes: the discovery of type 1 diabetes," *Diabetes*, vol. 50, no. 2, pp. 217–226, 2001.

[14] J. R. Johnson, G. Williams, and R. Pazdur, "End points and United States Food and Drug Administration approval of oncology drugs," *Journal of Clinical Oncology*, vol. 21, no. 7, pp. 1404–1411, 2003.

[15] S. M. Hewitt, J. Dear, and R. A. Star, "Discovery of protein biomarkers for renal diseases," *Journal of the American Society of Nephrology*, vol. 15, no. 7, pp. 1677–1689, 2004.

[16] D. W. Benson, "Advances in cardiovascular genetics and embryology: role of transcription factors in congenital heart disease," *Current Opinion in Pediatrics*, vol. 12, no. 5, pp. 497–500, 2000.

[17] F. Henschen, "On the term diabetes in the works of Aretaeus and Galen," *Medical History*, vol. 13, no. 2, pp. 190–192, 1969.

[18] H. P. Himsworth, "The syndrome of diabetes mellitus and its causes," *The Lancet*, vol. 253, no. 6551, pp. 465–473, 1949.

[19] J. F. Bach, "Insulin-dependent diabetes mellitus as an autoimmune disease," *Endocrine Reviews*, vol. 15, no. 4, pp. 516–542, 1994.

[20] J. J. Cook, I. Hudson, L. C. Harrison et al., "Double-blind controlled trial of azathioprine in children with newly diagnosed type I diabetes," *Diabetes*, vol. 38, no. 6, pp. 779–783, 1989.

[21] E. Ferrannini, "Insulin resistance versus insulin deficiency in non-insulin-dependent diabetes mellitus: problems and prospects," *Endocrine Reviews*, vol. 19, no. 4, pp. 477–490, 1998.

[22] A. J. Krentz and C. J. Bailey, "Oral antidiabetic agents: current role in type 2 diabetes mellitus," *Drugs*, vol. 65, no. 3, pp. 385–411, 2005.

[23] R. Noll, "The blood of the insane," *History of Psychiatry*, vol. 17, no. 4, pp. 395–418, 2006.

[24] P. F. Sullivan, "The psychiatric GWAS consortium: big science comes to psychiatry," *Neuron*, vol. 68, pp. 182–186, 2010.

[25] M. T. Tsuang, N. Nossova, T. Yager et al., "Assessing the validity of blood-based gene expression profiles for the classification of schizophrenia and bipolar disorder: a preliminary report," *American Journal of Medical Genetics: Part B*, vol. 133, no. 1, pp. 1–5, 2005.

[26] M. J. Romeo, V. Espina, M. Lowenthal, B. H. Espina, E. F. Petricoin III, and L. A. Liotta, "CSF proteome: a protein repository for potential biomarker identification," *Expert Review of Proteomics*, vol. 2, no. 1, pp. 57–70, 2005.

[27] R. Kaddurah-Daouk and K. R. R. Krishnan, "Metabolomics: a global biochemical approach to the study of central nervous system diseases," *Neuropsychopharmacology*, vol. 34, no. 1, pp. 173–186, 2009.

[28] A. J. Friedhoff and E. V. Winkle, "Isolation and characterization of a compound from the urine of schizophrenics," *Nature*, vol. 194, no. 4831, pp. 897–898, 1962.

[29] Editorial, "Lessons of the "Pink Spot"," *British Medical Journal*, vol. 18, p. 383, 1967.

[30] R. Freedman, R. Ross, S. Leonard et al., "Early biomarkers of psychosis," *Dialogues in Clinical Neuroscience*, vol. 7, no. 1, pp. 17–29, 2005.

[31] A. K. Tiwari, C. C. Zai, D. J. Muller, and Kennedy J. L., "Genetics in schizophrenia: where are we and what next?" *Dialogues in Clinical Neuroscience*, vol. 12, pp. 289–303, 2010.

[32] A. R. Jensen, "Estimation of the limits of heritability of traits by comparison of monozygotic and dizygotic twins," *Proceedings of the National Academy of Sciences of the United States of America*, vol. 58, no. 1, pp. 149–156, 1967.

[33] R. Sherrington, J. Brynjolfsson, H. Petursson et al., "Localization of a susceptibility locus for schizophrenia on chromosome 5," *Nature*, vol. 336, no. 6195, pp. 164–167, 1988.

[34] S. D. Detera-Wadleigh, L. R. Goldin, R. Sherrington et al., "Exclusion of linkage to 5q11-13 in families with schizophrenia and other psychiatric disorders," *Nature*, vol. 340, no. 6232, pp. 391–393, 1989.

[35] M. Gill, G. Donohoe, and A. Corvin, "What have the genomics ever done for the psychoses?" *Psychological Medicine*, vol. 40, no. 4, pp. 529–540, 2010.

[36] O. Blanc, G. Brousse, A. Meary, M. Leboyer, and P. M. Llorca, "Pharmacogenetic of response efficacy to antipsychotics in schizophrenia: pharmacodynamic aspects. Review and implications for clinical research," *Fundamental and Clinical Pharmacology*, vol. 24, no. 2, pp. 139–160, 2010.

[37] A. S. Bassett, S. W. Scherer, and L. M. Brzustowicz, "Copy number variations in schizophrenia: critical review and new perspectives on concepts of genetics and disease," *American Journal of Psychiatry*, vol. 167, no. 8, pp. 899–914, 2010.

[38] A. K. Malhotra, A. Breier, D. Goldman, L. Picken, and D. Pickar, "The apolipoprotein E $\varepsilon 4$ allele is associated with blunting of ketamine-Induced psychosis in schizophrenia: a preliminary report," *Neuropsychopharmacology*, vol. 19, no. 5, pp. 445–448, 1998.

[39] D. L. Liao, C. J. Hong, H. M. Chen et al., "Association of muscarinic M1 receptor genetic polymorphisms with psychiatric symptoms and cognitive function in schizophrenic patients," *Neuropsychobiology*, vol. 48, no. 2, pp. 72–76, 2003.

[40] K. E. Burdick, T. E. Goldberg, B. Funke et al., "DTNBP1 genotype influences cognitive decline in schizophrenia," *Schizophrenia Research*, vol. 89, no. 1–3, pp. 169–172, 2007.

[41] A. Mihaljević-Peleš, M. Šagud, N. Božina, M. Živković, and N. Jovanović, "Pharmacogenetics and antipsychotics in the light of personalized pharmacotherapy," *Psychiatria Danubina*, vol. 22, no. 2, pp. 335–337, 2010.

[42] N. Fleeman, Y. Dundar, R. Dickson et al., "Cytochrome P450 testing for prescribing antipsychotics in adults with schizophrenia: systematic review and meta-analyses," *Pharmacogenomics Journal*, vol. 11, no. 1, pp. 1–14, 2011.

[43] M. J. Arranz and J. De Leon, "Pharmacogenetics and pharmacogenomics of schizophrenia: a review of last decade of research," *Molecular Psychiatry*, vol. 12, no. 8, pp. 707–747, 2007.

[44] Y. Yamanouchi, N. Iwata, T. Suzuki, T. Kitajima, M. Ikeda, and N. Ozaki, "Effect of DRD2, 5-HT2A, and COMT genes on antipsychotic response to risperidone," *Pharmacogenomics Journal*, vol. 3, no. 6, pp. 356–361, 2003.

[45] F. P. Bymaster, S. K. Hemrick-Luecke, K. W. Perry, and R. W. Fuller, "Neurochemical evidence for antagonism by olanzapine of dopamine, serotonin, α-adrenergic and muscarinic receptors in vivo in rats," *Psychopharmacology*, vol. 124, no. 1–2, pp. 87–94, 1996.

[46] S. M. Stahl and H. Y. Meltzer, "The human platelet as a model for the dopaminergic neuron: kinetic and pharmacologic properties and the role of amine storage granules," *Experimental Neurology*, vol. 59, no. 1, pp. 1–15, 1978.

[47] W. B. Abrams and H. M. Solomon, "The human platelet as a pharmacologic model for the adrenergic neuron. The uptake and release of norepinephrine," *Clinical Pharmacology and Therapeutics*, vol. 10, no. 5, pp. 702–709, 1969.

[48] B. Arranz, P. Rosel, L. San et al., "Low baseline serotonin-2A receptors predict clinical response to olanzapine in first-episode schizophrenia patients," *Psychiatry Research*, vol. 153, no. 2, pp. 103–109, 2007.

[49] S. Sundram, B. Dean, and D. L. Copolov, "Typical and atypical neuroleptic drugs decrease platelet H-dopamine uptake in the rat," *Psychiatry Research*, vol. 62, no. 3, pp. 259–263, 1996.

[50] R. Reddy, M. Keshavan, and J. K. Yao, "Blunted serotonergic responsivity in neuroleptic-naïve patients at first-episode of schizophrenia," *Schizophrenia Research*, vol. 90, no. 1–3, pp. 81–85, 2007.

[51] M. Zucker, A. Valevski, A. Weizman, and M. Rehavi, "Increased platelet vesicular monoamine transporter density in adult schizophrenia patients," *European Neuropsychopharmacology*, vol. 12, no. 4, pp. 343–347, 2002.

[52] B. Dean, J. Kulkarni, D. L. Copolov, P. Shrikanthan, V. Malone, and C. Hill, "Dopamine uptake by platelets from subjects with schizophrenia: a correlation with the delusional state of the patient," *Psychiatry Research*, vol. 41, no. 1, pp. 17–24, 1992.

[53] H. Y. Meltzer and J. L. Zureick, "Relationship of auditory hallucinations and paranoia to platelet MAO activity in schizophrenics: sex and race interactions," *Psychiatry Research*, vol. 22, no. 2, pp. 99–109, 1987.

[54] P. Polister, "Reliability, decision rules, and the value of repeated tests," *Medical Decision Making*, vol. 2, no. 1, pp. 47–69, 1982.

[55] A. T. Weeraratna, J. E. Nagel, V. De Mello-Coelho, and D. D. Taub, "Gene expression profiling: from microarrays to medicine," *Journal of Clinical Immunology*, vol. 24, no. 3, pp. 213–224, 2004.

[56] K. Mirnics and J. Pevsner, "Progress in the use of microarray technology to study the neurobiology of disease," *Nature Neuroscience*, vol. 7, no. 5, pp. 434–439, 2004.

[57] T. J. Crow, "Is schizophrenia the price that Homo sapiens pays for language?" *Schizophrenia Research*, vol. 28, no. 2-3, pp. 127–141, 1997.

[58] B. Dean, "Is schizophrenia the price of human central nervous system complexity?" *Australian and New Zealand Journal of Psychiatry*, vol. 43, no. 1, pp. 13–24, 2009.

[59] B. Dean, D. Keriakous, E. Scarr, and E. A. Thomas, "Gene expression profiling in Brodmann's area 46 from subjetcs with schizophrenia," *Australian and New Zealand Journal of Psychiatry*, vol. 41, no. 4, pp. 308–320, 2007.

[60] S. Narayan, B. Tang, S. R. Head et al., "Molecular profiles of schizophrenia in the CNS at different stages of illness," *Brain Research*, vol. 1239, no. C, pp. 235–248, 2008.

[61] M. E. Kelley, G. L. Haas, and D. P. van Kammen, "Longitudinal progression of negative symptoms in schizophrenia: a new look at an old problem," *Schizophrenia Research*, vol. 105, no. 1–3, pp. 188–196, 2008.

[62] K. Mirnics, F. A. Middleton, G. D. Stanwood, D. A. Lewis, and P. Levitt, "Disease-specific changes in regulator of G-protein signaling 4 (RGS4) expression in schizophrenia," *Molecular Psychiatry*, vol. 6, no. 3, pp. 293–301, 2001.

[63] S. J. Glatt, I. P. Everall, W. S. Kremen et al., "Comparative gene expression analysis of blood and brain provides concurrent validation of SELENBP1 up-regulation in schizophrenia," *Proceedings of the National Academy of Sciences of the United States of America*, vol. 102, no. 43, pp. 15533–15538, 2005.

[64] N. A. Bowden, J. Weidenhofer, R. J. Scott et al., "Preliminary investigation of gene expression profiles in peripheral blood lymphocytes in schizophrenia," *Schizophrenia Research*, vol. 82, no. 2-3, pp. 175–183, 2006.

[65] M. Takahashi, H. Hayashi, Y. Watanabe et al., "Diagnostic classification of schizophrenia by neural network analysis of blood-based gene expression signatures," *Schizophrenia Research*, vol. 119, no. 1–3, pp. 210–218, 2010.

[66] T. Kanazawa, G. Chana, S. J. Glatt et al., "The utility of selenbp1 gene expression as a biomarker for major psychotic disorders: replication in schizophrenia and extension to bipolar disorder with psychosis," *American Journal of Medical Genetics, Part B*, vol. 147, no. 6, pp. 686–689, 2008.

[67] A. B. Niculescu, L. L. Lulow, C. A. Ogden et al., "PhenoChipping of psychotic disorders: a novel approach for deconstructing and quantitating psychiatric phenotypes," *American Journal of Medical Genetics, Part B*, vol. 141, no. 6, pp. 653–662, 2006.

[68] E. Scarr, T. F. Cowie, S. Kanellakis, S. Sundram, C. Pantelis, and B. Dean, "Decreased cortical muscarinic receptors define a subgroup of subjects with schizophrenia," *Molecular Psychiatry*, vol. 14, no. 11, pp. 1017–1023, 2009.

[69] H. Salah-Uddin, E. Scarr, G. Pavey et al., "Altered M Muscarinic Acetylcholine Receptor (CHRM1)-Gα Coupling in a Schizophrenia Endophenotype," *Neuropsychopharmacology*, vol. 34, no. 9, pp. 2156–2166, 2009.

[70] M. J. Cairns, N. Beveridge, E. Scarr, and B. Dean, "A potential role for gene directed microRNAs in the pathophysiology of muscarinic receptor deficit schizophrenia," *Australian and New Zealand Journal of Psychiatry*, vol. 44, supplement 1, p. A10, 2010.

[71] E. Schwarz and S. Bahn, "Biomarker discovery in psychiatric disorders," *Electrophoresis*, vol. 29, no. 13, pp. 2884–2890, 2008.

[72] S. I. Novikova, F. He, N. J. Cutrufello, and M. S. Lidow, "Identification of protein biomarkers for schizophrenia and bipolar disorder in the postmortem prefrontal cortex using SELDI-TOF-MS ProteinChip profiling combined with MALDI-TOF-PSD-MS analysis," *Neurobiology of Disease*, vol. 23, no. 1, pp. 61–76, 2006.

[73] J. Mei, D. Kolbin, H. T. Kao, and B. Porton, "Protein expression profiling of postmortem brain in schizophrenia," *Schizophrenia Research*, vol. 84, no. 2-3, pp. 204–213, 2006.

[74] Y. Levin, L. Wang, E. Schwarz, D. Koethe, F. M. Leweke, and S. Bahn, "Global proteomic profiling reveals altered proteomic signature in schizophrenia serum," *Molecular Psychiatry*, 2009.

[75] E. A. Thomas, B. Dean, G. Pavey, and J. G. Sutcliffe, "Increased CNS levels of apolipoprotein D in schizophrenic and bipolar subjects: implications for the pathophysiology of psychiatric disorders," *Proceedings of the National Academy of Sciences of the United States of America*, vol. 98, no. 7, pp. 4066–4071, 2001.

[76] S. P. Mahadik, M. M. Khan, D. R. Evans, and V. V. Parikh, "Elevated plasma level of apolipoprotein D in schizophrenia and its treatment and outcome," *Schizophrenia Research*, vol. 58, no. 1, pp. 55–62, 2002.
[77] J. T. J. Huang, L. Wang, S. Prabakaran et al., "Independent protein-profiling studies show a decrease in apolipoprotein A1 levels in schizophrenia CSF, brain and peripheral tissues," *Molecular Psychiatry*, vol. 13, no. 12, pp. 1118–1128, 2008.
[78] Y. J. La, C. L. Wan, H. Zhu et al., "Decreased levels of apolipoprotein A-I in plasma of schizophrenic patients," *Journal of Neural Transmission*, vol. 114, no. 5, pp. 657–663, 2007.
[79] Y. Yang, C. Wan, H. Li et al., "Altered levels of acute phase proteins in the plasma of patients with schizophrenia," *Analytical Chemistry*, vol. 78, no. 11, pp. 3571–3576, 2006.
[80] C. T. Wong, W. F. Tsoi, and N. Saha, "Acute phase proteins in male Chinese schizophrenic patients in Singapore," *Schizophrenia Research*, vol. 22, no. 2, pp. 165–171, 1996.
[81] E. Bock, B. Weeke, and O. J. Rafaelsen, "Serum proteins in acutely psychotic patients," *Journal of Psychiatric Research*, vol. 9, no. 1, pp. 1–9, 1971.
[82] L. Jiang, K. Lindpaintner, H. F. Li et al., "Proteomic analysis of the cerebrospinal fluid of patients with schizophrenia," *Amino Acids*, vol. 25, no. 1, pp. 49–57, 2003.
[83] E. Domenici, D. R. Willé, F. Tozzi et al., "Plasma protein biomarkers for depression and schizophrenia by multi analyte profiling of case-control collections," *PLoS ONE*, vol. 5, no. 2, article e9166, 2010.
[84] E. Van Cauter, R. Leproult, and D. J. Kupfer, "Effects of gender and age on the levels and circadian rhythmicity of plasma cortisol," *Journal of Clinical Endocrinology and Metabolism*, vol. 81, no. 7, pp. 2468–2473, 1996.
[85] K. P. McNatty, D. T. Baird, and A. Bolton, "Concentration of oestrogens and androgens in human ovarian venous plasma and follicular fluid throughout the menstrual cycle," *Journal of Endocrinology*, vol. 71, no. 1, pp. 77–85, 1976.
[86] P. C. Butler, J. Chou, W. B. Carter et al., "Effects of meal ingestion on plasma amylin concentration in NIDDM and nondiabetic humans," *Diabetes*, vol. 39, no. 6, pp. 752–756, 1990.
[87] F. D. Sistare, F. Dieterle, S. Troth et al., "Towards consensus practices to qualify safety biomarkers for use in early drug development," *Nature Biotechnology*, vol. 28, no. 5, pp. 446–454, 2010.
[88] B. Dean, D. Keriakous, E. A. Thomas, and E. Scarr, "Understanding the pathology of schizophenia: the impact of high-throughput screening of the genome and proteome in postmortem CNS," *Current Psychiatry Reviews*, vol. 1, pp. 1–9, 2005.
[89] P. F. Edgar, S. J. Schonberger, B. Dean, R. L. M. Faull, R. Kydd, and G. J. S. Cooper, "A comparative proteome analysis of hippocampal tissue from schizophrenic and Alzheimer's disease individuals," *Molecular Psychiatry*, vol. 4, no. 2, pp. 173–178, 1999.
[90] P. F. Edgar, J. E. Douglas, G. J. S. Cooper, B. Dean, R. Kydd, and R. L. M. Faull, "Comparative proteome analysis of the hippocampus implicates chromosome 6q in schizophrenia," *Molecular Psychiatry*, vol. 5, no. 1, pp. 85–90, 2000.
[91] J. A. English, K. Pennington, M. J. Dunn, and D. R. Cotter, "The neuroproteomics of schizophrenia," *Biological Psychiatry*, vol. 69, no. 2, pp. 163–172, 2011.
[92] E. Scarr, L. Gray, D. Keriakous, P. J. Robinson, and B. Dean, "Increased levels of SNAP-25 and synaptophysin in the dorsolateral prefrontal cortex in bipolar I disorder," *Bipolar Disorders*, vol. 8, no. 2, pp. 133–143, 2006.
[93] L. Gray, E. Scarr, and B. Dean, "N-Ethylmaleimide sensitive factor in the cortex of subjects with schizophrenia and bipolar I disorder," *Neuroscience Letters*, vol. 391, no. 3, pp. 112–115, 2006.
[94] B. Dean, L. Gray, and E. Scarr, "Regionally specific changes in levels of cortical S100β in bipolar 1 disorder but not schizophrenia," *Australian and New Zealand Journal of Psychiatry*, vol. 40, no. 3, pp. 217–224, 2006.
[95] B. Dean, S. A. Boer, A. Mackinnon, and M. Berk, "CNS 14-3-3ζ: changes with sex but not psychiatric diagnoses or psychotropic drug treatment," *Schizophrenia Research*, vol. 93, no. 1–3, pp. 51–57, 2007.
[96] N. Rifai, M. A. Gillette, and S. A. Carr, "Protein biomarker discovery and validation: the long and uncertain path to clinical utility," *Nature Biotechnology*, vol. 24, no. 8, pp. 971–983, 2006.
[97] I. Rudan, "New technologies provide insights into genetic basis of psychiatric disorders and explain their co-morbidity," *Psychiatria Danubina*, vol. 22, no. 2, pp. 190–192, 2010.
[98] D. D. Licatalosi and R. B. Darnell, "RNA processing and its regulation: global insights into biological networks," *Nature Reviews Genetics*, vol. 11, no. 1, pp. 75–87, 2010.
[99] B. Dean, G. Pavey, and A. I. Smith, "Using differential solubilization and 2-D gel electrophoresis to visualize increased numbers of proteins in the human cortex and caudate nucleus and putamen," *Proteomics–Clinical Applications*, vol. 2, no. 9, pp. 1281–1289, 2008.
[100] E. Cerasoli, P. D. Rakowska, A. Horgan et al., "MiS-MALDI: microgel-selected detection of protein biomarkers by MALDI-ToF mass spectrometry," *Molecular BioSystems*, vol. 6, no. 11, pp. 2214–2217, 2010.
[101] M. Ndao, A. Rainczuk, M. C. Rioux, T. W. Spithill, and B. J. Ward, "Is SELDI-TOF a valid tool for diagnostic biomarkers?" *Trends in parasitology*, vol. 26, pp. 561–567, 2010.
[102] J. De Leon, S. C. Armstrong, and K. L. Cozza, "Clinical guidelines for psychiatrists for the use of pharmacogenetic testing for CYP450 2D6 and CYP450 2C19," *Psychosomatics*, vol. 47, no. 1, pp. 75–85, 2006.

7

Parietal Lobes in Schizophrenia: Do They Matter?

Murat Yildiz,[1] Stefan J. Borgwardt,[2] and Gregor E. Berger[3]

[1] *Department of Neurology, Cantonal Hospital St. Gallen, 9007 St. Gallen, Switzerland*
[2] *Psychiatric Outpatient Clinic, University Hospital Basel, 4031 Basel, Switzerland*
[3] *Integrierte Psychiatrie Winterthur, Zurich Unterland, 8408 Winterthur, Switzerland*

Correspondence should be addressed to Murat Yildiz, yildizmur@yahoo.com

Academic Editor: Hugo Schnack

Objective. Despite observations that abnormal parietal lobe (PL) function is associated with psychotic-like experiences, our knowledge about the nature of PL involvement in schizophrenia is modest. The objective of this paper is to investigate the role of the PL in schizophrenia. *Method.* Medline databases were searched for English language publications using the following key words: parietal lobe, combined with schizophrenia, lesions, epilepsy, cognition, rare genetic disorders, MRI, fMRI, PET, and SPECT, respectively, followed by cross-checking of references. *Results.* Imaging studies in childhood onset schizophrenia suggest that grey matter abnormalities start in parietal and occipital lobes and proceed to frontal regions. Although, the findings are inconsistent, several studies with patients at risk to develop schizophrenia indicate early changes in the PL. *Conclusions.* We want to propose that in a proportion of individuals with emerging schizophrenia structural and functional alterations may start in the PL and progress to frontal regions.

1. Introduction

Despite observations that abnormal PL function is associated with psychotic-like experiences, our knowledge about the nature of PL involvement in schizophrenia (SZ) is relatively modest [1]. The PL is engaged in various neuropsychological functions which are affected in schizophrenic patients [2]. The PL supports the frontal lobe in storage and retrieval of verbal information [3]. Episodic memory encoding depends not only on recruiting prefrontal and medial temporal lobes but also on the activation of PL subregions [4]. The right inferior and medial parietal cortices have been associated with the ability to remember past events and arrange them in the right chronological order, consequently enabling us to conceive actions as controlled by ourselves and not a third person [5]. Finally, substantial processing for spatial perception, attention, and self-awareness takes place in the parietal lobes [6–8].

The PL forms strong anatomical connections with the frontal lobe [9]. Frontoparietal white matter maturation correlates with an increase in grey matter activity in both lobes during performance of a working memory (WM) task indicating the close functional connection [10]. Both lobes are frequently activated together while performing cognitive tasks [11]. Joint activation is characterised by a partially symmetrical anteroposterior ordering of activations in both lobes [12]. Croizé et al. demonstrated that although the frontoparietal network is activated in working memory (WM) tasks, both lobes perform distinctive processes [13].

First, we examine the neuropsychiatric manifestations of PL lesions, following a review of selected studies investigating the PL's contribution to SZ. The reevaluation of recent findings allows us to better understand the scope of the PL's influence in SZ. Finally, we propose a new disease model for SZ. A speculative hypothesis will be discussed suggesting that the timing and location of PL changes may differentiate one major pathway in the emergence and progression of SZ.

2. Method

Medline databases were searched for English language publications dating from 1966 to February 2011 using the following key words: parietal lobe combined with each of the following key words: schizophrenia, lesions, epilepsy, cognition, rare genetic disorders, MRI, fMRI, PET, and SPECT.

Cross-checking of references led to the identification of additional relevant references.

2.1. The Anatomical Structure. The parietal lobe can be divided into 3 subregions: the postcentral gyrus, the superior parietal gyrus, and the inferior parietal lobule, consisting of two distinct areas: the angular gyrus and the supramarginal gyrus. The postcentral sulcus separates the postcentral gyrus from the superior parietal gyrus and the inferior parietal lobule. The posteromedial part of the parietal lobe is called the precuneus. The boundaries of the medial surface of the parietal lobe are the frontal, occipital lobes, and the cingulate gyrus. The central sulcus separates the frontal from the parietal lobe. The parieto-occipital fissure lies between the parietal and occipital lobes, and the subparietal sulcus lies between the parietal lobe and cingulate gyrus. From the temporal lobe, the parietal lobe is separated anteriorly by the Sylvian fissure [37].

2.2. Parietal Lobe Lesions and Their Neuropsychiatric Manifestations

2.2.1. Stroke and Other Vascular Conditions. Lesions in the PL offer a unique opportunity to identify the consequences of altered PL function (see Table 1). In schizophrenic patients, dysfunctions can be seen which resemble symptoms seen in patients with PL lesions. Right PL injuries are often resulting in abnormal behaviour such as anosognosia [65]. This condition is associated with the denial of any impairment in the face of a hemiparetic limb [66, 67]. Unawareness of disease, lack of insight, is a phenomenon frequently seen in schizophrenic patients [68, 69]. Unawareness in SZ might occur in connection with deficits of executive functions [70] and thus be very similar to the concept of anosognosia in patients with detectable damage in the PL [71]. An association between structural damage in the frontal lobe and poor insight into illness could be established in schizophrenics [72]. The role of the PL in the phenomenon of unawareness in SZ has yet to be investigated in more detail in the context of the frontoparietal network.

A more obscure neuropsychiatric manifestations is alien hand syndrome (AHS) that may occur after damage of the PL as well as in other brain regions such as the frontal lobe or the corpus callosum [73]. The core symptom of AHS is the perceived loss of control over one's own body movements, that is, a limb. Patients suffer from the impression that an external force is responsible for movements of their own limbs; this symptom is seen occasionally in SZ as well [72]. Sporadically, patients with left PL ischemic lesions display ideomotor apraxia [73, 74] and have difficulties differentiating self-generated movements from foreign made movements [21]. Similar findings could be reproduced in healthy participants using transcranial magnetic stimulation of the superior parietal lobule [75]. These findings best correspond to passivity phenomena in SZ, which were associated with PL dysfunctions [76]. These patients report alien control of their limbs due to their inability to align the timing of motor actions internally [77].

Lesions in the posterior parietal cortex highlight the role of this region in disengaging attention from the current focus to a new one [78]. A deterioration of the ability to shift attention has been shown by several research groups in SZ [79]. Additionally, patients with PL lesions may experience difficulties to direct attention to the contralateral exterior world probably due to a disconnection of parieto-frontal networks [15, 80]. A lateralised defect in the control of attention was associated with the severity of symptoms in SZ [81]. Direct comparisons of the performances of schizophrenics and patients with neglect reveal qualitatively similar impairments [82]. Though, in some schizophrenics defects in spatial [83] and temporal perception are not as impressive as neglect seen in patients with PL lesions [84] and may be the reason that it has not attracted much attention so far.

2.2.2. Parietal Lobe Epilepsy. Focal epilepsy affecting the parietal lobe may also present itself with psychotic symptoms. In a retrospective Canadian study of patients with parietal lobe epilepsy, most patients experienced aurae, nearly all being somatosensory. Some patients described disturbances of body image, visual illusions, vertiginous sensations, and aphasia. A few patients expressed complex visual or auditory hallucinations [85]. Parietal lobe epilepsy often cooccurs with temporal lobe epilepsy which is often accompanied with psychotic like experiences. Marsh et al. described that grey matter volume in the temporal lobes and frontoparietal regions was significantly smaller not only in patients with epilepsy and chronic interictal psychosis but also in patients with unilateral temporal lobe epilepsy without chronic psychosis compared with healthy control subjects [86].

2.2.3. Rare Genetic Disorders with Parietal Involvement. Velocardiofacial (VCF) syndrome is associated with aberrant parietal and frontotemporal white matter tracts. The VCF syndrome is a rare genetic disorder with a prevalence estimated at 1 in 4,000 live births caused by deletion in chromosome 22q11.2 and characterized by cardiac and facial abnormalities. 25% of VCF cases present SZ-like symptoms [87] and visuospatial cognitive impairments in adulthood associated with posterior parietal abnormalities [88]. In VCF, autism spectrum disorders [79] and obsessive-compulsive disorder [89] occur frequently. Another rare genetic disorder, fragile X syndrome, is associated with impaired visual motion processing involving primarily the PL [90]. Mental retardation is the hallmark of fragile X syndrome caused by silencing of the fragile-X mental retardation (fraX) gene [91]. Interestingly, Rivera et al. demonstrated that the parietal region was more active in patients having a higher expression of fraX gene [92].

2.3. Parietal Lobes in SZ

2.3.1. Structural Imaging Studies with Parietal Involvement in Childhood-Onset Schizophrenia. Childhood onset schizophrenia (COS) is defined by its younger age of onset compared to its adult equivalent and may be a more homogeneous group [93]. Studies in COS are particularly important as they

Table 1: Studies reporting lesions in parietal lobe.

Investigator	Lesion site	Subjects	Affected function/impairment	Conclusion	Type of study
Danckert et al. 2002 [14]	Right PL	1 patient with visual neglect	Imagined movements did not show the same speed-accuracy trade-off observed for actual movements	Right parietal lobe may be important in the generation of internal models of motor movements	Case report
Doricchi and Tomaiuolo 2004 [15]	Right hemispheric damage	21 pts with neglect 10 ctrls	Neglect	Maximal overlap in supramarginal gyrus and superior longitudinal fasciculus; decisive role of parieto-frontal disconnection in neglect	Case series
Haaland et al. 2000 [16]	Left PL	41 pts with damage in left hemisphere	Ideomotor apraxia	Regions in the left hemisphere important for goal directed movements	Case series
Markowitsch et al. 1999 [17]	Left angular gyrus lesion	1 patient	Auditory working memory dysfunction	Calculation tasks were not affected	Case report
Paterson and Zangwill 1944 [18]	Penetrating head wound affecting the angular gyrus	1 patient		Neglect	Case report
Rosler et al. 1997 [19]	Ischemic lesion in the territory of the right middle cerebral artery	31 pts with right- or left- sided infarctions 31 ctrls	Facial recognition ability in pts with right-sided lesions was lessened compared with ctrls and with pts with left-sided infarctions	Graded impairment in patients with right middle cerebral artery infarcts	Cross-sectional case-control study
Rossetti et al. 2005 [20]	*First case*: bilateral parietal damage *Second case*: bilateral posterior parietal and upper and lateral occipital cortico-subcortical regions bilaterally through ischemic stroke	2 pts	*First case*: visual disorientation, simultanagnosia, and severe optic ataxia *Second case*: bilateral optic ataxia	Optic ataxia patients are impaired for immediate visuomotor processing but improve when required to delay before responding.	Case series
Sirigu et al. 1999 [21]	Left parietal cortex damage	3 pts with apraxia 6 ctrls with apraxia 2 nonapraxic neurological ctrs	pts were impaired in recognition of the viewed hand as the examiner's when it performed movements similar to their own movement	Parietal cortex is important for the perception of own movements as self-generated	Cross-sectional

PL: parietal lobe; pts: patients; ctrls: healthy controls.

are supposed to be more genetically determined than the adult onset form. As seen in the case of very early onset SZ more severe premorbid neurodevelopmental abnormalities, a higher rate of cytogenetic anomalies and familial SZ are observed than in later onset cases [42].

Thompson et al. described that a dynamic wave of grey matter loss occurs, beginning in the PL and proceeding to the temporal and finally to the prefrontal dorsolateral cortices [94, 95]. The latter findings suggest that the changes in the PL occur early on in the disease. Although serial brain MRI scans in healthy children over a ten-year period revealed a similar pattern of grey-matter loss beginning in the dorsal parietal and primary sensorimotor regions spreading laterally and caudally into temporal cortices and anteriorly into dorsolateral prefrontal areas [32]. The pattern matches the order of grey matter loss seen in *COS;* however, the extend of loss is larger in COS. Additionally, Kyriakopoulos et al. demonstrated that compared with healthy controls, individuals with adolescent-onset SZ showed fractional anisotropy decrease in parietal regions, in contrast to individuals with adult onset SZ who showed additional fractional anisotropy reductions in frontal and temporal regions [96]. Fractional anisotropy is measured with diffusion tensor imaging and is positively correlated with the degree of neuronal matura-tion and organisation of white matter tracts [97]. These findings support the concept of SZ as a neurodegenerative disease [29].

Table 2: Recent structural magnetic resonance imaging (MRI) and computerized tomography (CT) studies on psychosis and schizophrenia with relevance to the parietal lobe.

Investigators	Subject groups	Average age of first scan (years)	Average years of followup	Image slice thickness	methods of analysis	Brain regions showing significant change in patients	Correlations between brain changes and clinical variables
Buchanan et al. 2004 [22]	44 csz 34 ctrls	39 34	0	1.5 mm	ROI manual tracing	Smaller inferior prefrontal region vol. and reversal of the normal asymmetry of the inferior parietal cortex	
Cannon et al. 2002 [23]	20 MZ discordant pairs 20 DZ discordant pairs 20 MZ ctrls 20 DZ ctrls	48 49 48 47	0	1.2 mm	Three-dimensional cortical maps	Between patients and their MZ cotwins reduced grey matter in the superior *parietal lobule*, dorsolateral prefrontal cortex, Broca's area, premotor cortex and frontal eye fields, superior temporal gyrus.	Disease-related deficits in grey matter were correlated with measures of symptom severity and cognitive dysfunction
Dazzan et al. 2011 [24]	102 UHR	20	1	1.5 mm	VBM	Reductions in the frontal cortex in subjects who developed psychosis and the subgroup that subsequently developed SZ also showed smaller volumes in the *parietal cortex*	
Dubb et al. 2005 [25]	46 csz 92 ctrls	29 31	0	1.0 mm	VBM	Reduced vol. of the parietal and frontal lobe	
Foong et al. 2001[26]	25 csz 30 ctrls	37 35	0	5.0 mm	MTI	Frontal and temporal vol. reductions	Bilateral parieto-occipital cortex and genu of corpus callosum vol. reductions were associated with severity of negative symptoms in sz
Frederikse et al. 2000 [27]	15 male scz 15 female csz 15 male ctrls 15 female ctrls	39 40 39 38	0	1.5 mm	ROI of the inferior parietal lobule	Male csz had a reversal of the normal left greater than right male asymmetry and smaller left inferior parietal lobule grey matter vol. female csz did not differ from female ctrls	
Hubl et al. 2004 [28]	13 csz with to auditory hallucinations 13 csz without auditory hallucinations 13 ctrls	33 31 32	0	5.0 mm	DTI	pts with hallucinations had higher white matter directionality in the lateral parts of the temporoparietal section of the arcuate fasciculus and in parts of the anterior corpus callosum	Alterations of white matter fiber tracts in pts with frequent hallucinations lead to abnormal coactivation in regions related to the acoustical processing
Job et al. 2005 [29]	65 GHR 19 ctrls	21 21	2	1.9 mm	VBM	GHR with *right parietal grey matter*, temporal grey matter, right frontal grey matter reductions	GHR with psychotic symptoms and converters showed a different spatial pattern of reductions

TABLE 2: Continued.

Investigators	Subject groups	Average age of first scan (years)	Average years of followup	Image slice thickness	methods of analysis	Brain regions showing significant change in patients	Correlations between brain changes and clinical variables
Jung et al. 2009 [30]	29 UHR 31 SZ 29 ctrls	22 24 23	0	voxel size $0.45 \times 0.45 \times 0.9$ mm	VBM	UHR: cortical thinning in prefrontal cortex, anterior cingulate cortex, inferior parietal cortex, parahippocampal cortex, and superior temporal gyrus	Cortical thinning was more pronounced in SZ compared with UHR and ctrls
Kubicki et al. 2001 [31]	16 FE 16 affective psychosis 18 ctrls	26 23 24	0	1.5 mm	VBM	FE reduced volume of right inferior parietal lobule, right dorsolateral prefrontal cortex, left and right anterior cingulate gyrus, left and right insula	
Kyriakopoulos et al. 2009 [32]	17 adolescent-onset SZ 17 adolescent ctrls 17 adult-onset SZ 17 adult ctrls	17 16 24 24	0	2.5 mm	DTI	Individuals with adolescent onset SZ show fractional anisotropy decrease in parietal regionsindividuals with adult onset show additionally in frontal, temporal, and cerebellar regions	White matter abnormalities in SZ may depend on developmental stage at the time of illness onset
Minatogawa-Chang et al. 2009 [33]	88 FEP 86 ctrls	29 31	0	voxel size $2 \times 2 \times 2$ mm^3	MRI + controlled oral word association test + forward and backward digit span tests	Volume abnormalities in frontal and temporoparietal cortices	Cognitive deficits directly related to brain volume abnormalities in frontal and temporoparietal cortices in FEP subjects
Mitelman et al. 2009 [34]	17 csz with good outcome 17 csz with poor outcome 13 ctrls	37 47 42	4	1.2 mm	DTI	At baseline, csz had smaller frontal, temporal, and parietal gray matter volumes than ctrls	Grey matter volumes in poor-outcome patients decline more rapidly than in patients with good outcome
Narr et al. 2005 [35]	72 FE 78 ctrls	25 27	0	1.5 mm	MRI	Regional grey matter thinning in frontal, temporal and *parietal* heteromodal association cortices bilaterally	
Nierenberg et al. 2005 [36]	14 FE 14 ctrls	18–55	0	1.5 mm	ROI	Smaller left angular gyrus vol.	
Niznikiewicz et al. 2000 [37]	15 male right-handed csz 15 male right-handed ctrls	20–55	0	1.5 mm	ROI	Showed a reversed asymmetry in the inferior parietal lobule that was mainly seen in the angular gyrus	

Table 2: Continued.

Investigators	Subject groups	Average age of first scan (years)	Average years of followup	Image slice thickness	methods of analysis	Brain regions showing significant change in patients	Correlations between brain changes and clinical variables
Rowland et al. 2008 [38]	10 csz with neg. symptoms 10 csz without neg. symptoms 11 ctrls	46 40 37	0	2.2 mm	DTI	Reduced FA in the superior longitudinal fasciculus connecting parietal with frontal lobe	Support for altered frontal-parietal network in deficit SZ
Schultz et al. 2009 [39]	54 FE 54 ctrls	26 27	0	1 mm	MRI	Cortical thinning in: dorsolateral and frontopolar cortices, anterior cingulate cortex, superior temporal cortices, and superior parietal lobe	Widespread reduction of cortical thickness, mostly in heteromodal cortices of frontotemporal networks
Sun 2003 [40]	23 UHR-N 12 UHR-P	20 20	1	1.5 mm	MRI	*UHR-P* : reduction in dorsolateral prefrontal cortex and orbitofrontal cortex	High-risk psychosis subjects showed orbitofrontal cortex reduction compared to FE
Sun et al. 2005 [41]	23 FEP (16 FES) 11 csz 28 ctrls	22 33 26	2	1.5 mm	MRI	*FE versus ctrls*: whole brain, left (trend), and right motor-premotor, *left and right parietal*, left and right dorsal prefrontal *csz versus FE:* left and right dorsal prefrontal	FE brain surface retraction was similar to that of ctrls but significantly accelerated
Thompson et al. 2001 [42]	12 SZ 12 ctrls	14 14	4.6	1.2 mm	MRI	*Earliest scans:* deficits in parietal brain regions *Latest scans:* included dorsolateral prefrontal cortex and superior temporal gyri	Change patterns correlated with psychotic symptom severity
Whitford et al. 2005 [43]	31 FE 30 ctrls	19 19	0	1.5 mm	VBM	left prefrontal cortex, *left parietal* and temporal cortex, right cerebellum, *right parietal*, frontal, and cortex reductions	Reality distortion syndrome score correlates with grey matter reduction in FE
Whitford et al. 2006 [44]	41 FES followup: 25 FES 47 ctrls followup: 26 ctrls	19 19	2.6 2.4	1.5 mm	VBM	*Baseline:* grey matter reductions in the frontal, *parietal*, and temporal cortices and cerebellum *Followup interval:* especially in the *parietal* and temporal cortices further reductions	
Narr et al. 2001 [35]	48 csz 48 ctrls	33 32	0	0.9–1.4 mm	VBM	Left-dominant frontal, temporal, and insular grey matter reductions	Global assessment of functioning score correlated with grey matter vol. in the left inferior frontal and inferior parietal lobe
Zhou et al. 2006 [45]	53 csz 25 schizotypal disorder pts 59 ctrls	25 26 24	0	1 mm	ROI	csz: reduction in parietal lobe schizotypal subjects: postcentral gyrus volume reductions	

csz: chronic schizophrenic patients; ctrls: healthy controls; ROI: region of interest; vol.: volume; MZ: monozygotic twins; DZ: dizygotic twins; VBM: Voxel-Based Morphometry; MTI: magnetization transfer imaging; SZ: schizophrenia; DTI: diffusion tensor imaging; FE: first episode schizophrenia; FEP: first episode psychosis; FA: fractional anisotropy; GHR: subjects at genetically high risk; UHR: ultra-high-risk patients; UHR-P: ultra-high-risk subjects who became psychotic; UHR-N: ultra-high-risk subjects who did not became psychotic, VBM: voxel-based morphometry.

Table 3: Recent functional magnetic resonance imaging (MRI) and positron emission tomography (PET) studies on psychosis and schizophrenia with relevance to the parietal lobe.

Investigator	Subject groups	Average age	Paradigm	Tested brain function	Method of analysis	Main findings in patients compared with ctls	Conclusion
Arce et al. 2006 [46]	17 csz 17 ctrls	41 40	Visual Go/Nogo task with matched performance accuracy between csz and ctrls	Inhibition and cue processing	fMRI	*During cued inhibition*: greater activation in the left precuneus and left superior temporal gyrus *During inhibition*: less ACC and DLPFC activation *Implicit cue trials*: greater inferior frontal gyrus activation	Csz have difficulties with inhibition and clue processing
Braus et al. 2006 [47]	11 FE 11 ctrls	25 29	Simultaneous presentation of acoustical and optical inputs	Basic sensory input circuits	fMRI	Less activation of the PL, right thalamus, the right prefrontal cortex	Already at disease onset deficits in information processing are existing
Broome et al. 2009 [48]	17 UHR 10 FEP 15 ctrls	24 26 25	Verbal fluency task and an N-back	WM	fMRI	Activation pattern in UHR was during the N-back task different in dorsolateral prefrontal and parietal cortex compared to ctrls	The level of regional activation in the UHR group was intermediate between that in the FE group and ctrls
Franck et al. 2002 [49]	87 csz	31	Instructed to relax and not perform any tasks	Random episodic silent thought (REST)	PET	Schneiderian score positively correlated with rCBF in right superior parietal cortex and negatively correlated with rCBF in left posterior cingulate gyrus and in left lingual gyrus	Findings support hypothesis that cerebral pattern of activation is linked to symptoms of SZ
Henseler et al. 2010 [50]	12 csz 12 ctrls	33 32	Verbal item-recognition task and a visuospatial item-recognition task	WM	fMRI	SZ showed reduced connectivity of the prefrontal cortex with the intraparietal cortex and the hippocampus	Altered prefronto-hippocampal and parieto-occipital connectivity was found to be associated with higher positive symptoms
Hugdahl et al. 2004 [51]	csz depressed pts ctrls	32 33 31	First task: pressing a response button whenever a specific number was seen Second task: adding two consecutive numbers	Vigilance task Mental arithmetic task	fMRI	Less activation in prefrontal brain regions and greater parietal lobe activation relative compared to ctrls and patients with major depression.	In support double dissociation of parietal and frontal lobe activation between SZ and depression
Keedy et al. 2006 [52]	15 FE 24 ctrls	25 25	Eye movement tasks: visually guided saccade, smooth pursuit paradigms and oculomotor delayed response paradigm	Oculomotor function Spatial working memory	fMRI	Reduced activation in sensorimotor areas supporting eye movement control: parietal cortex, frontal eye fields, supplementary eye fields, and cingulated cortex	Generalized pattern of cortical dysfunction already present early SZ

Table 3: Continued.

Investigator	Subject groups	Average age	Paradigm	Tested brain function	Method of analysis	Main findings in patients compared with ctls	Conclusion
Keshavan et al. 2002 [53]	4 GHR 4 ctrls	13 13	Memory-guided saccade task	Spatial working memory	fMRI	Decreased activation in the inferior parietal cortex and the DLPFC	Dysfunction of prefrontal and parietal regions in GHR
Kim et al. 2003 [54]	12 csz 12 ctrls	26 26	n-back sequential picture task	WM	PET	Dorsolateral prefrontal, ventrolateral prefrontal and bilateral inferior parietal region activation abnormalities	Indicating that during working memory tasks there could be a parietofrontal disconnection
Öngür et al. 2006 [55]	20 csz 17 ctrls	40 38	Discrimination of previously seen and new pairs of visual stimuli	Relational memory	fMRI	While discriminating novel pairs decreased activation of the right parietal cortex and the anterior cingulate cortex	Deficit of relational memory connected to dysfunctional activation of the parietal cortex and the hippocampus
Ojeda et al. 2002 [56]	11 csz drug naive 10 ctrls	28 26	Auditory stimulation task Counting tasks with or without auditory stimulation	Attention tasks	PET	Inadequate activation of parietal and frontal regions during performance of cognitively emanding tasks	Evidence of compensatory mechanisms in frontoparietal regions
Paulus et al. 2003 [57]	15 scz 15 ctrls	42 41	Two-choice prediction task	Decision making with different degrees of uncertainty	fMRI	PL less activated in decision making in situations with high uncertain outcome	Inadequate processing in situations of uncertainty in the posterior parietal cortex
Quintana et al. 2003 [58]	8 sz 8 ctrls		Anticipatory task Retention task	WM	fMRI	Anticipatory task: decreased PFC and increased PPC activation Retention task: increased PFC activation	PFC shows more hypoactivation than PPC is able to compensate
Sanz et al. 2009 [59]	13 csz no information about ctrls included	20	verbal capacity task	verbal WM	fMRI	Lower levels of activation in frontal lobe, PL in the left hemisphere	Dysfunctional activation during WM processing related to the severity of negative and disorganized symptoms
Schneider et al. 2007 [60]	48 FE 57 ctrls	31 31	2- and 0-back tasks	WM attention connected processes	fMRI	*Working memory*: parietal hypoactivations, combined with hyperfrontality in VLPFC Attention-connected processes: hypoactivations in the VLPFC, superior temporal cortex, thalamus	Dysfunctional cerebral network not able to cope with required activation for attention and WM tasks
Sweeney et al. 2003 [61]	8 csz with auditory hallucinations 8 ctrls	31 29	Fast versus slow covert articulation of a word at two self-paced rates	Processing inner speech	fMRI	Reduced activation in the right superior temporal, inferior parietal, and parahippocampal regions	SZ patients with auditory hallucinations have aberrant activation pattern of brain regions

Table 3: Continued.

Investigator	Subject groups	Average age	Paradigm	Tested brain function	Method of analysis	Main findings in patients compared with ctls	Conclusion
Spence et al. 1997 [1]	7 d-scz 6 nd-scz 6 ctrls	Not stated	Performing movement task Second PET 4–6 weeks after first PET	Movement	PET	Increased right parietal and cingulate activation in csz with delusions of control but in d-scz with decreased passivity delusion in second scan hyperactivation of right parietal and cingulate remitted	Certain brain regions involved in generating delusions of passivity
Thermenos et al. 2005 [62]	14 SZ 22 ctrls	38 38	Visual letter 2-back task	WM	fMRI	Greater activation in the right medial frontal gyrus and left inferior parietal lobule/medial temporal gyrus region	Heteromodal association cortices show higher activation in SZ during performance of WoM task
Whalley et al. 2006 [63]	4 GHP-S 26 GHR-P 27 GHR-N 21 ctrls	23 26 27 27	Hayling sentence completion test	Word retrieval	fMRI and ROI	GHR-N showed increased activation of the PL and the anterior cingulate	PL and the lingual gyrus could be used to discriminate between converts and nonconverts
Whalley et al. 2004 [64]	21 GHR-P 48 GHR-N 21 ctrls	25 27 27	Part of Hayling sentence completion test	Verbal initiation	fMRI	GHR-P: increased activation in the left inferior parietal lobule GHR-N: less activity in medial prefrontal, thalamic and cerebellar regions	Soonest changes in patients with symptoms may be connected to hyperactivation in the parietal lobe

csz: patients with SZ; ctrls: healthy controls; fMRI: functional magnetic resonance imaging; ACC: anterior cingulate cortex; DLPFC: dorsolateral prefrontal cortex; FE: patients with first-episode schizophrenia; PL: parietal lobe; UHR: ultra-high risk patients with prodromal symptoms of schizophrenia; FEP: first episode psychosis; WM: working memory; PET: positron emission tomography; rCBF: regional cerebral blood flow; pts: patients; GHR: genetically defined high-risk for schizophrenia; PFC: prefrontal cortex; PPC: posterior parietal cortex; VLPC: ventrolateral prefrontal cortex; GHR-N: ultrahigh-risk subjects who remain nonpsychotic; GHR-P: ultra-high-risk subjects who became psychotic; GHP-S: ultra-high-risk subjects who became schizophrenic; nd-scz: schizophrenic patients without delusion of control; d-scz: schizophrenic patients with delusion of control; ROI: region of interest; SZ: schizophrenia.

2.3.2. Structural Imaging Studies with Parietal Involvement in High-Risk Patients. In a longitudinal study over two years with a genetically defined high-risk (GHR) cohort from Edinburgh a significant decline in grey matter density was found in the right parietal, right frontal, and temporal lobes [30]. In another study, patients at ultra-high risk (UHR) experiencing prodromal symptoms showed significant cortical thinning in the inferior parietal cortex compared to healthy controls [98]. Borgwardt et al. observed that UHR subjects who later developed psychosis (converters) showed volume reductions in the medial and superior parietal, in the frontal and inferior temporal cortex and in the cerebellum. There were no longitudinal volumetric changes in UHR subjects who did not develop psychosis (nonconverters) [99]. These findings suggest that PL changes may occur prior to the first psychotic episode. However, a previous study from Pantelis et al. could not trace over one year significant changes in the PL of converters. Instead, they demonstrated that converters compared to nonconverters show a longitudinal reduction in the grey matter of the right medial temporal, lateral temporal, inferior frontal, and cingulate cortex bilaterally [39].

2.3.3. Structural Imaging Studies with Parietal Involvement in First-Episode Psychosis and Established Schizophrenia. Reduced cortical thickness in the parietal and frontal regions is already evident in first-episode SZ patients (FE) [40]. It should be noted that a longitudinal surface contraction in frontal and parietal regions of the cortex was found in FE, but not in chronic schizophrenics [33, 100]. Prefrontal and temporoparietal grey matter volume reductions correlate significantly with cognitive performance in FE, indicating the clinical importance of such alterations [84].

Converging evidence suggests that chronic schizophrenics display PL structural abnormalities (see Table 2). Rowland et al. demonstrated with diffusion tensor imaging (DTI) a de-clined fractional anisotropy of white matter tracts connecting frontal and parietal regions in schizophrenics with negative symptoms [34]. Intriguingly, in the longitudinal four-year followup conducted by Mitelman et al., grey matter volumes in the parietal, frontal, and temporal lobes in schizophrenics with a poor clinical outcome continued to decline more rapidly compared to patients with a good clinical outcome [101]. Using three-dimensional cortical surface maps, a comparison between schizophrenics compared to their unaffect-ed monozygotic cotwins revealed deficits in the superior parietal lobe, dorsolateral prefrontal cortex, and superior temporal gyrus [102]. Additionally, a previous study by the same research group demonstrated that frontal lobe grey matter deficits were present in affected and nonaffected twins [48].

2.4. Functional Parietal Lobe Abnormalities

2.4.1. Functional Imaging Studies with Parietal Involvement in at Risk Mental States. Functional MRI (fMRI) studies indicate that UHR individuals display abnormal activation in the prefrontal and parietal cortex during performance of WM tasks [63]. Whalley et al. reported promising results from a recent longitudinal fMRI study in GHR individuals. fMRI data of converters compared to nonconverters showed increased activation of the PL and decreased activation of the anterior cingulate. However, the PL activation only had high predictive power if the lingual gyrus was also activated [64]. The study was limited as only 4 out of 62 at risk individuals developed SZ. Nevertheless, this study might demonstrate that parietal functional abnormalities are present in high-risk subjects who later become psychotic.

The same study group found in GHR individuals increased connectivity between the left parietal and left prefrontal regions compared to healthy controls. The authors interpreted the hyperactivation of the PL as compensatory, since there were no differences in performance between the groups [64]. These results underline that many PL findings are reported in connection with the frontoparietal network.

2.4.2. Functional Imaging Studies with Parietal Involvement in First-Episode Psychosis and in Chronic Schizophrenia. Prefrontal cortex dysfunctions have been identified as a key factor in SZ [103]. The role of PL dysfunctions still remains ambiguous in SZ. Parietal hypoactivation and ventrolateral prefrontal hyperactivity during WM tasks in FE patients indicate that frontoparietal networks are impaired early in the course of the illness [60]. Correspondingly, in patients with chronic SZ, parietal and frontal cortex activation deficits were described in WM tasks [104]. There is an increasing body of studies associating PL dysfunctions with a variety of symptoms in chronic SZ [105]. For instance, a PET study correlated positively regional cerebral blood flow in right superior parietal cortex with the severity of Schneiderian first-rank symptoms (voices conversing or commenting; thought broadcasting, withdrawal or insertion; made actions and thoughts) [49]. Moreover, Menon et al. demonstrated that thinking disturbance was correlated with deficits in activation in the parietal and the right frontal cortices [104]. In fact, overactivity in the right inferior parietal cortex was associated with the presence of delusions of control in a study with acute psychotic schizophrenics performing movement tasks. Interestingly, the activity in this region returned to normal levels when patients were symptom-free [1]. Lower levels of activation during verbal WM task performance in the left hemisphere across frontal and parietal regions were associated with poorer role functioning and greater severity of negative and disorganised symptoms [59]. A recent study identified disturbed parieto-occipital functional connectivity as related with positive symptoms of SZ [50]. These findings underline that two core symptoms of SZ, cognitive deficits and delusions, may be related to malfunctions in the parietal lobe [106].

3. Discussion

The nature of the pathological processes underlying progressive structural and functional changes in SZ and their exact timing in the brains remains unclear. Our paper provides a selection of studies indicating that PL lesions and epilepsy may cause psychotic-like symptoms and supports the concept that PL abnormalities could be important for SZ and related disorders. Structural brain irregularities in PL were found in imaging studies in COS suggesting that grey matter abnormalities start in parietal and occipital lobes and proceed in a dynamic wave to frontal cortices [42, 94]. This illustrates that PL structural alterations may occur early in the course of illness and points to genetic influences, yet to be determined [93]. The contribution of genetic factors to parietal involvement in SZ is further supported by a significant decline in grey matter found over time in GHR subjects [29]. The brain-derived neurotrophic factor (BDNF) could be one of the candidate genes for parietal lobe alterations seen in SZ. Indeed, there was decreased activity in the bilateral posterior parietal regions in GHR patients with BDNF Val homozygote versus BDNF Met carriers [107].

There is evidence that parietal lobe abnormalities may be only partially genetically determined as parietal lobe alterations were seen in monozygotic twins with SZ but not in their nonaffected twins [101]. There are studies indicating parietal structural alterations in the early phase of psychosis [99]. However, a reduction in the parietal volume was not found in the UHR sample from Melbourne [98]. This inconsistency could be explained by major methodological differences of both studies: the study by Borgwardt et al. spanned a time period of 3-4 years and the analysed MRI slices were 1 mm thick, whereas the Melbourne group observed their sample over 1 year and acquired MRI slices that were 3 mm thick [98, 99]. In a recent UHR study from Melbourne applying voxel-based morphometry methodology in 1.5 mm thick MRI slices, reductions in frontal and parietal cortices were detected in the UHR group who later converted to a psychotic disorder compared to those who did not convert [24].

The neurodevelopmental hypothesis suggests that early insults in pregnancy and infancy combined with genetic factors render the brain vulnerable for later development of SZ [108]. However, symptoms usually occur many years after the implied first damage [100, 109], hence a second insult was proposed to explain for the long delay [100]. Here, we want to propose that in a proportion of patients subsequently developing SZ, structural and functional alterations may start in parietal lobes progressing to frontal regions. The "parietal type" of SZ development may clinically present initially with working memory deficits [50, 56, 58, 60] and disturbed self-conceptualization [1, 84]. The "parietal type" may be more relevant for early onset forms of psychotic disorders in adolescents, with COS being the most extreme variant. In this model, genetic influences would play a more prominent role. Additional causative factors, yet to be identified, interacting with brain maturational processes in late adolescence and early adulthood may be decisive in the transition to a full-blown psychotic disorder [110]. Such an approach may enable us to characterise subtypes of SZ based on structural and functional brain processes and not merely on pure phenomenology.

The functional interdependency of the parietal and frontal cortices was revealed in GHR subjects with isolated psychotic symptoms. They displayed compensatory activation in the left inferior parietal lobule while performing the Hayling sentence completion task [40]. Additionally, Quintana et al. reported parietal cortex activation in schizophrenics as compensatory mechanism for prefrontal cortex dysfunction while performing a working memory task [58]. However, Schneider et al. described parietal hypoactivation combined with hyperfrontality in first-episode schizophrenia patients with poorer performance [60]. In contrast to the study by Schneider and colleagues, in the studies conducted by Whalley and Quintana no statistical differences in performance accuracy were found between patients and controls. The hyperactivation of the PL may compensate for frontal hypoactivity, then the network between the frontal and parietal cortices is sufficient; hence tasks can be performed adequately. But in case of a disconnection in the frontoparietal network [50], the PL is not recruited to support the frontal lobe. This could lead to an inadequate hyperactivation of the frontal lobe leading to poor performance. This hypothesis warrants confirmation in carefully planned studies.

Finally, some voxel-based morphometry studies have not found PL volume reductions in FEP [61, 111] and chronic SZ [108, 112]. More research is required to explore parietal lobe functions and volumes across different stages of SZ. Whether the pattern of parietal lobe changes is suitable for identifying a more homogeneous subgroup of patients with emerging SZ remains to be determined. Further longitudinal data are necessary from the earliest stages of SZ, particularly in prepsychotic individuals, to resolve this issue. A better understanding of the time course of structural and functional brain changes across different stages of psychotic disorders [109] will finally help us to distinguish between those individuals at incipient risk for a major mental illness and those with merely a transient crisis in life.

Acknowledgment

Murat Yildiz has received travel Grants from Merck Serono, Bayer AG, and Biogen Idec.

References

[1] S. A. Spence, D. J. Brooks, S. R. Hirsch, P. F. Liddle, J. Meehan, and P. M. Grasby, "A PET study of voluntary movement in schizophrenic patients experiencing passivity phenomena (delusions of alien control)," *Brain*, vol. 120, no. 11, pp. 1997–2011, 1997.

[2] E. Antonova, T. Sharma, R. Morris, and V. Kumari, "The relationship between brain structure and neurocognition in schizophrenia: a selective review," *Schizophrenia Research*, vol. 70, no. 2-3, pp. 117–145, 2004.

[3] J. Jonides, E. H. Schumacher, E. E. Smith et al., "The role of parietal cortex in verbal working memory," *Journal of Neuroscience*, vol. 18, no. 13, pp. 5026–5034, 1998.

[4] A. E. Cavanna and M. R. Trimble, "The precuneus: a review of its functional anatomy and behavioural correlates," *Brain*, vol. 129, no. 3, pp. 564–583, 2006.

[5] K. Vogeley, R. Tepest, T. Schneider-Axmann et al., "Automated image analysis of disturbed cytoarchitecture in Brodmann area 10 in schizophrenia," *Schizophrenia Research*, vol. 62, no. 1-2, pp. 133–140, 2003.

[6] M. F. S. Rushworth, A. Ellison, and V. Walsh, "Complementary localization and lateralization of orienting and motor attention," *Nature Neuroscience*, vol. 4, no. 6, pp. 656–661, 2001.

[7] D. Thoenissen, K. Zilles, and I. Toni, "Differential involvement of parietal and precentral regions in movement preparation and motor intention," *Journal of Neuroscience*, vol. 22, no. 20, pp. 9024–9034, 2002.

[8] J. Gottlieb, "From thought to action: the parietal cortex as a bridge between perception, action, and cognition," *Neuron*, vol. 53, no. 1, pp. 9–16, 2007.

[9] B. Seltzer and D. N. Pandya, "Further observations on parieto-temporal connections in the rhesus monkey," *Experimental Brain Research*, vol. 55, no. 2, pp. 301–312, 1984.

[10] P. J. Olesen, Z. Nagy, H. Westerberg, and T. Klingberg, "Combined analysis of DTI and fMRI data reveals a joint maturation of white and grey matter in a fronto-parietal network," *Cognitive Brain Research*, vol. 18, no. 1, pp. 48–57, 2003.

[11] J. M. Gurd, K. Amunts, P. H. Weiss et al., "Posterior parietal cortex is implicated in continuous switching between verbal fluency tasks: an fMRI study with clinical implications," *Brain*, vol. 125, no. 5, pp. 1024–1038, 2002.

[12] O. Simon, F. Kherif, G. Flandin et al., "Automatized clustering and functional geometry of human parietofrontal networks for language, space, and number," *NeuroImage*, vol. 23, no. 3, pp. 1192–1202, 2004.

[13] A. C. Croizé, R. Ragot, L. Garnero et al., "Dynamics of parietofrontal networks underlying visuospatial short-term memory encoding," *NeuroImage*, vol. 23, no. 3, pp. 787–799, 2004.

[14] J. Danckert, S. Ferber, T. Doherty, H. Steinmetz, D. Nicolle, and M. A. Goodale, "Selective, non-lateralized impairment of motor imagery following right parietal damage," *Neurocase*, vol. 8, no. 3, pp. 194–204, 2002.

[15] F. Doricchi and F. Tomaiuolo, "The anatomy of neglect without hemianopia: a key role for parietal-frontal disconnection?" *NeuroReport*, vol. 14, no. 2, pp. 239–243, 2003.

[16] K. Y. Haaland, D. L. Harrington, and R. T. Knight, "Neural representations of skilled movement," *Brain*, vol. 123, no. 11, pp. 2306–2313, 2000.

[17] H. J. Markowitsch, E. Kalbe, J. Kessler, H. M. Von Stockhausen, M. Ghaemi, and W. D. Heiss, "Short-term memory deficit after focal parietal damage," *Journal of Clinical and Experimental Neuropsychology*, vol. 21, no. 6, pp. 784–797, 1999.

[18] A. Paterson and O. L. Zangwill, "Disorders of visual space perception associated with lesions of the right cerebral hemisphere," *Brain*, vol. 67, no. 4, pp. 331–358, 1944.

[19] A. Rosler, S. Lanquillon, and O. Dippel, "Impairment of facial recognition in patients with right cerebral infarcts quantified by computer aided morphing," *Journal of Neurology, Neurosurgery & Psychiatry*, vol. 62, pp. 261–264, 1997.

[20] Y. Rossetti, P. Revol, R. McIntosh et al., "Visually guided reaching: bilateral posterior parietal lesions cause a switch from fast visuomotor to slow cognitive control," *Neuropsychologia*, vol. 43, no. 2, pp. 162–177, 2005.

[21] A. Sirigu, E. Daprati, P. Pradat-Diehl, N. Franck, and M. Jeannerod, "Perception of self-generated movement following left parietal lesion," *Brain*, vol. 122, no. 10, pp. 1867–1874, 1999.

[22] R. W. Buchanan, A. Francis, C. Arango et al., "Morphometric assessment of the heteromodal association cortex in Schizophrenia," *American Journal of Psychiatry*, vol. 161, no. 2, pp. 322–331, 2004.

[23] T. D. Cannon, P. M. Thompson, T. G. M. Van Erp et al., "Cortex mapping reveals regionally specific patterns of genetic and disease-specific gray-matter deficits in twins discordant for schizophrenia," *Proceedings of the National Academy of Sciences of the United States of America*, vol. 99, no. 5, pp. 3228–3233, 2002.

[24] P. Dazzan, B. Soulsby, A. Mechelli et al., "Volumetric abnormalities predating the onset of schizophrenia and affective psychoses: an MRI study in subjects at ultrahigh risk of psychosis," *Schizophrenia Bulletin*. In press.

[25] A. Dubb, Z. Xie, R. Gur, R. Gur, and J. Gee, "Characterization of brain plasticity in schizophrenia using template deformation," *Academic Radiology*, vol. 12, no. 1, pp. 3–9, 2005.

[26] J. Foong, M. R. Symms, G. J. Barker et al., "Neuropathological abnormalities in schizophrenia: evidence from magnetization transfer imaging," *Brain*, vol. 124, no. 5, pp. 882–892, 2001.

[27] M. Frederikse, A. Lu, E. Aylward, P. Barta, T. Sharma, and G. Pearlson, "Sex differences in inferior parietal lobule volume in schizophrenia," *American Journal of Psychiatry*, vol. 157, no. 3, pp. 422–427, 2000.

[28] D. Hubl, T. Koenig, W. Strik et al., "Pathways that make voices: white matter changes in auditory hallucinations," *Archives of General Psychiatry*, vol. 61, no. 7, pp. 658–668, 2004.

[29] D. E. Job, H. C. Whalley, E. C. Johnstone, and S. M. Lawrie, "Grey matter changes over time in high risk subjects developing schizophrenia," *NeuroImage*, vol. 25, no. 4, pp. 1023–1030, 2005.

[30] W. H. Jung, J. S. Kim, J. H. Jang et al., "Cortical thickness reduction in individuals at ultra-high-risk for psychosis," *Schizophrenia Bulletin*, vol. 37, no. 4, pp. 839–849, 2011.

[31] M. Kubicki, M. E. Shenton, D. F. Salisbury et al., "Voxel-based morphometric analysis of gray matter in first episode schizophrenia," *NeuroImage*, vol. 17, no. 4, pp. 1711–1719, 2002.

[32] M. Kyriakopoulos, R. Perez-Iglesias, J. B. Woolley et al., "Effect of age at onset of schizophrenia on white matter abnormalities," *British Journal of Psychiatry*, vol. 195, no. 4, pp. 346–353, 2009.

[33] T. M. Minatogawa-Chang, M. S. Schaufelberger, A. M. Ayres et al., "Cognitive performance is related to cortical grey matter volumes in early stages of schizophrenia: a population-based study of first-episode psychosis," *Schizophrenia Research*, vol. 113, no. 2-3, pp. 200–209, 2009.

[34] S. A. Mitelman, E. L. Canfield, R. E. Newmark et al., "Longitudinal assessment of gray and white matter in chronic schizophrenia: a combined diffusion-tensor and structural magnetic resonance imaging study," *The Open Neuroimaging Journal*, vol. 3, pp. 31–47, 2009.

[35] K. L. Narr, R. M. Bilder, A. W. Toga et al., "Mapping cortical thickness and gray matter concentration in first episode schizophrenia," *Cerebral Cortex*, vol. 15, no. 6, pp. 708–719, 2005.

[36] J. Nierenberg, D. F. Salisbury, J. J. Levitt, E. A. David, R. W. McCarley, and M. E. Shenton, "Reduced left angular gyrus volume in first-episode schizophrenia," *American Journal of Psychiatry*, vol. 162, no. 8, pp. 1539–1541, 2005.

[37] M. Niznikiewicz, R. Donnino, R. W. McCarley et al., "Abnormal angular gyrus asymmetry in schizophrenia," *American Journal of Psychiatry*, vol. 157, no. 3, pp. 428–437, 2000.

[38] L. M. Rowland, E. A. Spieker, A. Francis, P. B. Barker, W. T. Carpenter, and R. W. Buchanan, "White matter alterations in deficit schizophrenia," *Neuropsychopharmacology*, vol. 34, no. 6, pp. 1514–1522, 2009.

[39] C. C. Schultz, K. Koch, G. Wagner et al., "Reduced cortical thickness in first episode schizophrenia," *Schizophrenia Research*, vol. 116, no. 2-3, pp. 204–209, 2010.
[40] D. Sun, G. W. Stuart, S. J. Wood et al., "Progressive frontal lobe reduction in first episode psychosis," *Schizophrenia Research*, vol. 60, p. 208, 2003.
[41] D.-Q. Sun, *Longitudinal brain changes in early psychosis: a magnetic resonance imaging study*, Ph.D. dissertation, University of Melbourne, 2005.
[42] P. M. Thompson, C. Vidal, J. N. Giedd et al., "Mapping adolescent brain change reveals dynamic wave of accelerated gray matter loss in very early-onset schizophrenia," *Proceedings of the National Academy of Sciences of the United States of America*, vol. 98, no. 20, pp. 11650–11655, 2001.
[43] T. J. Whitford, T. F. D. Farrow, L. Gomes, J. Brennan, A. W. F. Harris, and L. M. Williams, "Grey matter deficits and symptom profile in first episode schizophrenia," *Psychiatry Research*, vol. 139, no. 3, pp. 229–238, 2005.
[44] T. J. Whitford, S. M. Grieve, T. F. D. Farrow et al., "Progressive grey matter atrophy over the first 2-3 years of illness in first-episode schizophrenia: a tensor-based morphometry study," *NeuroImage*, vol. 32, no. 2, pp. 511–519, 2006.
[45] S. Y. Zhou, M. Suzuki, T. Takahashi et al., "Parietal lobe volume deficits in schizophrenia spectrum disorders," *Schizophrenia Research*, vol. 89, no. 1-3, pp. 35–48, 2007.
[46] E. Arce, D. S. Leland, D. A. Miller, A. N. Simmons, K. C. Winternheimer, and M. P. Paulus, "Individuals with schizophrenia present hypo- and hyperactivation during implicit cueing in an inhibitory task," *NeuroImage*, vol. 32, no. 2, pp. 704–713, 2006.
[47] D. F. Braus, W. Weber-Fahr, H. Tost, M. Ruf, and F. A. Henn, "Sensory information processing in neuroleptic-naive first-episode schizophrenic patients: a functional magnetic resonance imaging study," *Archives of General Psychiatry*, vol. 59, no. 8, pp. 696–701, 2002.
[48] M. R. Broome, P. Matthiasson, P. Fusar-Poli et al., "Neural correlates of executive function and working memory in the 'at-risk mental state'," *British Journal of Psychiatry*, vol. 194, no. 1, pp. 25–33, 2009.
[49] N. Franck, D. S. O'Leary, M. Flaum, R. D. Hichwa, and N. C. Andreasen, "Cerebral blood flow changes associated with Schneiderian first-rank symptoms in Schizophrenia," *Journal of Neuropsychiatry and Clinical Neurosciences*, vol. 14, no. 3, pp. 277–282, 2002.
[50] I. Henseler, P. Falkai, and O. Gruber, "Disturbed functional connectivity within brain networks subserving domain-specific subcomponents of working memory in schizophrenia: relation to performance and clinical symptoms," *Journal of Psychiatric Research*, vol. 44, no. 6, pp. 364–372, 2010.
[51] K. Hugdahl, B. R. Rund, A. Lund et al., "Brain activation measured with fMRI during a mental arithmetic task in Schizophrenia and major depression," *American Journal of Psychiatry*, vol. 161, no. 2, pp. 286–293, 2004.
[52] S. K. Keedy, C. L. Ebens, M. S. Keshavan, and J. A. Sweeney, "Functional magnetic resonance imaging studies of eye movements in first episode schizophrenia: smooth pur-suit, visually guided saccades and the oculomotor delayed response task," *Psychiatry Research*, vol. 146, no. 3, pp. 199–211, 2006.
[53] M. S. Keshavan, V. A. Diwadkar, S. M. Spencer, K. A. Harenski, B. Luna, and J. A. Sweeney, "A preliminary functional magnetic resonance imaging study in offspring of schizophrenic parents," *Progress in Neuro-Psychopharmacology and Biological Psychiatry*, vol. 26, no. 6, pp. 1143–1149, 2002.
[54] J. J. Kim, J. S. Kwon, J. P. Hae et al., "Functional disconnection between the prefrontal and parietal cortices during working memory processing in schizophrenia: a [15(O)] H2O PET study," *American Journal of Psychiatry*, vol. 160, no. 5, pp. 919–923, 2003.
[55] D. Öngür, T. J. Cullen, D. H. Wolf et al., "The neural basis of relational memory deficits in schizophrenia," *Archives of General Psychiatry*, vol. 63, no. 4, pp. 356–365, 2006.
[56] N. Ojeda, F. Ortuno, J. Arbizu et al., "Functional neuroanatomy of sustained attention in schizophrenia: contribution of parietal cortices," *Human Brain Mapping*, vol. 17, pp. 116–130, 2002.
[57] M. P. Paulus, L. Frank, G. G. Brown, and D. L. Braff, "Schizophrenia subjects show intact success-related neural activation but impaired uncertainty processing during decision-making," *Neuropsychopharmacology*, vol. 28, no. 4, pp. 795–806, 2003.
[58] J. Quintana, T. Wong, E. Ortiz-Portillo et al., "Prefrontal-posterior parietal networks in schizophrenia: primary dysfunctions and secondary compensations," *Biological Psychiatry*, vol. 53, no. 1, pp. 12–24, 2003.
[59] J. H. Sanz, K. H. Karlsgodt, C. E. Bearden et al., "Symptomatic and functional correlates of regional brain physiology during working memory processing in patients with recent onset schizophrenia," *Psychiatry Research*, vol. 173, no. 3, pp. 177–182, 2009.
[60] F. Schneider, U. Habel, M. Reske et al., "Neural correlates of working memory dysfunction in first-episode schizophrenia patients: an fMRI multi-center study," *Schizophrenia Research*, vol. 89, no. 1-3, pp. 198–210, 2007.
[61] J. A. Sweeney, T. Li, Q. Gong et al., "Association of cerebral deficits with clinical symptoms in antipsychotic-naive first-episode schizophrenia: an optimized voxel-based morphometry and resting state functional connectivity study," *American Journal of Psychiatry*, vol. 166, no. 2, pp. 196–205, 2009.
[62] H. W. Thermenos, J. M. Goldstein, S. L. Buka et al., "The effect of working memory performance on functional MRI in schizophrenia," *Schizophrenia Research*, vol. 74, no. 2-3, pp. 179–194, 2005.
[63] H. C. Whalley, E. Simonotto, W. Moorhead et al., "Functional imaging as a predictor of schizophrenia," *Biological Psychiatry*, vol. 60, no. 5, pp. 454–462, 2006.
[64] H. C. Whalley, E. Simonotto, S. Flett et al., "fMRI correlates of state and trait effects in subjects at genetically enhanced risk of schizophrenia," *Brain*, vol. 127, no. 3, pp. 478–490, 2004.
[65] G. Berlucchi and S. Aglioti, "The body in the brain: neural bases of corporeal awareness," *Trends in Neurosciences*, vol. 20, no. 12, pp. 560–564, 1997.
[66] J. W. Cooney and M. S. Gazzaniga, "Neurological disorders and the structure of human consciousness," *Trends in Cognitive Sciences*, vol. 7, no. 4, pp. 161–165, 2003.
[67] V. S. Ramachandran, D. Rogers-Ramachandran, and S. Cobb, "Touching the phantom limb," *Nature*, vol. 377, no. 6549, pp. 489–490, 1995.
[68] E. Kraepelin, *Dementia Praecox*, Churchill Livingston, New York, NY, USA, 1919.
[69] X. F. Amador and J. M. Gorman, "Psychopathologic domains and insight in schizophrenia," *Psychiatric Clinics of North America*, vol. 21, no. 1, pp. 27–42, 1998.
[70] S. Sevy, K. Nathanson, H. Visweswaraiah, and X. Amador, "The relationship between insight and symptoms in schizophrenia," *Comprehensive Psychiatry*, vol. 45, no. 1, pp. 16–19, 2004.

[71] L. Pia and M. Tamietto, "Unawareness in schizophrenia: neuropsychological and neuroanatomical findings," *Psychiatry and Clinical Neurosciences*, vol. 60, no. 5, pp. 531–537, 2006.
[72] M. U. Shad, S. Muddasani, K. Prasad, J. A. Sweeney, and M. S. Keshavan, "Insight and prefrontal cortex in first-episode Schizophrenia," *NeuroImage*, vol. 22, no. 3, pp. 1315–1320, 2004.
[73] M. A. Kikkert, G. M. Ribbers, and P. J. Koudstaal, "Alien hand syndrome in stroke: a report of 2 cases and review of the literature," *Archives of Physical Medicine and Rehabilitation*, vol. 87, no. 5, pp. 728–732, 2006.
[74] L. J. Buxbaum, S. H. Johnson-Frey, and M. Bartlett-Williams, "Deficient internal models for planning hand-object interactions in apraxia," *Neuropsychologia*, vol. 43, no. 6, pp. 917–929, 2005.
[75] P. A. MacDonald and T. Paus, "The role of parietal cortex in awareness of self-generated movements: a transcranial magnetic stimulation study," *Cerebral Cortex*, vol. 13, no. 9, pp. 962–967, 2003.
[76] J. Danckert, M. Saoud, and P. Maruff, "Attention, motor control and motor imagery in schizophrenia: implications for the role of the parietal cortex," *Schizophrenia Research*, vol. 70, no. 2-3, pp. 241–261, 2004.
[77] P. Maruff, P. Wilson, and J. Currie, "Abnormalities of motor imagery associated with somatic passivity phenomena in schizophrenia," *Schizophrenia Research*, vol. 60, no. 2-3, pp. 229–238, 2003.
[78] M. I. Posner, J. A. Walker, F. J. Friedrich, and R. D. Rafal, "Effects of parietal injury on covert orienting of attention," *Journal of Neuroscience*, vol. 4, no. 7, pp. 1863–1874, 1984.
[79] S. Jazbec, C. Pantelis, T. Robbins, T. Weickert, D. R. Weinberger, and T. E. Goldberg, "Intra-dimensional/extra-dimensional set-shifting performance in schizophrenia: impact of distractors," *Schizophrenia Research*, vol. 89, no. 1-3, pp. 339–349, 2007.
[80] G. Vallar, "Extrapersonal visual unilateral spatial neglect and its neuroanatomy," *NeuroImage*, vol. 14, no. 1, pp. S52–S58, 2001.
[81] S. A. Harvey, E. Nelson, J. W. Haller, and T. S. Early, "Lateralization attentional abnormality in schizophrenia is correlated with severity of symptoms," *Biological Psychiatry*, vol. 33, no. 2, pp. 93–99, 1993.
[82] C. Cavézian, Y. Rossetti, J. Danckert, T. d'Amato, J. Dalery, and M. Saoud, "Exaggerated leftward bias in the mental number line of patients with schizophrenia," *Brain and Cognition*, vol. 63, no. 1, pp. 85–90, 2007.
[83] C. Cavézian, J. Danckert, J. Lerond, J. Daléry, T. d'Amato, and M. Saoud, "Visual-perceptual abilities in healthy controls, depressed patients, and schizophrenia patients," *Brain and Cognition*, vol. 64, no. 3, pp. 257–264, 2007.
[84] C. Cavezian, C. Striemer, M. Saoud, Y. Rossetti, and J. Danckert, "Schizophrenia and the neglect syndrome: parietal contributions to cognitive dysfunction in schizophrenia," *Current Psychiatry Reviews*, vol. 2, no. 4, pp. 439–451, 2006.
[85] V. Salanova, F. Andermann, T. Rasmussen, A. Olivier, and L. F. Quesney, "Parietal lobe epilepsy. Clinical manifestations and outcome in 82 patients treated surgically between 1929 and 1988," *Brain*, vol. 118, no. 3, pp. 607–627, 1995.
[86] L. Marsh, E. V. Sullivan, M. Morrell, K. O. Lim, and A. Pfefferbaum, "Structural brain abnormalities in patients with schizophrenia, epilepsy, and epilepsy with chronic interictal psychosis," *Psychiatry Research*, vol. 108, no. 1, pp. 1–15, 2001.
[87] N. Barnea-Goraly, V. Menon, B. Krasnow, A. Ko, A. Reiss, and S. Eliez, "Investigation of white matter structure in velocardiofacial syndrome: a diffusion tensor imaging study," *American Journal of Psychiatry*, vol. 160, no. 10, pp. 1863–1869, 2003.
[88] J. Burn and J. Goodship, "Developmental genetics of the heart," *Current Opinion in Genetics and Development*, vol. 6, no. 3, pp. 322–325, 1996.
[89] C. S. Kogan, A. Bertone, K. Cornish et al., "Integrative cortical dysfunction and pervasive motion perception deficit in fragile X syndrome," *Neurology*, vol. 63, no. 9, pp. 1634–1639, 2004.
[90] G. Turner, T. Webb, S. Wake, and H. Robinson, "Prevalence of fragile X syndrome," *American Journal of Medical Genetics*, vol. 64, no. 1, pp. 196–197, 1996.
[91] S. M. Rivera, V. Menon, C. D. White, B. Glaser, and A. L. Reiss, "Functional brain activation during arithmetic processing in females with fragile X syndrome is related to FMRI protein expression," *Human Brain Mapping*, vol. 16, no. 4, pp. 206–218, 2002.
[92] B. Childs and C. R. Scriver, "Age at onset and causes of disease," *Perspectives in Biology and Medicine*, vol. 29, no. 3, pp. 437–460, 1986.
[93] R. Nicolson and J. L. Rapoport, "Childhood-onset schizophrenia: rare but worth studying," *Biological Psychiatry*, vol. 46, no. 10, pp. 1418–1428, 1999.
[94] A. W. Toga, P. M. Thompson, and E. R. Sowell, "Mapping brain maturation," *Trends in Neurosciences*, vol. 29, no. 3, pp. 148–159, 2006.
[95] N. Gogtay, A. Sporn, L. S. Clasen et al., "Structural brain MRI abnormalities in healthy siblings of patients with childhood-onset schizophrenia," *American Journal of Psychiatry*, vol. 160, no. 3, pp. 569–571, 2003.
[96] C. Beaulieu, "The basis of anisotropic water diffusion in the nervous system—a technical review," *NMR in Biomedicine*, vol. 15, no. 7-8, pp. 435–455, 2002.
[97] I. Feinberg, "Schizophrenia: caused by a fault in programmed synaptic elimination during adolescence?" *Journal of Psychiatric Research*, vol. 17, no. 4, pp. 319–334, 1982.
[98] C. Pantelis, M. Yücel, S. J. Wood, P. D. McGorry, and D. Velakoulis, "Early and late neurodevelopmental disturbances in schizophrenia and their functional consequences," *Australian and New Zealand Journal of Psychiatry*, vol. 37, no. 4, pp. 399–406, 2003.
[99] S. J. Borgwardt, P. K. McGuire, J. Aston et al., "Reductions in frontal, temporal and parietal volume associated with the onset of psychosis," *Schizophrenia Research*, vol. 106, no. 2-3, pp. 108–114, 2008.
[100] C. Pantelis, M. Yücel, S. J. Wood et al., "Structural brain imaging evidence for multiple pathological processes at different stages of brain development in schizophrenia," *Schizophrenia Bulletin*, vol. 31, no. 3, pp. 672–696, 2005.
[101] S. J. Borgwardt, M. M. Picchioni, U. Ettinger, T. Toulopoulou, R. Murray, and P. K. McGuire, "Regional gray matter volume in monozygotic twins concordant and discordant for schizophrenia," *Biological Psychiatry*, vol. 67, no. 10, pp. 956–964, 2010.
[102] T. D. Cannon, M. O. Huttunen, J. Lonnqvist et al., "The inheritance of neuropsychological dysfunction in twins discordant for schizophrenia," *American Journal of Human Genetics*, vol. 67, no. 2, pp. 369–382, 2000.
[103] D. R. Weinberger, "Prefrontal function in schizophrenia: confounds and controversies," *Philosophical Transactions of the Royal Society B*, vol. 351, no. 1346, pp. 1495–1503, 1996.

[104] V. Menon, R. T. Anagnoson, D. H. Mathalon, G. H. Glover, and A. Pfefferbaum, "Functional neuroanatomy of auditory working memory in schizophrenia: relation to positive and negative symptoms," *NeuroImage*, vol. 13, no. 3, pp. 433–446, 2001.

[105] A. P. Weiss, C. B. Ellis, J. L. Roffman et al., "Aberrant fronto-parietal function during recognition memory in schizophrenia: a multimodal neuroimaging investigation," *Journal of Neuroscience*, vol. 29, no. 36, pp. 11347–11359, 2009.

[106] G. D. Pearlson, R. G. Petty, C. A. Ross, and A. Y. Tien, "Schizophrenia: a disease of heteromodal association cortex?" *Neuropsychopharmacology*, vol. 14, no. 1, pp. 1–17, 1996.

[107] B. J. Baig, H. C. Whalley, J. Hall et al., "Functional magnetic resonance imaging of BDNF val66met polymorphism in unmedicated subjects at high genetic risk of schizophrenia performing a verbal memory task," *Psychiatry Research*, vol. 183, no. 3, pp. 195–201, 2010.

[108] J. M. Segall, J. A. Turner, T. G. M. Van Erp et al., "Voxel-based morphometric multisite collaborative study on schizophrenia," *Schizophrenia Bulletin*, vol. 35, no. 1, pp. 82–95, 2009.

[109] P. D. McGorry, I. B. Hickie, A. R. Yung, C. Pantelis, and H. J. Jackson, "Clinical staging of psychiatric disorders: a heuristic framework for choosing earlier, safer and more effective interventions," *Australian and New Zealand Journal of Psychiatry*, vol. 40, no. 8, pp. 616–622, 2006.

[110] H. Sakata, M. Taira, M. Kusunoki, A. Murata, and Y. Tanaka, "The TINS lecture: the parietal association cortex in depth perception and visual control of hand action," *Trends in Neurosciences*, vol. 20, no. 8, pp. 350–357, 1997.

[111] A. K. Malla, M. Bodnar, R. Joober, and M. Lepage, "Duration of untreated psychosis is associated with orbital-frontal grey matter volume reductions in first episode psychosis," *Schizophrenia Research*, vol. 125, no. 1, pp. 13–20, 2011.

[112] W. Y. Chan, M. Y. Chia, G. L. Yang et al., "Duration of illness, regional brain morphology and neurocognitive correlates in schizophrenia," *Annals of the Academy of Medicine Singapore*, vol. 38, no. 5, pp. 388–395, 2009.

8

Long-Acting Injectable Antipsychotics for First-Episode Schizophrenia: The Pros and Cons

Borah Kim,[1] Sang-Hyuk Lee,[1] Yen Kuang Yang,[2] Jong-Il Park,[3] and Young-Chul Chung[3,4]

[1] *Department of Psychiatry, CHA Bundang Medical Center, CHA University, 59 Yatap-ro, Bundang-gu, Seongnam-si 463-712, Gyeonggi-do, Republic of Korea*
[2] *Department of Psychiatry, National Cheng Kung University Hospital, College of Medicine, National Cheng Kung University, 138 Sheng Li Road, Tainan 70428, Taiwan*
[3] *Department of Psychiatry, Chonbuk National University Medical School, 567 Baekje-daero, Deokjin-gu, Jeonju-si 561-756, Jeollabuk-do, Republic of Korea*
[4] *Research Institute of Clinical Medicine of Chonbuk National University, Biomedical Research Institute of Chonbuk National University Hospital, 20 Geonjiro, Deokjin-gu, Jeonju-si 561-712, Jeollabuk-do, Republic of Korea*

Correspondence should be addressed to Young-Chul Chung, chungyc@jbnu.ac.kr

Academic Editor: Eduard Parellada

Clinical and psychosocial deterioration associated with schizophrenia occurs within the first few years following the onset of the illness. Therefore, to improve the long-term prognosis, it is important to provide schizophrenia patients with intensive treatment following their first episode. Relapse is highly associated with partial medication adherence or nonadherence in patients with first-episode schizophrenia. Recent studies suggest that long-acting injectable (LAI) antipsychotics compared with oral antipsychotics are more effective for medication adherence and relapse prevention. Moreover, some clinical guidelines for the treatment of schizophrenia suggested that LAI antipsychotics should be considered when patients are nonadherent "at any stage." Decreased compliance is a common cause of relapse during the initial stages of the disease. Therefore, LAI antipsychotics should be highly considered when treating patients with first-episode schizophrenia. In the present paper, clinical trial data and current guidelines on the use of LAI antipsychotics for first-episode schizophrenia are discussed as well as the pros and cons of this treatment option.

1. Introduction

Schizophrenia is a chronic disorder characterized by periods of illness alternating with periods of full or partial remission. Previous studies [1, 2] suggest that schizophrenia is a neurodegenerative disease associated with frequent relapses. This alternating nature of the illness causes neurotoxicity in the brain, thereby resulting in structural abnormalities, including ventricular enlargement and cortical atrophy. Recent evidence further suggests that progressive structural changes in the brain occur within the initial years following a diagnosis [3–5]. Moreover, with each subsequent relapse after the first episode, it usually takes longer time to reach remission [6]. The primary clinical and psychosocial deterioration associated with schizophrenia occurs within the first 5 years following the onset of the illness, called the critical period [7, 8]. Therefore, it is important to provide intensive biopsychosocial interventions during the critical period in an effort to improve the long-term prognosis.

The primary goal of treatment during the critical period is to prevent a subsequent relapse and to restore socio-occupational functioning to the premorbid level. The relapse rate in patients with first-episode schizophrenia is relatively low during the first year of the illness but substantially rises to rates of 53.7% and 74%–81.9% after 2 and 5 years, respectively [9, 10]. The most common cause of relapse in patients with schizophrenia is a lack of adherence to oral medication [11, 12]. The discontinuation of antipsychotics in patients with first-episode schizophrenia or schizoaffective disorder increases the risk of relapse by approximately five times [9]. The rate of medication discontinuation in individuals with first-episode psychosis ranges from 26% [13] to 44% [14]

during the first year. Coldham et al. [15] reported a 59% rate of poor adherence (39% nonadherent and 20% inadequately adherent) within the year after the first episode. None of the interventions currently used to improve adherence have been completely reliable in the treatment of schizophrenia. Long-acting injectable (LAI) antipsychotics, however, may improve medication adherence and possibly reduce relapse in patients with schizophrenia [16]. The Texas Medication Algorithm Project Antipsychotic Algorithm for schizophrenia [17] recommended that clinicians should assess contributing factors and consider LAI antipsychotic preparations in patients who are inadequately adherent at any stage. Previous studies have suggested that LAI antipsychotics may be more effective for maintaining medication adherence [18] and preventing relapse [19] in first-episode schizophrenia compared with oral antipsychotics. Clinically, however, the majority of psychiatrists use LAI antipsychotics very conservatively [20, 21]. Moreover, very few psychiatrists offer LAI antipsychotics after a patient's first psychotic episode [22]. Recently, Osborne et al. (2012) reported that society associates a higher utility with increasing time between injections, with 4-weekly and 3-monthly administration of an antipsychotic LAI representing an advance over 2-weekly administration in the health-related quality of life (HRQoL) of patients with schizophrenia [23]. They discussed that participants from the general population preferred less frequent injections given the psychological stress and pain associated with injections as well as the burden related to the requirement of travel to outpatient clinics for their administration. In this regard, currently available option of LAI antipsychotic with one month injection interval would add substantial value to the improvement of quality of life in patients with schizophrenia and their family members. Optimal therapeutic outcomes associated with first-episode psychosis are often compromised by early treatment discontinuation and poor treatment adherence; therefore, LAI antipsychotics should be more actively considered with first-episode schizophrenia.

The present paper reviews the relevant literature including clinical drug trials, survey studies, and clinical guidelines on the use of LAI antipsychotics in patients with first-episode or recent-onset schizophrenia. Moreover, the pros and cons of LAI antipsychotic used with first-episode schizophrenia are discussed.

2. Overview of Clinical Studies on the Effectiveness of Long-Acting Injectable Risperidone Treatment for First-Episode or Recent-Onset Schizophrenia (Table 1)

In a study by Parellada et al. [24], 382 patients received long-acting injectable risperidone (RLAI) treatment during the early stages of their disease (i.e., within 3 years of diagnosis). The study, conducted in Europe, evaluated the efficacy and safety of RLAI. It was an open-label, nonrandomized, and single-arm, multicenter study that consisted of a 6-month treatment period. Significant improvements in total Positive and Negative Syndrome Scale (PANSS) scores were noted at the first visit and continued to improve through the end of the study. At the end of the study, 148 patients (40%) displayed an improvement in total PANSS and subscale scores. Functioning is also improved from baseline to endpoint, with a mean Global Assessment of Functioning (GAF) score of 57.6 (±6.5) at baseline and a mean GAF score of 65.3 (±18.3) at the end of the study. Adverse events were reported by 263 patients (69%), including extrapyramidal symptoms. These symptoms, however, improved significantly over the 6-month treatment period. Parellada [25] also reported that individuals treated with RLAI, including patients with first-episode schizophrenia, demonstrated improvement in symptom severity and compliance as well as a reduction in the rate of relapse and a favorable tolerability profile.

According to a study that compared RLAI and oral risperidone for the treatment of first-episode schizophrenia [19], significant improvements in PANSS, GAF, and Clinical Global Impression (CGI) were noted in the RLAI group compared with the oral risperidone group. No significant differences in extrapyramidal symptoms or frequency of prolactin-related adverse effects were noted in either group. Moreover, medication adherence was higher, and the relapse rates at 1 and 2 years were significantly lower in the RLAI group. The oral risperidone group showed significantly greater nonadherence. In the study, the amount of time to nonadherence predicted the relapse in patients with first-episode schizophrenia. The authors proposed that RLAI may be effective in preventing relapse through maintaining medication adherence. The authors [30] also emphasized that psychosocial interventions for relapse prevention may be effective for maintaining medication compliance in patients with schizophrenia who receive RLAI.

A single-site open-label study of 50 patients with first-episode schizophrenia who were treated with RLAI [26] found that 32 patients (64%) achieved remission. Of the 32 patients, 31 (97%) maintained remission throughout the study. The remission and nonremission groups were compared based on clinical, functional, and quality-of-life outcome measures. The remission group showed significantly greater improvements on the CGI-Severity (CGI-S) scale and PANSS total score and also displayed improvements in extrapyramidal symptoms. Remission patients received lower doses of RLAI and showed greater improvement in social functioning compared with the nonremission group in the study. Multivariate level analyses showed that the chance of remission increased in females. Early symptom improvement was also significantly associated with remission. Moreover, less decline in the PANSS score was associated with a reduced likelihood of remission. The remission rate in this study compared favorably with that reported in previously published studies could be benefit of assured antipsychotic delivery and better adherence of treatment of RLAI. In another study conducted at the same site [26], compared with patients treated with oral risperidone or haloperidol, RLAI-treated patients had significantly fewer all-cause discontinuations (26% versus 70% at 24 months), greater symptom reduction according to PANSS total score (−39.7 versus −25.7), higher remission rates (64% versus 40%), lower relapse rates (9.3% versus 42%), and lower extrapyramidal symptoms [27].

Table 1: Overview of clinical studies on the effectiveness of long-acting injectable antipsychotics for the treatment of first-episode or recent-onset schizophrenia.

Study	No. of patients (female/male)	No. of previous episodes	Duration of illness	Study duration	Design	Dosage	Reduction of total PANSS (%)	Reduction of CGI-S (%)	Functional improvement (%)	Tolerability	Adherence	Long-term outcome
Parellada et al. [24]	382 (117/265)	ns	1.5 (1.1) yr	6 mo	Open, 1-arm, mc	25–50 mg	18.3%	ns	GAF 13.4%	ESRS 53.8% ↓ PRL-related 0.3% wt gain 4%	ns	ns
Kim et al. [19]	RLAI: 22 (14/8) Oral: 28 (17/11)	1	1.5 (1.5) yr	2 yr	Open, C	25–50 mg	RLAI: 10.0% Oral: 2.0%	RLAI: 10.0 Oral: 2.5	GAF RLAI: 26.9% Oral: 0.5%	ns	RLAI: GA (>70%) 68% Oral: GA 32%	2-yr relapse RLAI: 23% Oral: 75%
Emsley et al. [26]	50 (18/32)	1	≤1 yr	2 yr	Open, 1-arm	25–50 mg	Remission: 45.0% No remission: 29.7%	Remission: 73.1% No remission: 34.4%	SOFAS remission: 85.2% No remission: 43.2%	ESRS 53.3% ↓ in remission; 55.0% ↑ in no remission	ns	2-yr remission 62%
Emsley et al. [27]	RLAI: 50 (18/32) Oral: 47 (20/27)	≤2 adm	≤ 1yr	2 yr	Post hoc comparison RLAI: Open, 1-arm Oral: R, C (ris versus hal)	25–50 mg	RLAI: 44.0% Oral: 28.8%	ns	ns	Total maximum changes of *ESRS* RLAI: 1.40 (2.60) Oral: ris 5.61 (5.22) hal 9.04 (6.21)	ns	2-yr remission RLAI: 64.0% Oral: 40.4%
Weiden et al. [18]	RLAI: 19 Oral: 11	1	≤16 wk of lifetime AP exposure	12 wk	Open, R, C	25–37.5 mg	ns	ns	ns	ns	RLAI: 89% Oral: 59%	ns
Napryeyenko et al. [28]	294 (116/178)	2.4 (0.7)	≤2 yr	26 wk	Open, 1-arm, mc	25–50 mg	18.6%	20.5%	GAF 16.9%	EPS 5.6% PRL-related 4.3% wt gain 3.0%	NC, $n = 3$	1-yr remission 59.5%
Dubois et al. [29]	105 (79/26)	<4	3.0 (3.92) yr	12 mo	Open, 1-arm, mc	25–50 mg	ns	43.4%	GAF 71.1%	EPS 3.8% PRL-related 9.5% wt gain 18.1%	>80%	1-yr remission 34.1%

PANSS: Positive and Negative Syndrome scale; CGI-S: Clinical Global Impression-Severity scale; GAF: Global Assessment of Functioning; SOFAS: Social Occupational Functioning Assessment scale; ESRS: Extrapyramidal Symptom Rating scale. adm: hospital admissions for psychosis; AP: antipsychotics; C: controlled study; EPS: extrapyramidal symptoms; GA: good adherence (>70%) group; hal: haloperidol; mc: multicenter; mo: month; NC: noncompliance; ns: not specified; open: open-label; oral: oral risperidone; PRL: prolactin; pts: patients; R: randomized; ris: risperidone; RLAI: long-acting injectable risperidone; wk: week; wt: weight; yr: year; 1-arm: single arm.

A randomized controlled trial reported on acceptance and initial adherence outcomes with RLAI treatment in patients with first-episode schizophrenia [18]. According to the results, 73% of subjects (19 out of 26) randomly assigned to receive RLAI accepted. Individuals who took RLAI were significantly more likely to remain adherent at 12 weeks compared with patients treated with oral antipsychotics. The authors suggested that better adherence was achieved in patients who received RLAI through two possible explanations. One is that starting treatment with RLAI might have direct adherence benefits in preventing or delaying nonadherence in some individuals. The other one is that refusal of the RLAI recommendation is a sign that the patient plans to stop oral medication in the very near future, which means that the more important thing is not so much the RLAI itself but the will to stay on treatment with any antipsychotics. The researchers anticipated that some patients would refuse the RLAI recommendation; however, they found that about 73% of subjects accepted the recommendation for treatment with RLAI. This suggests the feasibility and acceptability of LAI antipsychotics as a treatment strategy during the early stages of schizophrenia.

According to an open-label noncomparative study of recent-onset schizophrenia [28], patients showed good progress as indicated by symptom reduction, improved functional outcomes, and improved health-related quality of life. Rabinowitz et al. [31] also demonstrated that improved premorbid functioning in patients with schizophrenia is predictive of increased treatment response with RLAI as measured by clinical rating scales of symptoms and functioning, health care-related quality of life, and remission.

A multicenter, nonintervention, observational study on the clinical effectiveness of RLAI administration was published in 2011 [29]. Treatment with RLAI for 12 months during the early stages of schizophrenia was associated with significant improvements in clinical and functional outcomes in patients. This investigation suggested the effectiveness of RLAI for treatment of patients early in the course of schizophrenia in a similar vein to previous studies [19, 26] with the result from relatively large subjects (n = 105).

A recent study by Bartzokis et al. [32] compared RLAI and oral risperidone treatment in subjects with first-episode schizophrenia. The study focused on changes in frontal lobe myelination and cognitive functioning. White matter (WM) volume remained stable in the RLAI group and decreased significantly in the oral risperidone group, resulting in a significant difference on the effects of treatment. RLAI seems to promote myelination and stabilizes frontal lobe WM volume compared with oral risperidone. Moreover, the changes in frontal lobe WM volume were positively associated with higher-order executive functioning, working memory, and mental flexibility. No significant volume changes were noted in the frontal lobe. The authors suggested that the changes in WM and gray matter (GM) represent a myelination-driven shift of the GM/WM boundary into or out of the cortex. The myelination trajectory was significantly quadratic (inverted U) and peaked at 1 year of antipsychotic treatment. This was followed by a premature decline compared with healthy subjects who do not decline until after the fifth decade of life. The nonsignificant increase in WM volume observed with RLAI suggests that the trajectory defined by oral antipsychotic treatment may be modifiable with RLAI. Therefore, the consistent medication levels that are achieved with RLAI may result in a higher WM volume, which may subsequently impact cognitive performance.

Although favorable results of LAI antipsychotics have been reported for patients with first-episode or recent-onset schizophrenia, the effectiveness of LAI treatment for patients with chronic schizophrenia remains controversial. A meta-analysis of depot antipsychotics was conducted in 2001 [33]. This report suggested that depot antipsychotics were statistically better for global improvements compared with oral antipsychotics. However, relapse, attrition, and adverse effects were not significantly different. In addition, a recent long-term randomized controlled trial that included patients with unstable schizophrenia [34] demonstrated that RLAI was not superior to oral treatment in terms of duration of adherence, time to rehospitalization, clinical symptoms, or improvement in functional outcome. Moreover, this study reported that RLAI treatment was associated with more local injectionsite and extrapyramidal adverse effects. On the other hand, the recent meta-analysis [35] comparing LAI with oral antipsychotics showed that a reduced risk for relapse was associated with LAI over oral antipsychotics. To clarify clinical issue related to the use of LAI antipsychotics in first-episode or recent-onset schizophrenia, further studies, especially randomized controlled trials, are warranted especially with regard to the effectiveness on relapse or rehospitalization.

3. The Pros and Cons of LAI Antipsychotics (Table 2)

The general attitude of psychiatrists toward depot antipsychotics is negative. Depot antipsychotics are considered old-fashioned, stigmatized, and less acceptable to patients. Many psychiatrists stated that first-generation depots are avoided because of the threat of extrapyramidal side effects, whereas second-generation LAI drugs are associated with high treatment costs [20]. It is of interest to see two opposing opinions about the use of LAI drugs in first episode of psychosis in the recent surveys. Over half of the psychiatrists in the UK who participated in a survey agreed that LAI drugs can be used in patients with first-episode psychosis [21]. In contrast, Heres et al. [20] reported that the majority of psychiatrists (64–71%) applied the "no depot in first-episode psychosis" rule. They also recently investigated factors associated with psychiatrist's negative attitude toward offering depot treatment to first-episode patients and found that three factors, limited availability of different second-generation antipsychotic depot drugs, the frequent rejection of the depot offer by the patients, and the patients' skepticism based on the lack in experience of a relapse, were of marked influence [36]. In a study conducted in Switzerland, fewer than 10% of psychiatrists offered depot treatments in response to the first psychotic episode [22]. Given that psychiatrists are relatively conservative in offering

TABLE 2: The pros and the cons of using long-acting injectable (LAI) antipsychotics for the treatment of first-episode schizophrenia.

Pros	Cons
High relapse caused by poor compliance could be prevented	Because of uncertainty of diagnosis for those in first-episode psychosis, prescribing LAI drugs may be stigmatizing and may hamper therapeutic relationships
Some high-functioning individuals may prefer depot formulations	Discourage patient's motive to recover because of the general perception that an injectable treatment means a more severe condition with respect to the illness
Favorable side effect profile due to low variation in the peak and trough levels would have positive effects on drug compliance	For those with first-episode schizophrenia showing a positive outcome, the goal of treatment is to gradually reduce the dosage of antipsychotics, which does not fit the traditional goals of LAI drugs
Best time to prescribe LAI drugs may be just before discharge	It is difficult to adjust the dosage of LAI drugs quickly in response to side effects; therefore, LAI treatment may negatively affect subsequent treatment compliance during the critical period

information about depot antipsychotics [22] and that some patients feel positively toward treatment with depot medication [37, 38], more patients with first-episode psychosis may accept LAI medication if psychiatrists provided them with adequate information. The best rationale for using LAI antipsychotics in first episode of psychosis comes from the fact that frequent relapses occur during first few years of the illness, and there is evidence for decreased rate of relapse with LAI medication compared to oral antipsychotic drug in first-episode schizophrenia [19, 30, 39]. Another advantage may be that LAI antipsychotics can improve patient's quality-of-life overtime with more possibilities to meet friends and family, to live a more stable and independent life, outside the psychiatric hospital [40]. Patients with schizophrenia are more sensitive to adverse drug effects during the first few years of the illness [41–43]; therefore, the low incidence of adverse events caused by low variation in peak and trough levels of LAI antipsychotics may have additional benefits for pharmacological compliance during the critical period. Some people argued that the best time to prescribe LAI antipsychotics is just prior to discharge. One argument against the use of LAI antipsychotics for the treatment of first-episode psychosis may be related to the uncertainty of the diagnosis. If brief psychotic disorder, not otherwise specified (NOS) psychotic disorder, or schizophreniform disorder is suspected, the recommended duration of treatment should be much shorter, and a greater portion of patients may have a chance of recovery than in case of schizophrenia. For such cases, the patient's autonomy is even more important in the process of treatment decision. Because of negative association of injection with coercion, recommending LAI antipsychotics by treating doctors would hamper therapeutic relationship. Moreover, it would discourage patient's motive to recover because of the general perception that injection treatment option usually means severe condition of the illness. Moreover, due to the difficulty of adjusting the dose of LAI drugs quickly in response to side effects, treatment compliance may be negatively affected during the critical period. To improve the conservative attitude of psychiatrists with respect to LAI antipsychotic treatment for patients with first-episode schizophrenia, several issues must be tackled. First, the development of more accurate subjective or objective measures that predict or detect drug compliance in patients with first-episode schizophrenia should be pursued. Second, more diverse second-generation depot formulations should be available for the current clinical practice, like paliperidone palmitate, olanzapine pamoate, aripiprazole, or iloperidone depot. The development of completely different formulae, such as a patch drug containing olanzapine [44] or risperidone [45], would have wide applicability for patients with first-episode schizophrenia because one of the primary reasons why individuals reject LAI drugs is the fear of needles. Third is about using financial incentives may improve adherence to antipsychotic maintenance medication [46]. This applies not only to first-episode schizophrenia but also to multiple-episode chronic schizophrenia and raises its ethical issues [47]. In Japan, counseling and management fees have been used for depot antipsychotics since 1990 to promote the use of depot antipsychotics for schizophrenia (personal communication). It remains to be seen how financial incentives will unfold especially in relation to first-episode schizophrenia.

4. Guidelines for the Treatment of First-Episode Schizophrenia with LAI Antipsychotics

According to the American Psychiatric Association [48], LAI antipsychotic medication is recommended for patients with recurrent relapses related to partial or full nonadherence. Also, the Canadian clinical practice [49] recommends LAI formulations to reduce nonadherence in multiple-episode patients or patients with persistent positive symptoms. The International Psychopharmacology Algorithm Projects (IPAPs) schizophrenia algorithm (http://www.ipap.org/schiz/) suggested that depot antipsychotics were recommended in patients with partial or complete noncompliance. However, there was no mention of LAI for the treatment of first-episode schizophrenia. These guidelines, therefore, limit the use of LAI to patients characterized as multiple episodes or noncompliance.

However, there have been subtle changes in more recent guidelines. For example, the procedural manual by the Texas Medication Algorithm Project [17] recommends that the clinicians assess contributing factors and consider LAI antipsychotics in patients who are inadequately adherent "at any stage." It means that LAI could be used even in first-episode schizophrenia if the patients are not enough adherent to their medications. Similarly, in 2009, the National Institute for Health and Clinical Excellence (NICE) guidelines regarding schizophrenia (http://www.nice.org.uk/CG82) stated that clinicians should consider offering depot/LAI antipsychotic medications to patients with schizophrenia who would *"prefer such treatment after an acute episode and where avoiding covert nonadherence to antipsychotic medication is a clinical priority"* within the treatment plan. Kane and Garcia-Ribera [50] also mentioned that LAI can be indicated to *"any schizophrenia"* patients requiring long-term treatment, nonadherent, or having risk of relapse. They further suggested that even if patients refuse this option, it would be better to help them understand the potential advantages. On the other hand, recent guidelines from the British Association for Psychopharmacology [51] described that the place of antipsychotic depot/long-acting injections for first-episode schizophrenia remains uncertain on account of the absence of long-term data comparing LAI with oral antipsychotics after first-episode schizophrenia.

It is still true that LAI has a conservative position in treating first-episode schizophrenia according to the majority of the current guidelines. Nevertheless, considering the results from LAI studies in first-episode psychosis previously, future guidelines might be needed to update a treatment option to recommend LAI antipsychotics for any patients with schizophrenia who showed poor adherence attitude and behavior including first-episode schizophrenia.

5. Conclusions

With the availability of the different second-generation LAI antipsychotics, there are improved treatment options for schizophrenia in terms of duration of action and side effects. Psychiatrists, however, seem to conservatively use depot formulations and mostly introduce them after several episodes. The acceptability of prescribing LAI antipsychotics to patients with first-episode psychosis is currently under debate. Many clinical and technical issues should be addressed to encourage increased acceptability of LAI antipsychotics for the treatment of patients with first-episode schizophrenia. Nevertheless, given that low compliance is a frequent cause of relapse in the early course of schizophrenia, more active consideration of LAI drugs should be encouraged, and patients should be informed about the different types of medication that are available during the early stages of the illness. Further studies, especially randomized controlled trials, are urgently needed to clarify the advantages of second-generation LAI antipsychotics in patients with first-episode schizophrenia.

Disclosure

The English in this document has been checked by at least two professional editors, both are native speakers of English. For a certificate, please see http://www.textcheck.com/certificate/Wh824O.

Conflict of Interests

The authors declare that they have no conflict of interests with any commercial or other associations in connection with this paper.

References

[1] V. Molina, J. Sanz, F. Sarramea, C. Benito, and T. Palomo, "Lower prefrontal gray matter volume in schizophrenia in chronic but not in first episode schizophrenia patients," *Psychiatry Research*, vol. 131, no. 1, pp. 45–56, 2004.

[2] J. A. Lieberman, "Pathophysiologic mechanisms in the pathogenesis and clinical course of schizophrenia," *Journal of Clinical Psychiatry*, vol. 60, supplement 12, pp. 9–12, 1999.

[3] W. Cahn, H. E. Hulshoff Pol, E. B. Lems et al., "Brain volume changes in first-episode schizophrenia: a 1-year follow-up study," *Archives of General Psychiatry*, vol. 59, no. 11, pp. 1002–1010, 2002.

[4] B. C. Ho, N. C. Andreasen, P. Nopoulos, S. Arndt, V. Magnotta, and M. Flaum, "Progressive structural brain abnormalities and their relationship to clinical outcome: a longitudinal magnetic resonance imaging study early in schizophrenia," *Archives of General Psychiatry*, vol. 60, no. 6, pp. 585–594, 2003.

[5] D. Sun, G. W. Stuart, M. Jenkinson et al., "Brain surface contraction mapped in first-episode schizophrenia: a longitudinal magnetic resonance imaging study," *Molecular Psychiatry*, vol. 14, no. 10, pp. 976–986, 2009.

[6] J. A. Lieberman, J. M. Alvir, A. Koreen et al., "Psychobiologic correlates of treatment response in schizophrenia," *Neuropsychopharmacology*, vol. 14, no. 3, supplement, pp. 13S–21S, 1996.

[7] M. Birchwood, P. Todd, and C. Jackson, "Early intervention in psychosis: the critical period hypothesis," *British Journal of Psychiatry*, vol. 172, no. 33, supplement, pp. 53–59, 1998.

[8] J. A. Lieberman, D. Perkins, A. Belger et al., "The early stages of schizophrenia: speculations on pathogenesis, pathophysiology, and therapeutic approaches," *Biological Psychiatry*, vol. 50, no. 11, pp. 884–897, 2001.

[9] D. Robinson, M. G. Woerner, J. M. Alvir et al., "Predictors of relapse following response from a first episode of schizophrenia or schizoaffective disorder," *Archives of General Psychiatry*, vol. 56, no. 3, pp. 241–247, 1999.

[10] T. S. S. R. Group, "The Scottish first episode schizophrenia study VIII. Five-year follow-up: clinical and psychosocial findings," *British Journal of Psychiatry*, vol. 161, pp. 496–500, 1992.

[11] P. Thieda, S. Beard, A. Richter, and J. Kane, "An economic review of compliance with medication therapy in the treatment of schizophrenia," *Psychiatric Services*, vol. 54, no. 4, pp. 508–516, 2003.

[12] P. J. Weiden and M. Olfson, "Cost of relapse in schizophrenia," *Schizophrenia Bulletin*, vol. 21, no. 3, pp. 419–429, 1995.

[13] D. G. Robinson, M. G. Woerner, J. M. Alvir, R. M. Bilder, G. A. Hinrichsen, and J. A. Lieberman, "Predictors of medication discontinuation by patients with first-episode schizophrenia and schizoaffective disorder," *Schizophrenia Research*, vol. 57, no. 2-3, pp. 209–219, 2002.

[14] H. Verdoux, J. Lengronne, F. Liraud et al., "Medication adherence in psychosis: predictors and impact on outcome. A 2-year follow-up of first-admitted subjects," *Acta Psychiatrica Scandinavica*, vol. 102, no. 3, pp. 203–210, 2000.

[15] E. L. Coldham, J. Addington, and D. Addington, "Medication adherence of individuals with a first episode of psychosis," *Acta Psychiatrica Scandinavica*, vol. 106, no. 4, pp. 286–290, 2002.

[16] J. M. Kane, "Review of treatments that can ameliorate non-adherence in patients with schizophrenia," *Journal of Clinical Psychiatry*, vol. 67, supplement 5, pp. 9–14, 2006.

[17] T. R. Argo, M. L. Crimson, A. L. Miller et al., "The Texas Medication Algorithm Project antipsychotic algorithm for schizophrenia," The Texas Department of State Health Services, 2007.

[18] P. J. Weiden, N. R. Schooler, J. C. Weedon, A. Elmouchtari, A. Sunakawa, and S. M. Goldfinger, "A randomized controlled trial of long-acting injectable risperidone vs continuation on oral atypical antipsychotics for first-episode schizophrenia patients: initial adherence outcome," *Journal of Clinical Psychiatry*, vol. 70, no. 10, pp. 1397–1406, 2009.

[19] B. Kim, S. H. Lee, T. K. Choi et al., "Effectiveness of risperidone long-acting injection in first-episode schizophrenia: in naturalistic setting," *Progress in Neuro-Psychopharmacology and Biological Psychiatry*, vol. 32, no. 5, pp. 1231–1235, 2008.

[20] S. Heres, J. Hamann, W. Kissling, and S. Leucht, "Attitudes of psychiatrists toward antipsychotic depot medication," *Journal of Clinical Psychiatry*, vol. 67, no. 12, pp. 1948–1953, 2006.

[21] M. X. Patel, P. M. Haddad, I. B. Chaudhry, S. McLoughlin, and A. S. David, "Psychiatrists' use, knowledge and attitudes to first- and second-generation antipsychotic long-acting injections: comparisons over 5 years," *Journal of Psychopharmacology*, vol. 24, no. 10, pp. 1473–1482, 2010.

[22] M. Jaeger and W. Rossler, "Attitudes towards long-acting depot antipsychotics: a survey of patients, relatives and psychiatrists," *Psychiatry Research*, vol. 175, no. 1-2, pp. 58–62, 2010.

[23] R. H. Osborne, A. Dalton, J. Hertel, R. Schrover, and D. K. Smith, "Health-related quality of life advantage of long-acting injectable antipsychotic treatment for schizophrenia: a time trade-off study," *Health and Quality of Life Outcomes*, vol. 10, article 35, 2012.

[24] E. Parellada, R. Andrezina, V. Milanova et al., "Patients in the early phases of schizophrenia and schizoaffective disorders effectively treated with risperidone long-acting injectable," *Journal of Psychopharmacology*, vol. 19, no. 5, supplement, pp. 5–14, 2005.

[25] E. Parellada, "Long-acting injectable risperidone in the treatment of schizophrenia in special patient populations," *Psychopharmacology Bulletin*, vol. 40, no. 2, pp. 82–100, 2007.

[26] R. Emsley, P. Oosthuizen, L. Koen, D. J. H. Niehaus, R. Medori, and J. Rabinowitz, "Remission in patients with first-episode schizophrenia receiving assured antipsychotic medication: a study with risperidone long-acting injection," *International Clinical Psychopharmacology*, vol. 23, no. 6, pp. 325–331, 2008.

[27] R. Emsley, P. Oosthuizen, L. Koen, D. J. Niehaus, R. Medori, and J. Rabinowitz, "Oral versus injectable antipsychotic treatment in early psychosis: post hoc comparison of two studies," *Clinical Therapeutics*, vol. 30, no. 12, pp. 2378–2386, 2008.

[28] O. Napryeyenko, B. Burba, G. Martinez et al., "Risperidone long-acting injectable in recent-onset schizophrenia examined with clinician and patient self-report measures," *Journal of Clinical Psychopharmacology*, vol. 30, no. 2, pp. 200–202, 2010.

[29] V. Dubois, J. Megens, C. Mertens et al., "Long-acting risperidone in early-episode schizophrenia," *Acta Psychiatrica Belgica*, vol. 111, no. 1, pp. 9–21, 2011.

[30] S. H. Lee, T. K. Choi, S. Suh et al., "Effectiveness of a psychosocial intervention for relapse prevention in patients with schizophrenia receiving risperidone via long-acting injection," *Psychiatry Research*, vol. 175, no. 3, pp. 195–199, 2010.

[31] J. Rabinowitz, O. Napryeyenko, B. Burba et al., "Premorbid functioning and treatment response in recent-onset schizophrenia: prospective study with risperidone long-acting injectable," *Journal of Clinical Psychopharmacology*, vol. 31, no. 1, pp. 75–81, 2011.

[32] G. Bartzokis, P. H. Lu, C. P. Amar et al., "Long acting injection versus oral risperidone in first-episode schizophrenia: differential impact on white matter myelination trajectory," *Schizophrenia Research*, vol. 132, no. 1, pp. 35–41, 2011.

[33] C. E. Adams, M. K. Fenton, S. Quraishi, and A. S. David, "Systematic meta-review of depot antipsychotic drugs for people with schizophrenia," *British Journal of Psychiatry*, vol. 179, pp. 290–299, 2001.

[34] R. A. Rosenheck, J. H. Krystal, R. Lew et al., "Long-acting risperidone and oral antipsychotics in unstable schizophrenia," *The New England Journal of Medicine*, vol. 364, no. 9, pp. 842–851, 2011.

[35] C. Leucht, S. Heres, J. M. Kane, W. Kissling, J. M. Davis, and S. Leucht, "Oral versus depot antipsychotic drugs for schizophrenia-a critical systematic review and meta-analysis of randomised long-term trials," *Schizophrenia Research*, vol. 127, no. 1–3, pp. 83–92, 2011.

[36] S. Heres, T. Reichhart, J. Hamann, R. Mendel, S. Leucht, and W. Kissling, "Psychiatrists' attitude to antipsychotic depot treatment in patients with first-episode schizophrenia," *European Psychiatry*, vol. 26, no. 5, pp. 297–301, 2011.

[37] S. Pereira and R. Pinto, "A survey of the attitudes of chronic psychiatric patients living in the community toward their medication," *Acta Psychiatrica Scandinavica*, vol. 95, no. 6, pp. 464–468, 1997.

[38] B. Svedberg, G. Backenroth-Ohsako, and K. Lützén, "On the path to recovery: patients' experiences of treatment with long-acting injections of antipsychotic medication," *International Journal of Mental Health Nursing*, vol. 12, no. 2, pp. 110–118, 2003.

[39] J. Tiihonen, J. Haukka, M. Taylor, P. M. Haddad, M. X. Patel, and P. Korhonen, "A nationwide cohort study of oral and depot antipsychotics after first hospitalization for schizophrenia," *American Journal of Psychiatry*, vol. 168, no. 6, pp. 603–609, 2011.

[40] A. Viala, F. Cornic, and M. Vacheron, "Treatment adherence with early prescription of long-acting injectable antipsychotics in recent-onset schizophrenia," *Schizophrenia Research and Treatment*, vol. 2012, Article ID 368687, 5 pages, 2012.

[41] M. Álvarez-Jiménez, C. González-Blanch, B. Crespo-Facorro et al., "Antipsychotic-induced weight gain in chronic and first-episode psychotic disorders: a systematic critical reappraisal," *CNS Drugs*, vol. 22, no. 7, pp. 547–562, 2008.

[42] S. M. Francey, B. Nelson, A. Thompson et al., "Who needs antipsychotic medication in the earliest stages of psychosis? A reconsideration of benefits, risks, neurobiology and ethics in the era of early intervention," *Schizophrenia Research*, vol. 119, no. 1–3, pp. 1–10, 2010.

[43] D. L. Kelly, R. R. Conley, and W. T. Carpenter, "First-episode schizophrenia: a focus on pharmacological treatment and safety considerations," *Drugs*, vol. 65, no. 8, pp. 1113–1138, 2005.

[44] G. Aggarwal, S. Dhawan, and S. L. Harikumar, "Formulation, in vitro, and in vivo evaluation of matrix-type transdermal patches containing olanzapine," *Pharmaceutical Development and Technology*, vol. 2011, Article ID 108374, 2011.

[45] G. Aggarwal, S. Dhawan, and S. L. Harikumar, "Formulation, in vitro and in vivo evaluation of transdermal patches containing risperidone," *Drug Development and Industrial Pharmacy*, vol. 2012, Article ID 036390, 2012.

[46] S. Priebe, A. Burton, D. Ashby et al., "Financial incentives to improve adherence to anti-psychotic maintenance medication in non-adherent patients—a cluster randomised controlled trial (FIAT)," *BioMedCentral Psychiatry*, vol. 9, article 61, 2009.

[47] D. Claassen, "Financial incentives for antipsychotic depot medication: ethical issues," *Journal of Medical Ethics*, vol. 33, no. 4, pp. 189–193, 2007.

[48] A. F. Lehman, J. A. Lieberman, L. B. Dixon et al., "Practice guideline for the treatment of patients with schizophrenia, second edition," *American Journal of Psychiatry*, vol. 161, no. 2, supplement, pp. 1–56, 2004.

[49] C. P. Association, "Clinical practice guidelines. Treatment of schizophrenia," *Canadian Journal of Psychiatry*, vol. 50, no. 13, supplement 1, pp. 7S–57S, 2005.

[50] J. M. Kane and C. Garcia-Ribera, "Clinical guideline recommendations for antipsychotic long-acting injections," *British Journal of Psychiatry*, vol. 195, supplement, pp. S63–S67, 2009.

[51] T. R. Barnes and Schizophrenia Consensus Group of British Association for Psychopharmacology, "Evidence-based guidelines for the pharmacological treatment of schizophrenia: recommendations from the British Association for Psychopharmacology," *Journal of Psychopharmacology*, vol. 25, no. 5, pp. 567–620, 2011.

9

Hospitalisation Utilisation and Costs in Schizophrenia Patients in Finland before and after Initiation of Risperidone Long-Acting Injection

Christian Asseburg,[1] Michael Willis,[2] Mickael Löthgren,[3] Niko Seppälä,[4] Mika Hakala,[4] and Ulf Persson[2]

[1] *ESiOR Oy, Tulliportinkatu 2, 70100 Kuopio, Finland*
[2] *The Swedish Institute for Health Economics (IHE), 22002 Lund, Sweden*
[3] *Amgen (Europe) GmbH Dammstrasse 23, P.O. Box 1557, CH-6301 Zug, Switzerland*
[4] *Department of Psychiatry, Satakunta Hospital District, 29200 Harjavalta, Finland*

Correspondence should be addressed to Michael Willis, mw@ihe.se

Academic Editor: Dawn I. Velligan

Objectives. Quantify changes in hospital resource use in Finland following initiation of risperidone long-acting injection (RLAI). *Materials and Methods.* A retrospective multi-center chart review (naturalistic setting) was used to compare annual hospital bed-days and hospital episodes for 177 schizophrenia patients (mean age 47.1 years, 52% female, 72% hospitalized) before and after initiation of RLAI (between January 2004 and June 2005) using the within-patient "mirror-image" study design. The base case analytical approach allocated hospital episodes overlapping the start date entirely to the preinitiation period. In order to investigate the impact of inpatient care ongoing at baseline, the change in bed-days was also estimated using an alternative analytical approached related to economic modelling. *Results.* In the conventional analysis, the mean annual hospitalisation costs declined by €11,900 and the number of bed-days was reduced by 40%, corresponding to 0.19 fewer hospital episodes per year. The reductions in bed-days per patient-year were similar for patients switched to RLAI as inpatients and as outpatients. In the modelling-based analysis, an 8% reduction in bed-days per year was observed. *Conclusion.* Despite uncertainty in the choice of analytic approach for allocating inpatient episodes that overlapping this initiation, consistent reductions in resource use are associated with the initiation of RLAI in Finland.

1. Introduction

Schizophrenia is a serious mental illness causing significant social or occupational dysfunction. With an annual global incidence of 8 to 40 individuals per 100,000 per year [1], the total costs of treating schizophrenia are high [2] and may be as much as 3% of all health expenditures [3]. Most of the direct costs of schizophrenia (79%) result from hospitalisation or other residential care [3], thus a principal aim of treatment in schizophrenia patients is to prevent relapse, reduce the requirements for in-hospital treatment, and enable patients to lead near-normal lives.

Pharmacological treatments for schizophrenia have been available since the mid-1950s. The first class of medication, "typical antipsychotics," is effective at treating psychotic symptoms but, while still used widely, is associated with problematic extrapyramidal side effects. The second generation of drugs, "atypical antipsychotics," became available in the 1990s and may cause fewer extrapyramidal side effects, though medication noncompliance continues to be common in schizophrenia patients in part because of serious metabolic concerns. Long-acting depot formulations of some first-generation antipsychotic agents have been developed to improve medication compliance by shifting responsibility from unpredictable patients to their health care providers [2], and the extent to which long-acting injectable medication can reduce rates of relapse and rehospitalisation is a topic of active research [4].

Risperidone long-acting injection (RLAI, available in many countries as RISPERDAL CONSTA) is the first long-acting depot formulation of an atypical antipsychotic and was introduced in Finland in February 2003. Administered once every two weeks by intramuscular injection, RLAI provides steadier plasma levels than oral formulations and hence a more consistent relief of symptoms and lower rates of side effects [3].

While the unit cost of RLAI is higher than the unit costs of alternative antipsychotics at comparable doses, RLAI may provide a number of potentially offsetting economic benefits (in particular, reduced healthcare costs related to relapse and hospitalisation [3]). Indeed, a number of studies have identified reductions in hospital admission rates following initiation of risperidone in a host of countries. For example, Eriksson and colleagues [5, 6] found a 65% reduction in annual inpatient bed-days in Sweden; Chue and colleagues [7] found that the number of patients requiring hospitalization decreased continuously from 38% in the 3 months prior to RLAI to 12% after 1 year of treatment in an international study; Fuller and colleagues [8] found reductions of 37% in psychiatric-related hospitalizations and 56% in psychiatric-related hospital bed-days in the USA; Niaz and Haddad [9] found roughly 50% reductions in both number of admission and hospital days per patient-year in the UK though Taylor et al. [10] found little difference; Su and colleagues [11] found reductions in hospital admissions of 55% and inpatient bed-days of 48% in Taiwan; Willis and colleagues [12] found reductions of 27% in hospitalization rate and 45% in hospital bed-day; Carswell and colleagues [13] found that patients in New Zealand had fewer hospital admissions but longer lengths of stay. Health care is setting specific, however, and the economic efficiency of interventions in one country is seldom generalizable to another. We are not aware of data for Finland.

2. Aims of the Study

This study aim is to estimate the change in resource usage, hospitalisation rates, and costs seen in actual practice in Finland for schizophrenia patients before and after initiation of treatment with RLAI.

3. Patients and Methods

3.1. Study Design. We collected data using a retrospective, observational review of patient charts for patients suffering from schizophrenia or schizoaffective disorders and treated with RLAI in Finland. To estimate the changes in resource use associated with RLAI treatment, data for the periods before and after initiation are compared on a patient-by-patient within-subject basis (sometimes labelled "mirror-image" analysis [14]).

3.2. Endpoints. Outcome measures include the differences in the mean number of inpatient hospital bed-days per year, the mean rate of hospitalisation per year, and the mean annual costs of inpatient hospital care related to schizophrenia (reported in 2007 €).

3.3. Ethics Approval. Ethics approval was sought from the ethics review board at the Joint Municipal Authority for Medical and Social Services in North Karelia and granted. Informed consent was not required.

3.4. Patient Selection. Based on participation in previous studies or because they were known to use RLAI, 10 Finnish psychiatry sites were selected to participate: Pohjois-Karjala central hospital (Paihola), Harjavalta psychiatric hospital (Harjavalta), Pori mental health care centre (Pori), Turku city psychiatry department (Turku), Kaivanto psychiatric hospital (Kangasala), TaUCH Pitkäniemi hospital (Pitkäniemi), Helsinki and Uusimaa hospital district area Kellokoski psychiatric hospital (Kellokoski) and Tammiharju psychiatric hospital (Tammisaari), Kitee mental health care centre (Kitee), and Helsinki city psychiatric department (Helsinki).

Patients who participated in any RLAI clinical trial were excluded from this study. The inclusion criteria were at least 18 years old, diagnosed with schizophrenia or schizoaffective disorder, first initiation of RLAI treatment between 1 January 2004 and 30 June 2005, and medical chart record covering at least two years prior to RLAI treatment and at least until 31 July 2006. At each study site, investigators aimed to enlist all eligible subjects up to a maximum of 40 (to prevent overrepresentation of some sites).

3.5. Data Analytic Procedures. Single hospital episodes were recorded in the data collection forms using dates of admission and discharge. Hospitalisations that involved changes in level of care (psychiatric, psychiatric intensive, and forensic) were recorded in the hospital charts as a sequence of separate "episodes" with individual dates of admission and discharge. We merged these into a single episode except when calculating hospital costs.

When attributing observed resource use to RLAI or the prior treatment, hospitalisation episodes that overlapped the index initiation RLAI must be allocated to the periods before and after the index initiation. Given the seriousness of schizophrenia, withdrawal effects associated with the previous drugs [15], and time to adequate blood serum levels for most depot formulations (RLAI reaches satisfactory blood serum levels first after 3 weeks, until which time additional antipsychotic treatment is required to maintain adequate control [16]), an improvement sufficient for discharge to occur instantaneously after RLAI initiation cannot be expected. An intent-to-treat definition based strictly on the day of initiation, thus, would artificially penalise the RLAI by attributing the consequences of the failure of previous medications (and consequent poor health requiring hospitalization) to the postinitiation treatment.

We adopt the simple allocation rule used by Fuller and colleagues [8], Niaz and Haddad [9], and others, who assigned the entire episode of hospitalisations ongoing at the time of initiation to the treatment ongoing at admission

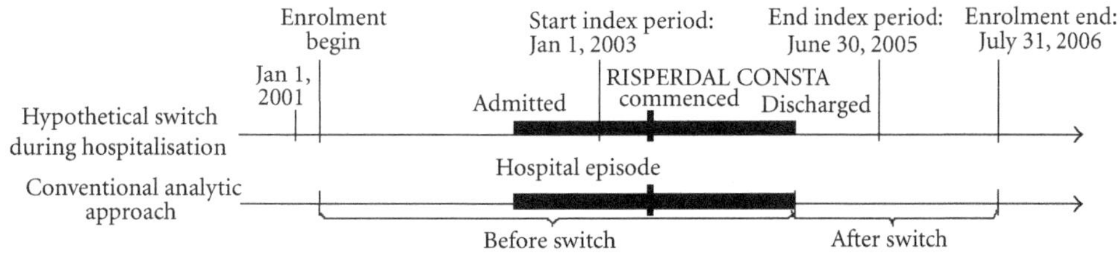

FIGURE 1: Illustration of the conventional allocation rule for hospitalisation episodes ongoing at the time of initiation. The start of the post-initiation period is adjusted so the entirety of hospitalisations episode overlapping the initiation date are included in the pre-switch period.

TABLE 1: Patient characteristics at time of initiation of RLAI.

Variable	N	Mean
Age (years)	177	47.1 (SD 13.6) Range 22–84
Female (%)	177	92 (52.0%)
Disease duration		
Years	137*	15.3 (SD 12.5)
% less than 4 years	137*	31 (17.5%)
% 4 to 10 years	137*	44 (24.8%)
% more than 10 years	137*	102 (57.7%)
GAF (raw score)	21*	22.5 (SD 13.9) Range 5–60
GAS (raw score)	49*	35.2 (SD 9.6) Range 19–58
CGI-S (%)		
Normal	177	0
Borderline or mildly Ill	177	1 (0.6%)
Moderately Ill	177	2 (1.1%)
Markedly Ill	177	16 (9.0%)
Severely or among most extensively Ill	177	8 (4.5%)
Unknown	177	150 (84.7%)
Occupational status (%)		
Full time	177	2 (1.1%)
Part time	177	0
Sheltered work	177	1 (0.6%)
Unemployed	177	13 (7.3%)
Retired	177	121 (68.4%)
Long-term sick leave	177	33 (18.7%)
Other	177	7 (4.0%)
Unknown	177	0
Accommodation status (%)		
Psychiatric nursing home	177	15 (8.5%)
Sheltered living	177	5 (2.8%)
With parents or relatives	177	20 (11.3%)
Own apartment	177	125 (70.6%)
Other	177	12 (6.8%)
Unknown	177	0

*Missing information resulted in reduced sample sizes.

("conventional analytic approach," Figure 1). This approach seems reasonable because hospital resource use is more likely attributable to the treatment that was ongoing and failing at admission (possibly due to insufficient efficacy, sideeffects, or low adherence) than to a treatment that was begun after admission to hospital. The start of the exposure period to RLAI in a patient hospitalised when initiating RLAI is then adjusted to the date of hospitalisation episode discharge. Conservatively, patients who were initiated on RLAI as outpatients are assumed to start the post-initiation period at the actual time of initiation. The end of the exposure period is at death or study completion (31 July 2006), whether or not the patient was still taking RLAI. The control period runs from 2 years prior to treatment initiation with RLAI to the start of the treatment exposure period.

By allocating to the prior treatment the entirety of the hospitalisation episodes that overlap the initiation, the conventional analytic approach may bias the results in favour of RLAI. This bias is stronger in proportion to the prevalence and length of overlapping hospitalisation episodes and ameliorated by longer study follow-up durations. Because this allocation affects only measures of resource use on-going at the time of initiation (bed-days and hospital costs), whereas a hospitalisation event is clearly before or after initiation, this source of bias does not apply to the endpoint of hospitalisation rates.

To investigate the sensitivity of study results to this allocation rule, we conducted two additional analyses. First, the primary endpoints are presented separately for patients who were hospitalised and were not hospitalised at the time of initiation. Results for the subgroup who started RLAI as outpatients are unaffected by this bias. Second, we present an alternative approach in which we model the change based on the fact that the number of bed-days per year is the product of annual hospitalisation rate and average length of inpatient stay per episode. Specifically, we multiply the empirical estimates of hospitalisation rates before and after the initiation of RLAI by the average lengths of stay per hospitalisation episode *strictly before* and *strictly after* initiation. This modelling-based estimate of resource use eliminates the effect of hospitalisation episodes ongoing at the time of initiation.

In analyses of inpatient bed-days, number of episodes, and hospitalisation costs, the unit of analysis is the patient. Results are presented as mean, standard error, and two-sided 95% confidence intervals. A difference was interpreted as statistically significant if the confidence interval for the estimated mean difference did not contain 0. To estimate the costs of hospital resource use, the recorded durations of episodes were multiplied by unit costs for bed-days in the different levels of inpatient service [17, 18]. Adjusted to 2007 € prices using Finnish price indices, the costs per bed-day are

Table 2: Length of follow-up and of hospitalisation episodes.

Variable	N	Mean	Standard deviation	Min	Max
Follow-up prior to initiation of RLAI (years)	177	2.00	—	—	—
Follow-up following initiation of RLAI (years)	177	1.80	0.45	0.43	2.56
Proportion of patients hospitalised at initiation of RLAI	177	127 (72%)	—	—	—
Hospital length of stay (days per episode)					
All Episodes	576	65.0	95.4	0*	816
Episodes strictly before RLAI initiation	227	45.6	53.2	1	405
Episodes overlapping RLAI initiation	128	120.1	145.0	9	816
Episodes strictly after RLAI initiation	221	53.0	80.3	0*	638

* Inpatient hospitalisation episodes that recorded discharge on the day of admissions were assigned a duration of zero days.

€280.46 for standard psychiatric care, €542.48 for psychiatric intensive care, and €510.00 for forensic care.

Additional subgroup analyses were carried out with regard to type of previous antipsychotic treatment based on recorded treatments on the day of initiation of RLAI or the previous day. Patients are classified into the following five mutually exclusive categories: typical oral only, typical depot only, atypical oral only, combination of any of these, or untreated (which does not necessarily imply drug-naïve).

4. Results

4.1. Descriptive Results. Data were collected for 199 patients. Twenty-two subjects were excluded from analysis because they were hospitalised before the start of RLAI and not discharged before the end of follow-up (2 patients), the start date of RLAI could not be established ($n = 6$), their RLAI prescription record was incomplete or inconsistent ($n = 5$), they started RLAI before 1 January 2004 ($n = 2$), or the number and duration of hospitalisation episodes could not be clearly established ($n = 9$). Multiple exclusion criteria applied to 2 patients. The analysis sample, thus, consists of 177 patients.

Descriptive statistics for the patient population at the time of initiation to RLAI are presented in Table 1. Mean age at initiation of RLAI therapy was 47.1 years, 52% of the sample was female, and mean disease duration was 15.3 years. Patient functioning was poorly documented in hospital charts. Indeed, only 21 had a recorded Global Assessment of Functioning (GAF) score, only 49 had a recorded Global Assessment Scale (GAS) score, and only 27 had a recorded Clinical Global Impressions Scale (CGIS) score, and 92 patients had neither.

The lengths of the coverage periods and hospitalisations are presented in Table 2. By definition, two years of data on each patient are available prior to the initiation. Postinitiation data coverage ranges from 0.43 years (five patients died during study follow-up) to 2.56 years, with a mean of 1.80 years. 576 hospitalisation episodes were recorded during the study, of which 227 were entirely before the initiation of RLAI and 221 were entirely after the initiation. 128 patients (72%) were hospitalised when initiated on RLAI therapy. The mean duration of hospitalisations overlapping the index initiation was 120 days, considerably longer than the mean duration of hospital episodes observed strictly before (46 days) or strictly after initiation (53 days).

Statistics on the use of RLAI are detailed in Table 3. The most frequently cited reasons for initiating therapy with RLAI were noncompliance on other medications (63%), lack of efficacy on other medications (34%), and relapse (27%). The average duration of RLAI treatment observed during the study period was 1.33 years, ranging from 0 days (i.e., first and last dose occurring on the same day) to 2.56 years. For 66 patients, RLAI therapy was discontinued during the study follow-up, primarily for the following reasons: lack of efficacy (35%), non-compliance (35%), and patient choice (33%). Table 4 shows the distribution of RLAI dosing over time. Seventy-six percent of patients started at 25 mg, doses above 50 mg were rarely observed.

4.2. Main Analysis. The results of the conventional analytic approach are shown in Table 5. The mean number of bed-days per patient per year was reduced by 24.89 bed-days (40%), from 62.89 to 38.00 per patient-year, a statistically significant difference. The mean number of hospitalisations per year was reduced by 0.19 episodes (20%), a statistically significant reduction from 0.93 episodes per year before initiation of RLAI to 0.74 episodes after. Statistically significant reductions in total hospitalisation costs are also associated with the initiation of RLAI therapy. Mean hospital costs per patient-year decreased by €11,948 (43%), from €28,046 per year before initiation of RLAI to €16,098 after initiation.

Table 6 presents results for the subgroups of patients who were initiated on RLAI during a hospitalization ($n = 128$) or on an outpatient basis ($n = 49$). Statistically significant reductions of 21.81 (36%) and 32.93 (48%) in the mean number of bed-days per year were observed in the inpatient and outpatient cohorts, respectively. A statistically significant reduction of 0.24 episodes (24%) in the mean number of hospitalisations per patient-year was observed in the inpatient subgroup; a reduction of 0.06 episodes (8%) in the outpatient subgroup did not reach statistical significance due to small sample size. For the modelling-based approach, the estimates of episodes per year in the two periods (0.93 and 0.74 episodes per patient-year, resp.) are multiplied with the average lengths of stay associated with hospitalisation in the two periods, excluding any hospitalisation episodes ongoing at the time of initiation (45.6 and 53.0 days, resp.). This complementary approach estimates a reduction in the mean

TABLE 3: Use of RLAI.

Variable	*N*	Mean
Reasons for initiation to RLAI* (%)		
Adverse event: weight gain	177	3 (1.7%)
Adverse event: extrapyramidal symptoms	177	14 (7.9%)
Adverse event: other	177	11 (6.2%)
Lack of efficacy	177	61 (34.5%)
Relapse	177	47 (26.6%)
Patient choice	177	26 (14.7%)
Noncompliance	177	112 (63.3%)
Unknown	177	0
Duration of RLAI use (days)	177	485.5 (SD 287.4)range 0–936
RLAI persistence (proportion of patients known to continue therapy during)		
at least 6 months	175†	134 (76.6%)
at least 12 months	172†	122 (70.9%)
at least 18 months	128†	87 (68.0%)
at least 24 months	68†	45 (66.2%)
Reasons for stopping RLAI* (%)		
Adverse event: weight gain	66	2 (3.0%)
Adverse event: extrapyramidal	66	3 (4.5%)
Adverse event: other	66	10 (15.2%)
Lack of efficacy	66	23 (34.8%)
Relapse	66	2 (3.0%)
Patient choice	66	22 (33.3%)
Noncompliance	66	23 (34.8%)
Unknown	66	0

* Multiple answers were allowed. † Reduced sample size reflects follow-up durations.

TABLE 4: RLAI dose distributions in patients beginning with RLAI, and every 6 months onwards. for each patient, the last known observation on dose was carried forward to the time point. Two patients were excluded from the analysis of dose changes at later time points because of missing information.

	At treatment beginning	6 months later	12 months later	18 months later	24 months later
N (patients)	177 (100%)	132 (100%)	121 (100%)	87 (100%)	45 (100%)
25 mg	134 (76%)	41 (31%)	33 (27%)	24 (28%)	17 (38%)
37.5 mg	24 (14%)	40 (30%)	35 (29%)	26 (30%)	13 (29%)
50 mg	19 (11%)	48 (36%)	49 (40%)	34 (39%)	14 (31%)
62.5 mg	0	1 (1%)	1 (1%)	0	0
75 mg	0	2 (2%)	3 (2%)	3 (3%)	1 (2%)
100 mg	0	0	0	0	0

number of bed-days per patient per year by 3.2 (i.e., 8%), from 42.4 to 39.2 bed-days per patient-year.

Results by previous treatment are presented in Table 7. The results are suppressed for patients treated exclusively with typical antipsychotic agents just prior to the initiation as sample sizes were small. The combination therapy subgroup is made up predominantly of patients who receive atypical and typical oral agents in combination.

In the large subgroups of patients with previous atypical oral agent (alone or in combination), results are generally similar to the overall results, for example a reduction of 0.22 episodes in the single atypical oral subgroup, from 0.90 episodes per year before initiation to 0.69 episodes per year after the initiation of RLAI. For the small subgroup of patients untreated at the time of initiation ($n = 9$), the annual number of hospitalisation episodes before the initiation is estimated to be higher (1.18 per year) than the overall average, and a larger reduction by 0.77 is seen with the initiation to a postinitiation mean annual number of 0.41 hospitalisations. Resource use as measured by bed-days per year is, however, below average for this subgroup, with mean 50 days per year prior to the initiation and 18 days after initiation.

5. Discussion

Results suggest that RLAI is associated with sizeable and statistically significant reductions in resource use. The mean number of hospitalisations per year decreased by 20%. This

TABLE 5: Results of the main analysis. Hospitalisation episodes overlapping the date of RLAI initiation are allocated to the period before initiation. Sample unit (N) is the patient.

Endpoints	Before initiation		After initiation		Difference	
	Mean (SE)	95% CI	Mean (SE)	95% CI	Mean (SE)	95% CI
Inpatient bed-days per patient-year ($N = 177$)	62.89 (4.16)	(54.74; 71.04)	38 (5.19)	(27.83; 48.17)	−24.89 (5.93)	(−36.51; 13.26)
No. hospitalizations per patient-year ($N = 177$)	0.93 (0.05)	(0.83; 1.03)	0.74 (0.09)	(0.57; 0.91)	−0.19 (0.09)	(−0.36; −0.01)
Hospital costs per patient-year, € ($N = 177$)	28,046 (1,782)	(24,554; 31,539)	16,098 (2,117)	(11,949; 20,248)	−11,948 (2,555)	(−16,995; −6,941)
Cost of other antipsychotic agents, € per patient-year ($N = 177$)	907 (148)	(617; 1,197)	1,130 (174)	(788; 1,471)	233 (135)	(−43; 488)
Cost of RLAI per patient-year, € ($N = 177$)	—	—	4,193 (196)	(3,809; 4,576)	—	—

TABLE 6: Results of the subgroup analysis for the endpoints: inpatient bed-days per patient and year, and number of hospitalisations per patient and year. Results are presented for subgroups of patients who are in- or outpatients at the time of initiating RLAI.

Endpoints	Before initiation		After initiation		Difference	
	Mean (SE)	95% CI	Mean (SE)	95% CI	Mean (SE)	95% CI
Inpatient bed-days per patient-year						
Inpatient ($N = 128$)	60.88 (4.03)	(52.97; 68.79)	39.07 (6.13)	(27.06; 51.09)	−21.81 (7.21)	(−35.94; −7.68)
Outpatient ($N = 49$)	68.13 (10.76)	(47.05; 89.22)	35.2 (9.82)	(15.96; 54.44)	−32.93 (10.23)	(−52.98; −12.98)
No. hospitalizations per patient-year						
Inpatient ($N = 128$)	0.99 (0.06)	(0.87; 1.11)	0.76 (0.11)	(0.54; 0.97)	−0.24 (0.11)	(−0.45; −0.02)
Outpatient ($N = 49$)	0.77 (0.09)	(0.59; 0.95)	0.71 (0.14)	(0.43; 0.98)	−0.06 (0.14)	(−0.34; 0.21)

translated into reduced inpatient bed-days and corresponding costs, but the magnitude is sensitive to the method of allocating hospitalisation episodes on-going at the time of initiation. The conventional approach resulted in a reduction in bed-days per patient-year by 40% and a corresponding cost-saving of over €16,000 per patient-year, while the alternative modelling-based approach found a reduction in inpatient days of 8%. The subgroup of patients who were initiated on RLAI on an outpatient basis (and which does not suffer from uncertainty about the appropriate allocation of hospital episodes overlapping the initiation) experienced a 48% reduction of bed-days per patient-year (similar to the conventional approach). Despite variation in the magnitude of this reduction between the three approaches, all analyses point to a consistent and considerable reduction in resource use associated with the initiation to RLAI.

5.1. Study Strengths and Weaknesses. This study has some important strengths. First, the use of a noninterventional design allowed us to answer questions about "real-world" resource use in a timely manner. Through the use of chart review, resource use in schizophrenia patients could be observed as it occurred in actual practice rather than in the context of controlled clinical trials with corresponding protocol bias [11]. Moreover, the study endpoints are highly likely to be captured in patient charts, resulting in data integrity on hospitalisation episodes and costs.

Second, the retrospective study design was chosen to ensure recruitment of a reasonably-sized patient sample within the time constraints imposed by demands of the Finnish Pharmaceuticals Pricing Board (Lääkkeiden Hintalautakunta), which would have been impossible to achieve in a prospective study. With a relatively long patient follow-up of, on average, 1.8 years after initiation of RLAI, this study may also be more likely to capture the effects of treatment persistence and compliance, which a shorter study is likely to underestimate [4]. The "mirror-image" design, moreover, provides a within-group comparison that controls for time-invariant individual patient covariates.

Third, informed consent was not required. This may have avoided the selection bias related to willingness to participate in clinical studies [19] and facilitated the recruitment of a

TABLE 7: Results of the subgroup analysis for the endpoints: inpatient bed-days per patient and year, number of hospitalisations per patient and year, and hospital costs per patient and year. Results are presented for previous therapy subgroups containing more than 5 patients.

Endpoints	Before initiation		After initiation		Difference	
	Mean (SE)	95% CI	Mean (SE)	95% CI	Mean (SE)	95% CI
Inpatient bed-days per patient-year						
Atypical oral only ($N = 129$)	61.63 (4.30)	(53.20; 70.05)	37.69 (6.03)	(25.87; 49.51)	−23.94 (7.21)	(−38.07; −9.81)
Atypical oral combination ($N = 32$)	70.76 (12.80)	(45.67; 95.86)	38.95 (13.27)	(12.95; 64.95)	−31.81 (14.35)	(−59.93; −3.98)
Untreated ($N = 9$)	50.06 (15.94)	(18.82; 81.30)	17.8 (6.65)	(4.77; 30.84)	−32.26 (16.19)	(−63.99; −0.54)
No. hospitalizations per patient-year						
Atypical oral only ($N = 129$)	0.9 (0.06)	(0.80; 1.01)	0.69 (0.09)	(0.51; 0.86)	−0.22 (0.09)	(−0.40; −0.03)
Atypical oral combination ($N = 32$)	0.96 (0.14)	(0.69; 1.24)	0.78 (0.23)	(0.32; 1.24)	−0.18 (0.17)	(−0.51; 0.15)
Untreated ($N = 9$)	1.18 (0.30)	(0.59; 1.78)	0.41 (0.14)	(0.13; 0.68)	−0.77 (0.29)	(−1.34; −0.21)
Hospital costs per patient-year, €						
Atypical oral only ($N = 129$)	27,560 (1,934)	(23,770; 31,351)	16,177 (2,546)	(11,187; 21,167)	−11,383 (3,007)	(−17,276; −5,491)
Atypical oral combination ($N = 32$)	32,415 (5,439)	(21,755; 43,075)	15,666 (5,027)	(5,812; 25,519)	−16,749 (6,782)	(−30,041; −3,457)
Untreated ($N = 9$)	20,561 (6,633)	(7,561; 33,562)	8,435 (3,379)	(1,812; 15,059)	−12,126 (7,735)	(−27,28; 3,035)

relatively large sample. Moreover, because the data before the initiation of RLAI are compared with data from the same patients after initiation, the study design controls for biases due to time-invariant individual covariates, irrespective of whether these are recorded in the study.

There are also several important study limitations. First, "mirror-image" studies are subject to inherent biases [14]. Because the treatment under investigation (RLAI) is typically initiated during an acute episode when patient health was sufficiently poor to necessitate a treatment initiation, gravitation to the mean [20] may have contributed to optimistic estimates in this study. The asymmetrical definition of treatment periods may have introduced a conservative bias because the dose titration period is included in the estimation of the RLAI treatment effect. The strict temporal sequence of periods before and after the initiation of RLAI may have caused biases relating to disease progression or changes in the health-care system (period bias), such as the conservative bias associated with the worsening severity status in schizophrenia patients over time. While the lack of a concurrent control group precludes assessment of these biases, leading some authors to consider results from "mirror-image" studies inconclusive [21], this design is nonetheless often used in studies of health resource use [14].

Second, this study may not represent schizophrenia patients generally because it appears to have recruited, on average, quite severely ill schizophrenia patients. Indeed, a "first-wave" effect, in which severely ill patients are more likely than others to receive a novel drug, may have occurred because the recruitment index period began soon after the launch of RLAI in Finland. Seventy-two percent were initiated on RLAI while hospitalised, which indicates above-average severity in the sampled schizophrenia patients. Treatment success may be less likely in these difficult-to-treat patients, so the resource use reductions reported here for the subgroup of patients initiating RLAI as outpatients may be more representative of the broader population of schizophrenia patients than the overall results reported here.

Third, controversy exists regarding the appropriate definition of treatment periods. Gianfrancesco et al. [14] argue that a pure intent-to-treat principle cannot and should not be applied to "mirror-image" studies because the before-treatment period is not defined according to intent-to-treat. This is a clear deficit inherent in the "mirror-image" study design. Health-economic studies, however, aim to compare the patient outcomes resulting from the decision to start different therapies, rather than during a treatment-specific period in which treatment is considered "successful." It is therefore appropriate to follow the pragmatic, intent-to-treat principle when analysing health-economic datasets in general [22] and in schizophrenia [23]. The conventional analytic approach adjusts the initiation date in some patients and its results are thus, strictly speaking, not associated with the start of RLAI therapy. The subgroup results presented for patients initiating RLAI as outpatients are consistent with the intent-to-treat principle in the postinitiation period.

Fourth, there is no comparison with relevant treatment alternatives. Choosing a relevant comparator is difficult because typical depots differ from atypical depots in their sideeffects profile, atypical oral preparations differ in patient compliance with the treatment [24], and RLAI is the first-to-market atypical depot.

Fifth, there is methodological uncertainty about how to analyse hospitalisation episodes that are ongoing at initiation. Specifically, the entirety of these hospitalizations that overlapped the index initiation of RLAI could be allocated to the preinitiation treatment as in the conventional analytic approach in this study as well as elsewhere [5, 6, 8]. Other studies have excluded patients who initiated on an inpatient basis [10, 12] or carried out sensitivity analyses in which they were excluded ([5, 8] and here). The magnitude of treatment effect appears sensitive to analysis methods, which is significant here because nearly 75% of the sample falls into this category and because these hospital stays were longer (mean 120 days) than other stays on average (around 50 days).

Many of the above design weaknesses are due to a lack of consensus on the correct method for analysing resource use episodes that overlap the initiation date. Ideally, these limitations would be overcome in future studies by comparing data on the initiation of RLAI with data on the initiation of another therapy, suitably chosen to avoid introducing patient selection biases. The biases introduced by choice of method would then affect both arms equally so that the conclusions should be more robust to the chosen methods of analysis and allocation. Additionally, studies with longer follow-up durations would reduce the impact of the methodological uncertainty associated with attribution of the episode ongoing at initiation because its contribution to overall resource use will be smaller. Health-economic analysis would benefit from both innovations because long-term comparative results on the different consequences of relevant treatment options are of more use to decision makers than studies of single-treatment options.

5.2. Interpretation of Study Results. Several other studies have collected data on resource use in patients diagnosed with schizophrenia or schizoaffective disorder and treated with RLAI. The results of the conventional analytic approach in the present study appear generally consistent with other studies (accounting for some differences in the design and recruitment) [6, 8, 10–13]. The similarities with an identically designed study in neighbouring Sweden is striking, 40% fewer bed-days in the current study and 45% in Willis et al. [12].

While the present study was not designed to investigate the reasons for reduced resource use in patients being treated with RLAI, the large proportion of patients who were initiated on RLAI because of noncompliance with the previous treatment (63%) suggests that doctors choose RLAI to improve medication compliance, a likely benefit of RLAI compared to oral medication [3].

6. Conclusion

This study found consist evidence that sizable reductions in resource usage are associated with the initiation of RLAI in Finland. The choice of analytic approach for allocating inpatient episodes that are ongoing at the initiation of therapy affects estimates of the magnitude, however, and future work to evaluate a novel approach based on economic modelling is desired.

Acknowledgments

M. Löthgren was and M. Hakala is employee of Janssen-Cilag AB, the manufacturer of RISPERDAL CONSTA. C. Asseburg, M. Willis, and U. Persson have received funding for this study from Janssen-Cilag via the Swedish Institute for Health Economics. All authors have read and approved the final version of the paper. The authors wish to thank Katja Kettunen, Anu Ahonen and Leena Rahkamo at Janssen-Cilag Finland for the data collection, chart reviews, and unit cost estimates for Finland the investigators at the study sites, Maxim Cheine, Valeria Golovanova, Vjatcheslav Golovanov, Grigori Joffe, Tero Laiho, Ilkka Larmo, Henno Ligi, Antti Liuska, Mertsi Maaniitty, Oli-Pekka Mehtonen, Inkeri Mikkola, Teija Nummelin, Pekka Ollila, Katri Paganus, Maire Santala, Niko Seppälä, Matti Vaittinen, Mari Varga and Sanna Vähäkangas, for their collaboration and effort; and Sofie Persson at IHE Lund for entering the data into the electronic database.

References

[1] R. Tandon, R. H. Belmaker, W. F. Gattaz et al., "World Psychiatric Association Pharmacopsychiatry Section statement on comparative effectiveness of antipsychotics in the treatment of schizophrenia," *Schizophrenia Research*, vol. 100, no. 1–3, pp. 20–38, 2008.

[2] K. T. Mueser and S. R. McGurk, "Schizophrenia," *The Lancet*, vol. 363, no. 9426, pp. 2063–2072, 2004.

[3] P. Chue, "Long-acting risperidone injection: efficacy, safety, and cost-effectiveness of the first long-acting atypical antipsychotic," *Neuropsychiatric Disease and Treatment*, vol. 3, no. 1, pp. 13–39, 2007.

[4] J. M. Kane and S. Leucht, "Unanswered questions in schizophrenia clinical trials," *Schizophrenia Bulletin*, vol. 34, no. 2, pp. 302–309, 2008.

[5] L. Eriksson et al., "Reduction in need for institutional care in chronic schizophrenia subjects switched to long-acting risperidone," in *Proceedings of the 45th Annual Meeting of the Scandinavian College of Neuro-Psychopharmacology*, Juan-les-Pins, France, 2004.

[6] L. Eriksson, A. Almqvist, A. Mehnert et al., "Treatment with long acting risperidone significantly reduces the need for institutional psychiatric care regardless of previous treatment," in *Proceedings of the 45th Annual Meeting of the Scandinavian College of Neuro-Psychopharmacology*, Juan-les-Pins, France, 2004.

[7] P. Chue, P. M. Llorca, I. Duchesne, A. Leal, D. Rosillon, and A. Mehnert, "Hospitalization rates in patients during long-term treatment with long-acting risperidone injection," *Journal of Applied Research*, vol. 5, no. 2, pp. 266–274, 2005.

[8] M. Fuller, K. Shermock, and M. Secic, "Hospitalization and resource utilization in schizophrenia following initiation of risperidone long-acting injection in the Veterans Affairs Healthcare System (VISN 10)," in *Proceedings of the Collegium Internationale Neuro-Psychopharmacologium 25th Biennial Congress*, Chicago, Ill, USA, 2006.

[9] O. S. Niaz and P. M. Haddad, "Thirty-five months experience of risperidonelong-acting injection in a UK psychiatric service including a mirror-image analysis of in-patient care," *Acta Psychiatrica Scandinavica*, vol. 116, no. 1, pp. 36–46, 2007.

[10] M. Taylor, A. Currie, K. Lloyd, M. Price, and K. Peperell, "Impact of risperidone long acting injection on resource utilization in psychiatric secondary care," *Journal of Psychopharmacology*, vol. 22, no. 2, pp. 128–131, 2008.

[11] K.-P. Su, H.-C. Chang, S.-J. Tsai, F.-C. Yen, and C.-H. Tang, "Relapse and long-acting injectable risperidone: a 1-year mirror image study with a national claims database in Taiwan," *Value in Health*, vol. 12, supplement 3, pp. S118–S121, 2009.

[12] M. Willis, M. Svensson, M. Löthgren, B. Eriksson, A. Berntsson, and U. Persson, "The impact on schizophrenia-related hospital utilization and costs of switching to long-acting risperidone injections in Sweden," *European Journal of Health Economics*, vol. 11, no. 6, pp. 585–594, 2010.

[13] C. Carswell, A. Wheeler, J. Vanderpyl, and E. Robinson, "Comparative effectiveness of long-acting risperidone in New Zealand: a report of resource utilization and costs in a 12-month mirror-image analysis," *Clinical Drug Investigation*, vol. 30, no. 11, pp. 777–787, 2010.

[14] F. Gianfrancesco, R. H. Wang, R. Mahmoud, and R. White, "Methods for claims-based pharmacoeconomic studies in psychosis,," *PharmacoEconomics*, vol. 20, no. 8, pp. 499–511, 2002.

[15] A. J. Goudie and J. C. Cole, "Switching antipsychotics. Antipsychotic tolerance, withdrawal and relapse: unresolved issues and research implications," *Journal of Psychopharmacology*, vol. 22, no. 7, pp. 815–817, 2008.

[16] *Pharmaca Fennica*, Finnish Centre for Medicine Information (Lääketietokeskus), Helsinki, Finland, 2008.

[17] T. Hujanen, *Terveydenhuollon Yksikkökustannukset 2001*, Stakes, Helsinki, Finland, 2003.

[18] HYKS-Hinnasto, *Helsinki University Central Hospital*, 2006.

[19] A. Hofer, M. Hummer, R. Huber, M. Kurz, T. Walch, and W. W. Fleischhacker, "Selection bias in clinical trials with antipsychotics," *Journal of Clinical Psychopharmacology*, vol. 20, no. 6, pp. 699–702, 2000.

[20] V. Morton and D. J. Torgerson, "Regression to the mean: treatment effect without the intervention," *Journal of Evaluation in Clinical Practice*, vol. 11, no. 1, pp. 59–65, 2005.

[21] D. Robinson and N. Schooler, "Clinical study design—critical issues," in *Psychopharmacology: The Fourth Generation of Progress*, Raven Press, New York, NY, USA, 1995.

[22] S. Byford and S. Palmer, "Common errors and controversies in pharmacoeconomic analyses," *PharmacoEconomics*, vol. 13, no. 6, pp. 659–666, 1998.

[23] W. M. Glazer and B. M. Johnstone, "Pharmacoeconomic evaluation of antipsychotic therapy for schizophrenia," *Journal of Clinical Psychiatry*, vol. 58, supplement 10, pp. 50–54, 1997.

[24] J. M. Kane, "Strategies for improving compliance in treatment of schizophrenia by using a long-acting formulation of an antipsychotic: clinical studies," *Journal of Clinical Psychiatry*, vol. 64, supplement 16, pp. 34–40, 2003.

10

Examining the Factors Associated with Paid Employment of Clients Enrolled in First Episode of Psychosis Programs

Carolyn S. Dewa,[1,2] Lucy Trojanowski,[1] Chiachen Cheng,[1,3] and Desmond Loong[1]

[1] *Centre for Research on Employment and Workplace Health, Centre for Addition and Mental Health, 455 Spadina Avenue, Suite 300, Toronto, ON, Canada M5S 2G8*
[2] *Department of Psychiatry, University of Toronto, 250 College Street, Toronto, ON, Canada M5T 1R8*
[3] *Clinic & Resource Centre, Canadian Mental Health Association, 272 Park Avenue, Thunder Bay, ON, Canada P7B 1C5*

Correspondence should be addressed to Carolyn S. Dewa, carolyn_dewa@camh.net

Academic Editor: Eóin Killackey

Schizophrenia is one of the most debilitating mental disorders. For a significant portion of individuals who suffer from this disorder, onset occurs in young adulthood, arresting important social and educational development that is necessary for future successful labor force participation. The purpose of this paper is to contribute to the literature about clients enrolled in first episode psychosis programs and psychosocial outcomes by examining the factors associated with paid employment among young adults who have experienced their first psychotic episodes. In this paper, we consider the association of socioeconomic factors to employment. Our results suggest that in addition to treatment, socioeconomic factors such as receipt of public disability benefits and educational attainment are associated with employment status. These results can help to inform future directions for the enhancement of psychosocial programs in FEP models to promote paid employment.

1. Introduction

Schizophrenia is one of the most debilitating mental disorders. For a significant portion of individuals who suffer from this disorder, onset occurs in young adulthood, arresting important social and educational development that is necessary for future successful labor force participation. As a result, schizophrenia is often associated with an eventual downward spiral ending in poverty and isolation[1]. To avert this dismal future, the focus on the first psychotic episode (FEP) is becoming a priority for mental health care globally (e.g., Johannessen et al. [2]).

There is also growing evidence surrounding the low employment rates of people with FEP. Employment rate estimates range from 13 to 55% [3–5]. Reviews of the literature [3, 6] note that there are a number of factors associated with employment along a number of dimensions [7–9]. Along with cognitive impairment and symptoms, educational attainment, family socioeconomic status, social benefit structures, and labour market conditions also potentially affect employment of young adults with first episode psychosis [3]. There appears to be a complex mix of both individual and environmental factors linked to successful labour market participation. Although it is a multifaceted challenge, there is increasing evidence for the effectiveness of interventions such as Individual Placement and Support (IPS) programs and the interventions of vocational specialists for this population [4, 6, 10–13]. As such, the International First Episode Vocational Recovery (iFEVR) Group [14] released a consensus statement advocating for the "right to education, training and employment" for young people enrolled in early intervention programs.

The need for the iFEVR consensus statement is motivated by the mounting evidence that employment is often not a priority for providers who serve and support FEP clients. For example, Rinaldi and colleagues [6] note that few FEP studies have focused on employment and education outcomes. In fact, employment is often discouraged by well-intentioned medical professionals and family [6, 10, 15]. In addition, governments have been less than supportive of employment programs for people with mental illnesses [16].

The purpose of this paper is to contribute to the literature about clients enrolled in first episode psychosis programs and psychosocial outcomes by examining the factors associated with paid employment among young adults who have experienced their first psychotic episode. In this paper, we consider the association of socioeconomic factors with employment.

2. Background

2.1. Characteristics of FEP Programs. FEP programs are designed to facilitate recovery from psychotic illnesses that first arise during youth, most commonly schizophrenia and bipolar disorder, and have historically been most associated with very high levels of disability [17]. Programs are designed to provide services to both clients and their families. Services include comprehensive diagnostic assessment, treatment, psychosocial supports, as well as family education and support. There is emphasis on a multidisciplinary team approach that integrates medical treatment, counseling, case management, substance abuse treatment, cognitiv behavioural therapy, in addition to psychoeducation for families.

2.2. Characteristics of the Study FEP Programs. The six FEP programs included in this study were located in six regions throughout the province of Ontario, Canada. Each program accepted youth who were experiencing their first episode or early stages of psychosis. Each early intervention program was developed to exclusively provide outpatient services.

Five of the six FEP programs reported that nearly three-quarters of their clientele were males. Three of the FEP programs engaged clients aged 14 to 35 years old, while the remaining three programs limited access to people who were at least 16 years old. Two FEP programs engaged transitional aged youth 16 to 23 years old.

All but one of the six programs were located in established community mental health agencies. The exception was a community-based program that was part of an acute care hospital. The number of staff members in each of the six programs varied considerably, ranging from three part-time positions to 10 full-time equivalent positions. Each of the FEP programs was developed in accordance with the guidelines and standards set forth by the International Early Psychosis Association and other pioneers in the field [17–20].

2.3. FEP Programs and Vocational Outcomes. There is evidence that compared to FEP clients who receive usual care, those enrolled in early intervention programs have significantly better educational and vocational outcomes [21]. The relatively better vocational outcomes associated with FEP programs may be associated with the shorter duration of untreated psychosis for these clients. Norman et al. [22] found that shorter duration of untreated psychosis and greater social support were significantly associated with either more full-time competitive work or full-time enrollment in school at three-year followup.

In their review, Rinaldi and colleagues [6] note that when compared to those enrolled in community mental health teams, clients enrolled in FEP program seem to experience a relatively smaller decline in employment and education. They attribute this to a protective role played by FEP programs. Major et al. [5] observed a decrease in unemployment among FEP clients after 12 months even in the absence of a vocational focus.

However, there is less evidence regarding the long-run outcomes for FEP programs versus usual care. After 18 months, the LEO (Lambeth Early Onset team) study did not find [21] a significant difference between clients in specialize programs versus those who were not. After 5 years, the OPUS trial did not find significant differences in employment between clients who were in FEP versus usual care [23].

2.4. Work History and Employment. In the literature focusing on vocational outcomes in the adult population with severe and persistent mental disorders, it has been observed that work history is one of the most consistent predictors of employment [24]. However, because of their stage in life, young adults experiencing their first psychotic episode have not had the opportunity to accumulate labor force experience. This can place FEP clients at a disadvantage in finding paid employment.

2.5. Educational Attainment and Employment. The literature also indicates that educational attainment is significantly related to employment status. People who have no high school diploma are more likely to be unemployed [25, 26]. If young people have their education interrupted by their illness, they can be faced with another disadvantage in finding employment.

2.6. Disability Benefits and Employment. There is also an association between receipt of disability benefits and unemployment [10, 27]. The fear of losing disability benefits has been identified as one of the barriers to obtaining and maintaining employment for clients with severe mental illness [3, 24, 28]. As a result, those who receive benefits often have poorer employment experiences.

Thus, there is accumulating evidence suggesting that in addition to treatment in FEP programs, socioeconomic factors such as educational attainment and income sources also play a role in employment outcomes. This type of evidence can help to inform future directions for the enhancement of psychosocial programs in FEP models.

3. Methods

3.1. Data Collection. The study protocol was approved by the Centre for Addiction and Mental Health's Research Ethics Board. A cross-sectional data collection approach was used at three points in time during October 2005, 2006, and 2007 in six FEP programs located throughout Ontario, Canada's largest and most populous province.

Interview participation criteria included (1) willingness to be contacted by a study interviewer, (2) ability to understand and give informed consent to be interviewed, and (3) enrollment in one of the six participating FEP programs. Data were collected using face-to-face structured interviews

Table 1: Characteristics of FEP clients who did and did not have paid employment during previous 12 months.

Characteristics	Had paid employment during the previous 12 months		Did not have paid employment during the previous 12 months		Statistical tests for differences between characteristics of employed and unemployed
	% or mean	*n* or sd	% or mean	*n* or sd	
Sex					
Male	70.2%	59	72.2%	39	$\chi^2(1) = 0.063, P = 0.80$
Female	29.8	25	27.8	15	
Age (in years)	23.3	sd = 5.13	21.93	sd = 3.98	t-test (136) = −1.62, $P = 0.11$
No high school diploma	24.1%	20	44.4%	24	$\chi^2(1) = 6.21, P = 0.013$
Population density of region of residence					
≤100 people/km^2	52.4%	44	48.2%	26	$\chi^2(1) = 0.24, P = 0.63$
200–450 people/km^2	38.1	32	24.1	13	$\chi^2(1) = 2.94, P = 0.086$
≥3,929 people/km^2	9.5	8	27.8	15	$\chi^2(1) = 7.89, P = 0.0050$
Living with family	66.7%	56	66.7%	36	$\chi^2(1) = 0.0, P = 1.0$
Enrolled in school during the past 12 months	52.4%	44	40.7%	22	$\chi^2(1) = 1.78, P = 0.18$
Provincial disability-benefits main source of income	17.7%	14	59.2%	29	$\chi^2(1) = 23.31, P < 0.001$
Enrolled in FEP program >1 year	37.8%	31	28.3%	15	$\chi^2(1) = 1.29, P = 0.26$

administered by trained interviewers. Potential study participants were referred by program case managers.

In 2005, the participating FEP programs referred 45 clients (28%) of the total 161 enrolled, to be contacted by the study; of these, 33 (73%) were successfully interviewed. They represented 20% of the total clients enrolled. In 2006, 106 (32%) of 302 early intervention clients were eligible to be contacted by the study. There were 75 (71%) who were successfully interviewed. They represented 25% of the total clients. In 2007, 162 (44%) of 370 early intervention clients were eligible to be contacted for interviews. Of these, 107 (66%) were successfully interviewed. These clients constituted 29% of the total early intervention clients enrolled in the six programs.

3.2. Dependent Variable. An indicator variable was created to capture whether or not study participants had paid employment during the previous 12 months.

3.3. Study Participant Characteristics. Indicator variables were created to capture whether the respondent was living with family (i.e., parent(s), sibling(s), and spouse), education (completed high school: yes/no), gender (male: yes/no), age at time of interview, receipt of provincial disability benefits as the primary income source (yes/no) and enrolled in school during the previous 12 months (yes/no). An indicator variable was also created to capture whether participants were enrolled in their FEP program for more than a year.

Three region indicator variables were created to capture the population density of the region in which the participant lived. Region 1 indicated that the participant resided in a region in which the population density was less than 100 people/km^2. Region 2 indicated that the region of residence had a population density between 200 and 450 people/km^2. Finally, Region 3 indicated that the region of residence had 3,929 people/km^2.

3.4. Analyses. Descriptive statistics were used to test for significant differences in the characteristics of people who had paid employment during the previous 12 months. Chi-square and Fisher exact tests were used to test the differences between the categorical variables.

Logistic regression analysis was used to identify the factors associated with having had paid employment. The most parsimonious model was used based on the factors described in the literature that are associated with employment for people with serious mental illnesses.

4. Results

About 61% of the sample had paid employment during the previous 12 months. In Table 1, compared to those who did not have employment, among those who had employment, there was a significantly greater proportion of people with at least a high school diploma ($\chi^2(2) = 6.21$, $P = 0.013$) and a significantly lower proportion who identified provincial disability benefits as their primary income source ($\chi^2(2) = 23.31$, $P < 0.0001$).

Table 2 contains the results of the logistic regression analysis. The regression model produced 83.2% concordant and 16.6% discordant predicted probabilities and observed responses. The Hosmer and Lemeshow Goodness-of-Fit Test

Table 2: Logistic regression results: outcome = paid employment during past 12 months.

Variables	Odds ratio	P value
Male (reference group: females)	0.78	0.64
Age (in years)	1.12	0.10
No high school diploma (reference group: has high school diploma)	0.34	0.045
Population density of region of residence (Reference group: <100 people/km^2)		
200–450/km^2	2.73	0.062
≥3,929/km^2	1.21	0.78
Living with family (reference group: not living with family)	0.46	0.15
Enrolled in school during the past 12 months (reference group: not enrolled in school in past 12 months)	1.29	0.62
Provincial disability-benefits main source of income (reference group: provincial disability benefits not main source of income)	0.069	<0.0001
Enrolled in FEP program >1 year (Reference group: enrolled in FEP program ≤1 year)	3.014	0.045
$\chi^2(9) = 44.32, P < 0.0001$		
$R^2 = 0.30$		
$n = 124$		

was $\chi^2(8) = 10.99$, $P = 0.202$. These results indicate that the null hypothesis cannot be rejected; the model fits the data and the model has adequate goodness-of-fit.

The results suggest that the odds of having been employed in the past 12 months are significantly lower for people who have not completed high school (OR = 0.34, 95% CI = 0.12, 0.97) and for clients who identified provincial disability benefits as their primary income source (OR = 0.069, 95% CI = 0.022, 0.21). There is also a significant positive association between employment and being enrolled in the FEP program for more than a year (OR = 3.014, 95% CI = 1.027, 8.85).

5. Discussion

In our sample, 61% of respondents had paid employment during the previous 12 months. This proportion is greater than that reported in the literature. For example, Singh et al. [29] observed that among the cohort of FEP clients, the past year employment rate (either full or part time) was 31.3%. Similarly, Norman et al. [22] reported employment rates of 44%, while Turner et al. [30] reported an employment rate of 46%.

We also observed a significant difference between the educational attainment of those who were employed and those who were not. Educational attainment is a significant concern among FEP clients [10, 11]. Norman et al. [22] observed that 46% of clients in their sample had attained less than a high school education at time of program entry. Assessing the three-year outcomes of FEP clients, Singh et al. [29] reported that 53.6% participants had not attained their secondary education certificates.

Our regression results underscore one of the major problems associated with the lack of educational attainment; educational attainment is associated with the ability to attain employment. Our results indicate that those who did not complete high school were less likely to be employed. This association corroborates what has been reported in literature [5, 31]. These results echo the need highlighted by Cook [32] in her review of the literature that a significant proportion of people with serious and persistent mental disorders have their education interrupted by the onset of mental disorders. That is, people with severe mental illness are likely to have lower educational attainment than their counterparts who have not experienced a mental disorder. In turn, this places them at a disadvantage to successfully compete in the labor market.

One of the arguments for early labour market participation is because of its effect on future employment. In their longitudinal study of people with severe mental illness, Bush and colleagues [33] found that those who were employed at the beginning of a 10-year period were more likely to remain steadily employed throughout. In contrast, those who were not employed at the beginning were more likely to remain unemployed throughout the period. It should be noted that Bush et al. [33] looked at a group of people with severe mental illness. It will be important for future studies to examine effects of early employment in the FEP population.

Our regression results also indicate that enrollment in a FEP program for more than a year is significantly associated with employment. That is, clients who have been enrolled in a FEP program for more than a year are three times more likely to have been employed during the year than clients who were enrolled for less than a year. This is a trend that has been reported in the literature. After a three-year followup of FEP clients, Singh et al. [29] saw past 12-month employment rates increase from 25.3% at intake to 31.3% at followup. This could be reflective of the protective effect provided by FEP programs [6].

None of the FEP programs that participated in this study had vocational specialists. This suggests that vocational outcomes were not necessarily one of the main foci of the programs. Yet, there was improvement in vocational outcomes. At the same time, compared to FEP programs without a vocational focus, those with IPS programs and vocational specialists have reported relatively better vocational outcomes [4, 6, 10–13]. Thus, although FEP programs appear to provide a protective effect, there is evidence that with a vocational focus, they can be more than protective.

Finally, these results suggest that enrolment in a public disability benefit program also decreases the likelihood of being employed. Our results may reflect the fact that the people who receive disability benefits are too ill to be employed. Alternatively, the results could also be related to incentives associated with receipt of disability benefits. In her review of the literature, Cook [32] points out that few people leave public disability benefits due to employment. Our finding corroborates findings that disability benefits are inversely associated with employment rates. That is, as disability benefit levels decrease, employment rates increase, and the use of unemployment benefits decreases [34]. This suggests that publicly funded benefits may inadvertently create disincentives to work. For example, people might perceive that they will be penalized for working. In Ontario, the province in which this study was conducted, when people are employed and also receive benefits from the provincial disability support program, the program calculates half of the client's net monthly earnings, deducts part or all of his/her monthly child care and disability-related work costs, and subtracts this amount from the client's total income support [35]. Although in theory the earned income should substitute for income support, people who receive disability benefits and who work will see their disability income support decreased but not necessarily associate the decrease with their pay check.

At the same time, the provincial disability benefit program also seeks to create an incentive for paid employment by offering clients an additional monthly $100 work-related benefit [35] if they are employed in a paid position. Yet, the incentive to work may not be sufficient if people are unsure about their long-term ability to maintain employment. There may still be a fear that if they lose their disability benefits, they will be without a safety net if they lose their jobs [36–38]. It will be important for future research to explore the mechanisms of designing safety nets that ensure that when people are unable to work, they will have income while encouraging employment when it is possible. It will also be a challenge for FEP programs to design programs that help clients to receive training for jobs in business sectors in which they can earn a living wage [32] and that can accommodate episodes of illness so clients can accumulate successful employment histories.

Limitations. The results of this study should be considered in the light of its limitations. One of its major limitations relates to its generalizability. The clients who participated in these interviews may not necessarily be representative of all clients in FEP programs. Given that only clients who were able to provide informed consent were asked to participate, those who were the most sick would have been omitted. Thus, our results are a conservative estimate of the proportion who were unemployed if the most severely ill were more likely to be unemployed. Likewise, the regression results reflect associations for less severely ill people and may differ for the more severely ill; however, the latter group may also be less likely to be seeking employment.

In addition, the sample only included people who were enrolled in early intervention for psychosis programs. Results may be different for people experiencing their first psychotic episode who do not receive services from a program specializing in first psychotic episode cases.

6. Conclusions

There is little in the literature focusing on employment in the FEP population examining the contribution of socioeconomic factors to employment status. The results of our analyses indicate that receipt of public disability benefits and high school education are important factors related to employment. They also suggest that if paid employment is to be used as one measure of psychosocial outcomes, it is an outcome that may require cross-sector collaboration among health, education, and social services.

Acknowledgments

The authors are grateful for the excellent research assistance provided by the Matryoshka Coordinating team as well as all the interviewers and the Centre for Addiction and Mental Health's regional staff. The authors would also like to gratefully acknowledge the participation of the programs and interview participants who supported this project and who were willing to so generously share their experiences with them. This paper has also greatly benefited from the comments and suggestions of the anonymous reviewers. This project was funded by the Ontario Mental Health Foundation and the Social Sciences and Humanities Research Council of Canada. C. S. Dewa also gratefully acknowledges the support provided by her CIHR/PHAC Applied Public Health Chair. The Centre for Addiction and Mental Health receives funding from the Ontario Ministry of Health and Long-Term Care to support research infrastructure. Any remaining errors are the sole responsibility of the authors and do not reflect the views of any of the funders.

References

[1] W. Löffler and H. Häfner, "Ecological pattern of first admitted schizophrenics in two German cities over 25 years," *Social Science and Medicine*, vol. 49, no. 1, pp. 93–108, 1999.

[2] J. O. Johannessen, T. H. McGlashan, T. K. Larsen et al., "Early detection strategies for untreated first-episode psychosis," *Schizophrenia Research*, vol. 51, no. 1, pp. 39–46, 2001.

[3] S. Marwaha and S. Johnson, "Schizophrenia and employment: a review," *Social Psychiatry and Psychiatric Epidemiology*, vol. 39, no. 5, pp. 337–349, 2004.

[4] M. Rinaldi, K. McNeil, M. Firn, M. Koletsi, R. Perkins, and S. P. Singh, "What are the benefits of evidence-based supported

employment for patients with first-episode psychosis?" *Psychiatric Bulletin*, vol. 28, no. 8, pp. 281–284, 2004.

[5] B. S. Major, M. F. Hinton, A. Flint, A. Chalmers-Brown, K. McLoughlin, and S. Johnson, "Evidence of the effectiveness of a specialist vocational intervention following first episode psychosis: a naturalistic prospective cohort study," *Social Psychiatry and Psychiatric Epidemiology*, vol. 45, no. 1, pp. 1–8, 2010.

[6] M. Rinaldi, E. Killackey, J. Smith, G. Shepherd, S. P. Singh, and T. Craig, "First episode psychosis and employment: a review," *International Review of Psychiatry*, vol. 22, no. 2, pp. 148–162, 2010.

[7] A. D. Henry and A. M. Lucca, "Facilitators and barriers to employment: the perspectives of people with psychiatric disabilities and employment service providers," *Work*, vol. 22, no. 3, pp. 169–182, 2004.

[8] K. T. Mueser, R. E. Clark, M. Haines et al., "The Hartford study of supported employment for persons with severe mental illness," *Journal of Consulting and Clinical Psychology*, vol. 72, no. 3, pp. 479–490, 2004.

[9] S. R. McGurk and K. T. Mueser, "Cognitive functioning, symptoms, and work in supported employment: a review and heuristic model," *Schizophrenia Research*, vol. 70, no. 2-3, pp. 147–173, 2004.

[10] E. J. Killackey, H. J. Jackson, J. Gleeson, I. B. Hickie, and P. D. McGorry, "Exciting career opportunity beckons! Early intervention and vocational rehabilitation in first-episode psychosis: employing cautious optimism," *Australian and New Zealand Journal of Psychiatry*, vol. 40, no. 11-12, pp. 951–962, 2006.

[11] K. H. Nuechterlein, K. L. Subotnik, L. R. Turner, J. Ventura, D. R. Becker, and R. E. Drake, "Individual placement and support for individuals with recent-onset schizophrenia: integrating supported education and supported employment," *Psychiatric Rehabilitation Journal*, vol. 31, no. 4, pp. 340–349, 2008.

[12] M. Rinaldi, R. Perkins, E. Glynn, T. Montibeller, M. Clenaghan, and J. Rutherford, "Individual placement and support: from research to practice," *Advances in Psychiatric Treatment*, vol. 14, no. 1, pp. 50–60, 2008.

[13] E. Killackey, H. J. Jackson, and P. D. McGorry, "Vocational intervention in first-episode psychosis: individual placement and support v. treatment as usual," *British Journal of Psychiatry*, vol. 193, no. 2, pp. 114–120, 2008.

[14] E. Killackey, "Meaningful lives: supporting young people with psychosis in education, training and employment: an international consensus statement," *Early Intervention in Psychiatry*, vol. 4, no. 4, pp. 323–326, 2010.

[15] S. Marwaha and S. Johnson, "Views and experiences of employment among people with psychosis: a qualitative descriptive study," *International Journal of Social Psychiatry*, vol. 51, no. 4, pp. 302–316, 2005.

[16] G. R. Bond, D. R. Becker, R. E. Drake et al., "Implementing supported employment as an evidence-based practice," *Psychiatric Services*, vol. 52, no. 3, pp. 313–322, 2001.

[17] Ontario Ministry of Health and Long-Term Care, *Early Psychosis Intervention Program Standards*, Ontario Ministry of Health and Long-Term Care, Toronto, Canada, 2011.

[18] J. Bertolote and P. McGorry, "Early intervention and recovery for young people with early psychosis: consensus statement," *British Journal of Psychiatry*, vol. 187, no. 48, pp. s116–s119, 2005.

[19] J. Edwards and P. McGorry, "Developing an early psychosis service—'nuts and bolts'," in *Implementing Early Intervention in Psychosis: A Guide to Establishing Early Psychosis Services*, J. Edwards and P. McGorry, Eds., pp. 85–106, Martin Dunitz, London, UK, 2002.

[20] International Early Psychosis Association Writing Group, "International clinical practice guidelines for early psychosis," *British Journal of Psychiatry*, vol. 187, pp. 120–124, 2005.

[21] P. A. Garety, T. K. J. Craig, G. Dunn et al., "Specialised care for early psychosis: symptoms, social functioning and patient satisfaction—randomised controlled trial," *British Journal of Psychiatry*, vol. 188, pp. 37–45, 2006.

[22] R. M. G. Norman, A. K. Mallal, R. Manchanda et al., "Does treatment delay predict occupational functioning in first-episode psychosis?" *Schizophrenia Research*, vol. 91, no. 1–3, pp. 259–262, 2007.

[23] M. Bertelsen, P. Jeppesen, L. Petersen et al., "Five-year follow-up of a randomized multicenter trial of intensive early intervention versus standard treatment for patients with a first episode of psychotic illness : the OPUS trial," *Archives of General Psychiatry*, vol. 65, no. 7, pp. 762–771, 2008.

[24] K. Campbell, G. R. Bond, R. E. Drake, G. J. McHugo, and H. Xie, "Client predictors of employment outcomes in high-fidelity supported employment: a regression analysis," *Journal of Nervous and Mental Disease*, vol. 198, no. 8, pp. 556–563, 2010.

[25] L. Harvey, "New realities: the relationship between higher education and employment," *Tertiary Education and Management*, vol. 6, no. 1, pp. 3–17, 2000.

[26] Statistics Canada, *Employment Rates, Educational Attainment*, Statistics Canada, Ottawa, Canada, 2010.

[27] B. C. Ho, N. Andreasen, and M. Flaum, "Dependence on public financial support early in the course of schizophrenia," *Psychiatric Services*, vol. 48, no. 7, pp. 948–950, 1997.

[28] M. McQuilken, J. H. Zahniser, J. Novak, R. D. Starks, A. Olmos, and G. R. Bond, "The work project survey: consumer perspective on work," *Journal of Vocational Rehabilitation*, vol. 18, no. 1, pp. 59–68, 2003.

[29] S. P. Singh, T. Croudace, S. Amin et al., "Three-year outcome of first-episode psychoses in an established community psychiatric service," *British Journal of Psychiatry*, vol. 176, pp. 210–216, 2000.

[30] N. Turner, S. Browne, M. Clarke et al., "Employment status amongst those with psychosis at first presentation," *Social Psychiatry and Psychiatric Epidemiology*, vol. 44, no. 10, pp. 863–869, 2009.

[31] G. Waghorn, D. Chant, and H. Whiteford, "The strength of self-reported course of illness in predicting vocational recovery for persons with schizophrenia," *Journal of Vocational Rehabilitation*, vol. 18, no. 1, pp. 33–41, 2003.

[32] J. A. Cook, "Employment barriers for persons with psychiatric disabilities: update of a report for the president's commission," *Psychiatric Services*, vol. 57, no. 10, pp. 1391–1405, 2006.

[33] P. W. Bush, R. E. Drake, H. Xie, G. J. McHugo, and W. R. Haslett, "The long-term impact of employment on mental health service use and costs for persons with severe mental illness," *Psychiatric Services*, vol. 60, no. 8, pp. 1024–1031, 2009.

[34] E. Westerhout, "Disability risk, disability benefits, and equilibrium unemployment," *International Tax and Public Finance*, vol. 8, no. 3, pp. 219–243, 2001.

[35] Ontario Ministry of Community and Social Services, *Ontario Disability Benefits*, Ontario Ministry of Community and Social Services, Toronto, Canada, 2010.

[36] C. S. Dewa and D. McDaid, "Investing in the mental health of the labor force: epidemiological and economic impact of mental disorders in the workplace," in *Handbook of Job*

Accomodation on Mental Health, I. Schultz and E. Rogers, Eds., Springer, New York, NY, USA, 2009.

[37] K. L. MacDonald-Wilson, E. S. Rogers, M. L. Ellison, and A. Lyass, "A study of the social security work incentives and their relation to perceived barriers to work among persons with psychiatric disability," *Rehabilitation Psychology*, vol. 48, no. 4, pp. 301–309, 2003.

[38] S. Magura, "The role of work in substance dependency treatment: a preliminary overview," *Substance Use and Misuse*, vol. 38, no. 11–13, pp. 1865–1876, 2003.

11

Do People with Schizophrenia Lack Emotional Intelligence?

Sara Dawson,[1] Lisa Kettler,[1] Cassandra Burton,[2] and Cherrie Galletly[2,3,4,5]

[1] *School of Psychology, The University of Adelaide, Adelaide, SA 5000, Australia*
[2] *The Adelaide Clinic, Ramsay Health Care (SA) Mental Health Services, Gilberton, SA 5000, Australia*
[3] *Discipline of Psychiatry, School of Medicine, The University of Adelaide, Adelaide, SA 5000, Australia*
[4] *Northern Mental Health, Adelaide Metro Mental Health Directorate, Adelaide, SA 5000, Australia*
[5] *The Adelaide Clinic Consulting Suites, 33 Park Terrace, Gilberton, SA 5081, Australia*

Correspondence should be addressed to Cherrie Galletly, cherrie.galletly@adelaide.edu.au

Academic Editor: Robin Emsley

Social cognition is a domain of cognitive function that includes the ability to understand and manage social interactions. Emotional intelligence (EI) has been identified as a component of social cognition and is defined as the ability to identify, use, understand, and manage emotions. Neurocognitive impairments are known to be associated with poorer social function in people with schizophrenia, but less is known about the relationships between EI, neurocognition, and social function. The current study assessed EI using the Mayer-Salovey-Caruso Emotional Intelligence Test (MSCEIT) in 20 people with schizophrenia and 20 controls. The schizophrenia group had significantly lower scores on all measures of EI and demonstrated poorer neurocognition and social functioning than controls. The difference between schizophrenia and control groups was greatest for the Understanding Emotions Branch of the MSCEIT. The neurocognition score and total EI score accounted for 18.3% of the variance in social function in the control group and 9.1% of the variance in social function in the schizophrenia group. Our results suggest that a total EI score is not a useful predictor of overall social function and it may be more clinically useful to develop an individual profile of social cognitive abilities, including EI, to form a remediation program.

1. Introduction

Social cognition refers to aspects of cognition that are critical for social functioning and interpersonal relationships, such as accurate perception of the emotions of others, the ability to recognize important social cues, theory of mind (TOM), and the management of emotions in social situations [1]. Various components of social cognition have been found to be impaired in people with schizophrenia [2, 3]. Impaired social cognition may also be a risk factor for psychosis—Kim et al. [4] reported that poor performance on social cognition tasks was associated with higher rates of transition to psychosis in young people who were at ultra-high risk of psychosis.

Emotional intelligence (EI) is an important component of social cognition [5, 6]. EI is defined as the ability to process, understand, and manage emotions. EI is most commonly assessed using the Mayer-Salovey-Caruso Emotional Intelligence Test, Version 2.0 (MSCEIT) [7, 8]. Mayer and Salovey [6] identified four components (termed Branches) of EI. The four Branches are Identifying Emotions (the perception of emotion in the self and others); Facilitating or Using Emotions (the capacity to use and generate emotions, and to use emotions in cognitive tasks such as problem-solving and creativity); Understanding Emotions (the ability to comprehend complex information about emotions, including changes or degrees of emotion); and Managing Emotions (the ability to regulate emotions in ourselves and others, and use this information effectively in social interactions).

The MSCEIT has been widely used in normal populations and has been shown to have good face and content validity [8]. Factor analysis, utilising data from almost 2000 subjects, strongly supports the four-branch model of EI [8]. Higher levels of EI have been shown to be associated with better social engagement and quality of social interaction [9]. People with higher levels of EI are less likely to engage in aggressive behaviour and are less likely to use tobacco or drink excessively [10, 11]. Several studies have demonstrated small but positive correlations between EI and general intelligence [7, 12]. These findings suggest that EI is a useful construct that is reliably associated with real world functioning in normal subjects.

The National Institute of Mental Health Measurement and Treatment Research to Improve Cognition in Schizophrenia (MATRICS) initiative evaluated a number of tests of social cognition and selected the Managing Emotions branch of the MSCEIT for inclusion in the final MATRICS Consensus Cognitive Battery (MCCB) [13]. The MCCB, including the social cognition domain, has since been used extensively [14]. Whilst the Managing Emotions branch of the MSCEIT is widely used as part of the MCCB, there have been only two previous studies utilising the full MSCEIT battery in people with schizophrenia [15, 16]. Eack et al. [15] found that the MSCEIT has adequate internal consistency and reliability in people with schizophrenia. Kee et al. [16] reported that people with schizophrenia had lower total MSCEIT scores compared to controls, with significantly worse performance on the Identifying, Understanding, and Managing Emotions Branches of the MSCEIT.

Many people with schizophrenia experience difficulties in social functioning, including problems with independent living, employment, and interpersonal relationships [17]. Whilst negative symptoms and cognitive impairment have long been known to correlate with social outcomes, these associations are modest and do not explain all of the difficulties in social functioning evident in schizophrenia [18]. Recent research has addressed the possibility that impaired social cognition might also contribute to poor functional outcome. Brüne et al. [19] administered tests of general intelligence, executive function, mental state attribution, symptoms, and social behaviour to 38 people with schizophrenia. Mental state attribution scores accounted for almost half of the variance in social function. Similarly, a meta-analysis by Fett et al. [20] showed that social cognition accounted for 23% of the variance in functional outcome in schizophrenia. However, there has been less research specifically investigating the contribution of EI to social outcome. If EI is found to make a significant contribution to social function, interventions designed to remediate deficits in EI may improve outcomes for people with schizophrenia.

Kee et al. [16] assessed 50 people with schizophrenia using the MSCEIT. They found modest correlations between all Branches of the MSCEIT and independent living/self-care; between Identifying Emotions (Branch 1) and work productivity, relationships with family and spouse, and psychosocial adjustment and between Understanding Emotions (Branch 3) and psychosocial adjustment. Eack et al. [15] reported a significant association between total MSCEIT scores and the major role functioning subscale of the Social Adjustment Scale in 64 people with schizophrenia, but otherwise there was little relationship between MSCEIT scores and objective measures of functional outcome. A subgroup of these subjects undertook two years of intensive therapy designed to improve social cognition, attention, and memory. Improvements in Managing Emotions (Branch 4) of the MSCEIT were associated with improvements in functional outcome [21]. Improved neurocognition, and in particular improved executive function, was found to mediate the effects of cognitive enhancement therapy on functioning.

We developed a pilot study which compared EI, measured using the MSCEIT Version 2.0, in 20 people with schizophrenia and 20 controls matched for age, gender, and years of education. We assessed neurocognition and social functioning in both groups, and investigated the relationships between EI, neurocognition, and social functioning. We expected that total EI scores, as well as subscale (Branch) scores, would be significantly lower in the schizophrenia group compared to the control group. Specifically, it was hypothesised that after controlling for neurocognition, a significant positive correlation would be observed between EI and social functioning in both the schizophrenia and control groups. Given that a relationship between the Managing Emotions Branch (Branch 4) of the MSCEIT and social function has been demonstrated in previous studies [13, 21] we hypothesised that this particular branch of the MSCEIT would be most strongly associated with social function in our subjects with schizophrenia.

2. Methods

2.1. Participants. Twenty people meeting the diagnostic criteria for schizophrenia (DSM-IV-TR) [22] were recruited from public mental health services across metropolitan Adelaide, South Australia. The schizophrenia group were outpatients, living in the community, taking maintenance antipsychotic medication, and considered clinically stable by their treating clinicians. Control subjects matched by age, gender, and years of education were recruited by radio advertising. Potential control subjects were assessed using the Mini International Neuropsychiatric Interview (M.I.N.I) [23] and excluded if any symptoms of psychosis were present.

All subjects spoke fluent English and were screened for current major depression, alcohol abuse and dependence, and substance use disorders by a trained clinician, using the M.I.N.I [23]. They were excluded if these disorders were present. Other exclusion criteria for both groups included intellectual disability or neurological conditions that could interfere with psychological or cognitive functioning.

All subjects gave written informed consent after the study had been fully explained. The study was reviewed and approved by the Central Northern Adelaide Health Service Ethics of Human Research Committee and the University of Adelaide, School of Psychology Human Ethics Subcommittee. This research was carried out in accordance with the latest version of the Declaration of Helsinki.

2.2. Measures. Participants attended individual testing sessions that lasted for two to three hours. Demographic data was collected and screening measures administered. Participants who were eligible to participate in the study completed the measures of EI, neurocognition, and social functioning.

2.2.1. Emotional Intelligence Was Measured Using the MSCEIT V2.0 [8]. The MSCEIT is a self-administered test which consists of 8 tasks based on 141 items, with two tasks forming a single branch. Tasks range from identifying emotion in human faces to identifying strategies to manage emotions in social situations. The MSCEIT V2.0 provides an overall EI quotient and four subscale (Branch) scores.

(1) Identifying Emotions (Branch 1) refers to an individual's ability to recognise how they and those around them are feeling [24]. This involves attending to and decoding emotional signals in other people's facial expressions, tone of voice, or posture as well as the ability to accurately identify emotions within oneself.

(2) Using Emotions (Branch 2) includes an individual's knowledge of the link between emotions and thinking, and the ability to take feelings into account when reasoning and problem solving [24, 25].

(3) Understanding Emotions (Branch 3) refers to an individual's capacity to analyse emotions, appreciate their probable trends over time, and to understand their outcomes [25]. This includes the ability to recognise groups of related emotional terms and to understand the antecedents of different emotions, for example, that irritation and frustration might lead to anger [24].

(4) Managing Emotions (Branch 4) includes the knowledge that it is adaptive to regulate emotions to facilitate positive social interactions [24, 25].

There are two methods of scoring the MSCEIT V2.0 described in the literature. Responses can be scored according to either the general or the expert consensus method, where scores for each response are weighted according to either the proportion of a general population sample or the proportion of a panel of emotion experts that endorsed the same response [25]. For the current study, the expert consensus weighted scores were used to ensure that higher scores represented superior levels of EI [25].

2.2.2. Premorbid Intelligence Was Estimated Using the National Adult Reading Test (NART). (See [26].)

2.2.3. Current Neurocognitive Functioning Was Assessed Using the Brief Assessment of Cognition in Schizophrenia (BACS) [27, 28]. The BACS includes assessments of verbal memory and learning, working memory, motor function, verbal fluency, and executive function [27]. BACS scores were converted to Z scores for statistical analysis [28].

2.2.4. Social Functioning Was Assessed Using the Social Functioning Scale (SFS) [29]. The SFS is a 79-item scale which measures seven major domains of functioning thought to be crucial for successful community living for individuals with schizophrenia.

2.3. Statistical Analysis. Independent-samples t-tests were used to compare total EI scores, the scores on each Branch of the MSCEIT V2.0, and total BACS and SFS scores for the two groups. Pearson's bivariate correlations were used to determine the correlation between MSCEIT V2.0, BACS, and SFS scores for each group.

Separate linear regression analyses were performed to examine the relationship between MSCEIT V2.0 and SFS scores in each study group, with BACS scores as a potential mediator variable. To examine the relationships between variables, the following regression analyses were conducted.

(1) The potential mediator variable (BACS score) was regressed on the independent variable (MSCEIT V2.0 score);

(2) the dependent variable (SFS score) was regressed on the independent variable (MSCEIT V2.0 score);

(3) the dependent variable (SFS scores) was regressed on the potential mediator variable (BACS scores).

To further examine the relationship between EI and social functioning, multiple regressions were performed for each group. SFS scores were entered as the dependent variable in each analysis. To test whether any relationship between MSCEIT V2.0 and SFS scores was mediated by BACS scores, BACS scores were entered at Step 1 and total MSCEIT V2.0 scores were entered at Step 2.

We found that the schizophrenia group had greatest impairment on the Understanding Emotions Branch of the MSCEIT V2.0. Exploratory post hoc analyses, using Pearson's bivariate correlations, were undertaken to evaluate the correlations between scores on the Understanding Emotions Branch of the MSCEIT V2.0 and total and subscale scores on the BACS and the SFS. We expected that in the schizophrenia group, lower Understanding Emotions (Branch 3) MSCEIT V2.0 scores would be associated with poorer cognitive and social functioning, with a P value of less than 0.01 accepted as significant.

There was a significant difference in premorbid intelligence scores between groups; therefore, a post hoc ANCOVA was performed to determine differences in MSCEIT V2.0 scores between groups with NART scores as a covariate.

3. Results

Demographic characteristics are described in Table 1. The control group scored significantly better than the schizophrenia group on the NART.

Differences between the schizophrenia and the control group on measures of EI, neurocognition, and social function are presented in Table 2. The schizophrenia group had significantly lower scores than controls on all subscales of the MSCEIT V2.0. The greatest difference was found on Understanding Emotions (Branch 3). A post hoc ANCOVA with calculation of effect size showed that 12% of the difference in MSCEIT scores was explained by premorbid intelligence whilst 24% was explained by group (schizophrenia or control).

The schizophrenia group also had significantly lower scores on all of the BACS subtests. Their scores were lower than controls on all components of the SFS, and these

TABLE 1: Participant demographic and clinical characteristics.

Variable	Schizophrenia		Controls		t	Cohen's d	P
	N	Mean (SD)	N	Mean (SD)			
Age	20	43.25 (9.15)	20	38.60 (10.86)	1.47	0.46	0.15
NART score	20	107.45 (6.90)	20	114.00 (4.30)	−3.82	1.14	<0.001***
Age of illness onset	19	23.63 (7.52)					
Duration of illness (years)	19	19.42 (9.90)					
Education (years)	20	12.50 (1.99)	20	14.80 (2.50)	−3.22	1.02	0.19
	N	%	N	%		χ^2	P
Gender							
Male	10	50	10	50			
Female	10	50	10	50			
Marital status							
Married	3	15	9	45			
In relationship	3	15	4	20			
Single	14	70	7	35		5.48	0.07

***Indicates $P < 0.001$.

TABLE 2: MSCEIT, BACS, and SFS scores for schizophrenia and control groups.

	Schizophrenia mean (SD)	Control mean (SD)	t	95% CI	Cohen's d	P
MSCEIT scores						
Branch 1—Perceiving emotions	98.98 (15.57)	110.98 (14.16)	−2.55	−21.53, −2.48	0.81	0.02*
Branch 2—Using emotions	96.14 (14.53)	107.50 (15.79)	−2.37	−21.07, −1.64	0.75	0.02*
Branch 3—Understanding emotions	81.80 (11.63)	105.70 (12.59)	−6.23	−31.66, −16.14	1.97	<0.001***
Branch 4—Managing emotions	90.75 (12.41)	101.06 (14.74)	−2.39	−19.03, −1.59	0.76	0.02*
MSCEIT global score	86.15 (11.81)	109.45 (14.46)	−5.58	−31.76, −14.85	1.77	<0.001***
BACS Scores						
Verbal memory	−2.16 (1.39)	−0.20 (1.02)	−5.09	−2.75, −1.18	1.92	<0.001***
Digit sequencing	−0.41 (0.77)	0.54 (0.51)	−4.63	−1.37, −0.54	1.86	<0.001***
Token motor task	−1.21 (1.31)	−0.03 (0.68)	−3.58	−1.86, −0.51	1.74	0.001*
Verbal fluency	−0.55 (0.97)	0.62 (0.69)	−4.41	−1.71, −0.63	1.70	<0.001***
Symbol coding	−0.88 (0.45)	0.45 (0.59)	−7.97	−1.66, −0.99	2.25	<0.001***
Tower of london	−0.49 (1.04)	0.61 (0.74)	−3.82	−1.68, −0.51	1.49	0.001*
BACS total Z score	−1.32 (0.93)	0.52 (0.66)	−5.09	−2.36, −1.32	2.28	<0.001***
SFS scores						
Withdrawal/social engagement	106.18 (11.60)	111.58 (12.41)	−1.42	−13.09, 2.29	0.44	0.163
Interpersonal communication	123.95 (19.56)	137.40 (12.40)	−2.60	−24.00, −2.90	1.08	0.014*
Independence performance	107.53 (7.70)	119.80 (7.53)	−5.10	−17.15, −7.40	1.63	<0.001***
Independence competence	111.85 (7.44)	121.13 (4.02)	−4.90	−13.14, −5.40	2.31	<0.001***
Recreation	100.39 (26.63)	124.00 (11.66)	−3.63	−36.77, −10.45	2.02	0.001**
Prosocial	101.13 (15.38)	114.28 (27.23)	−1.88	−27.31, 1.01	0.48	0.068
Employment/occupation	106.43 (15.34)	119.85 (3.79)	−3.80	−20.76, −6.09	3.54	0.001**
SFS total score	108.21 (8.03)	121.80 (6.57)	−5.86	−18.28, −8.89	1.85	<0.001***

*Indicates $P < 0.05$, **indicates $P < 0.01$, ***indicates $P < 0.001$.

differences reached significance for five of the seven domains of social functioning.

The schizophrenia group did not show any significant correlation between MSCEIT V2.0, BACS, and SFS total scores (Table 3). The Understanding Emotions Branch of the MSCEIT V2.0 was significantly correlated with the BACS Total Z score, SFS independent performance score and the total SFS score. Managing Emotions (Branch 4) correlated with the SFS Recreation score. In addition, the BACS Total Z score correlated with the SFS Interpersonal Communication score.

In the control group, Using Emotions (Branch 2), Managing Emotions (Branch 4), and the total MSCEIT V2.0 score all correlated with the SFS withdrawal/social engagement subscale. Managing Emotions (Branch 4) also correlated with the total SFS score.

Table 3: Bivariate correlations for MSCEIT, BACS, and SFS scores.

	Perceiving emotions (Branch 1)	Using emotions (Branch 2)	Understanding emotions (Branch 3)	Managing emotions (Branch 4)	Global EI score	BACS total Z score
Schizophrenia Group						
BACS total Z score	−0.06	−0.08	0.52*	0.14	0.26	
SFS Withdrawal/social engagement score	−0.09	−0.11	−0.03	0.01	−0.09	−0.09
SFS interpersonal communication score	−0.20	−0.21	0.18	0.03	−0.04	0.48**
SFS independence performance score	−0.08	−0.04	0.44*	0.14	0.16	−0.02
SFS independence competence Score	0.09	0.21	0.31	0.32	0.32	0.07
SFS recreation score	−0.40	−0.43	−0.10	−0.60**	0.54*	−0.14
SFS prosocial score	−0.35	0.05	0.41	0.17	0.05	0.36
SFS occupation/employment score	−0.38	−0.20	0.15	0.18	−0.13	0.25
SFS total score	−0.18	−0.03	0.48*	0.25	0.02	0.28
Control group						
BACS Total Z Score	−0.16	0.12	0.38	0.28	0.17	
SFS withdrawal/social engagement score	0.27	0.65**	0.42	0.50*	0.57**	0.15
SFS interpersonal communication score	−0.21	0.34	0.35	0.30	0.23	0.15
SFS independence performance score	−0.26	0.29	0.28	0.14	0.14	−0.11
SFS independence competence score	−0.14	0.21	0.28	0.02	0.06	−0.16
SFS recreation score	0.00	0.27	−0.02	0.18	0.12	−0.07
SFS prosocial score	0.00	0.32	0.28	0.31	0.28	0.34
SFS occupation/employment score	−0.27	−0.02	0.06	−0.04	−0.10	−0.10
SFS total score	0.01	0.53**	0.29	0.50*	0.41	0.18

*Indicates $P < 0.05$, **indicates $P < 0.01$.

Regression analyses for the schizophrenia group revealed that total MSCEIT V2.0 scores were not a significant predictor of total BACS scores ($b = 0.26$, $P = 0.28$), with total MSCEIT V2.0 scores accounting for just 6.6% of the variance in total BACS scores. In addition, neither total MSCEIT V2.0 scores ($b = 0.18$, $P = 0.45$) nor total BACS scores ($b = 0.28$, $P = 0.23$) were significant predictors of total SFS scores, with each explaining just 7.9% and 3.2% of the variance in social functioning, respectively.

Together, the total BACS and MSCEIT V2.0 scores accounted for just 9.1% of the variance in the total SFS scores. In addition, once total BACS scores were statistically controlled for, total MSCEIT V2.0 scores accounted for just 1.2% of the variance in the total SFS scores ($b = 0.12$, $P = 0.64$).

Similarly, in the control group, total MSCEIT V2.0 scores did not significantly predict total BACS scores ($b = 0.17$, $P = 0.47$), with the total MSCEIT V2.0 scores accounting for just 2.4% of the variance in total BACS scores. Total MSCEIT V2.0 scores did not predict total SFS scores ($b = 0.41$, $P = 0.07$), and similarly total BACS scores did not predict total SFS scores ($b = 0.18$, $P = 0.45$). Hierarchical analyses for the control group participants showed that the combined influence of total BACS and total MSCEIT V2.0 scores explained 18.3% of the variance in total SFS scores. Once total BACS scores were controlled for, total MSCEIT V2.0 scores accounted for 15.1% of the variance ($b = 0.39$, $P = 0.10$).

Post hoc analysis showed that in the schizophrenia group, there was a positive correlation between the score for Understanding Emotions (Branch 3) of the MSCEIT V2.0 and the BACS verbal fluency score ($r = 0.646$, $P = 0.002$). There were no other significant correlations between scores on Understanding Emotions (Branch 3) of the MSCEIT V2.0 and BACS or SFS subtests scores, for either group.

4. Discussion

Our results replicate the findings of Kee et al. [16] in demonstrating that people with schizophrenia are impaired on all aspects of EI, compared to control subjects. Impairment was greatest for Understanding Emotions (Branch 3). Understanding Emotions is assessed using tasks which require the participant to imagine that a person may be experiencing a particular emotion, then to imagine that this emotion may evolve into another related emotion. This is consistent with the literature showing that people with schizophrenia have impaired performance on TOM tasks [2], which assess the ability to correctly infer the thoughts and feelings of other people.

We had expected that impaired EI would be associated with poorer cognitive function, and that both EI and neurocognition would predict social outcome. In the schizophrenia group, there was a correlation between Understanding Emotions (Branch 3), the total BACS score, and SFS scores, confirming that impairment in recognising and understanding the emotions of others, and being able to predict the likely course of these emotions in a given set of circumstances, is of particular importance in schizophrenia. The correlation between Understanding Emotions and the total BACS score may indicate that the capacity for abstract thought and prediction of complex emotions and behaviours, necessary for successful completion of TOM tasks, was lacking in those with more impaired cognitive function. In turn, lack of capacity for affective TOM (knowledge about other people's emotions) [30] and impaired executive function [31] are both linked to poor insight, which in turn tends to be associated with poor outcome [32].

Eack et al. [15] found a positive correlation between all four Branches of the MSCEIT and a composite neurocognitive score in people with schizophrenia. The composite neurocognitive score reflected a battery of tests including processing speed, working memory, verbal memory, and executive function. Improvements in neurocognition and in Managing Emotions (Branch 4) were associated with better functional outcome [31]. Similarly, we found that in the schizophrenia group that the Managing Emotions Branch of the MSCEIT correlated with the SFS Recreation score. Associations between EI and social function were stronger in the control group, where Using Emotions (Branch 2), Managing Emotions (Branch 4), and the total MSCEIT score all correlated with social function.

Fett et al. [20], in a meta-analysis of the associations between neurocognition, social cognition, and community functioning in schizophrenia, reported that an overall neurocognitive factor accounted for only 6% of the variance in community functioning. In the present study, the MSCEIT did not significantly predict neurocognition or social functioning individually and neurocognition and EI together accounted for only 9.1% of the variance in social functioning scores in the schizophrenia group. These findings suggest that whilst neurocognition and social cognition do make some contribution to outcome, there are other factors which have a more substantial impact.

We found that the associations between EI and social outcome were stronger in the control group than the schizophrenia group. This may reflect the presence of other factors specific to schizophrenia, such as poor insight or negative symptoms, modifying social outcome in the control group.

This study was limited by the small sample size, and the groups were not well matched for premorbid intelligence, thus the study may have been underpowered. However, our within group analyses, looking at associations between EI, neurocognition, and social functioning, were not affected by this potential confounding factor. The correlational design of the study means the direction of the relationship between variables cannot be accurately deduced. For example, in the control group where a significant correlation between EI and social functioning was found, it may be the case that poorer social functioning leads to lower levels of EI, as lack of social contact results in fewer opportunities for individuals to learn social norms and gain experience in understanding the emotional reactions in others.

5. Conclusion

EI has proven to be a very useful construct in the general population, and further research into EI could contribute to our understanding of the nature of deficits in social cognition in schizophrenia. Our findings provide a basis for further studies exploring the relationships between EI, general intelligence, the various domains of cognitive function, and functional outcome in schizophrenia. A deeper understanding of the scope and clinical correlations of social cognitive deficits may help to identify targets of new treatments to improve emotional processing and functional outcome.

Conflict of Interests

The authors have no conflict of interests to disclose.

Acknowledgment

The authors would like to thank Ms. Ashlee Rigby for her help with paper preparation and submission.

References

[1] M. F. Green, B. Olivier, J. N. Crawley, D. L. Penn, and S. Silverstein, "Social cognition in schizophrenia: recommendations from the measurement and treatment research to improve cognition in schizophrenia new approaches conference," *Schizophrenia Bulletin*, vol. 31, no. 4, pp. 882–887, 2005.

[2] E. Bora, M. Yucel, and C. Pantelis, "Theory of mind impairment in schizophrenia: meta-analysis," *Schizophrenia Research*, vol. 109, no. 1–3, pp. 1–9, 2009.

[3] P. Stratta, M. Bustini, E. Daneluzzo, I. Riccardi, M. D'Arcangelo, and A. Rossi, "Deconstructing theory of mind in Schizophrenia," *Psychiatry Research*, vol. 190, no. 1, pp. 32–36, 2011.

[4] H. S. Kim, N. Y. Shin, J. H. Jang et al., "Social cognition and neurocognition as predictors of conversion to psychosis in individuals at ultra-high risk," *Schizophrenia Research*, vol. 130, no. 1–3, pp. 170–175, 2011.

[5] G. Matthews, M. Zeidner, and R. D. Roberts, "Emotional intelligence: consensus, controversies, and questions," in *The Science of Emotional Intelligence*, Oxford University Press, New York, NY, USA, 2007.

[6] J. D. Mayer and P. Salovey, "What is emotional intelligence?" in *Emotional Development and Emotional Intelligence: Educational Implications*, Basic Books, New York, NY, USA, 1997.

[7] J. D. Mayer, P. Salovey, and D. R. Caruso, *Mayer-Salovey-Caruso Emotional Intelligence Test (MSCEIT) User's Manual*, MHS, Toronto, Canada, 2002.

[8] J. D. Mayer, P. Salovey, D. R. Caruso, and G. Sitarenios, "Measuring Emotional Intelligence with the MSCEIT V2.0," *Emotion*, vol. 3, no. 1, pp. 97–105, 2003.

[9] P. N. Lopes, P. Salovey, S. Côté, and M. Beers, "Emotion regulation abilities and the quality of social interaction," *Emotion*, vol. 5, no. 1, pp. 113–118, 2005.

[10] M. A. Brackett and J. D. Mayer, "Convergent, discriminant, and incremental validity of competing measures of emotional intelligence," *Personality and Social Psychology Bulletin*, vol. 29, no. 9, pp. 1147–1158, 2003.

[11] D. R. Trinidad and C. A. Johnson, "The association between emotional intelligence and early adolescent tobacco and alcohol use," *Personality and Individual Differences*, vol. 32, no. 1, pp. 95–105, 2002.

[12] N. R. Burns, V. A. Bastian, and T. Nettelbeck, "Emotional intelligence: more than personality and cognitive ability?" in *The Science of Emotional Intelligence*, Oxford University Press, New York, NY, USA, 2007.

[13] K. H. Nuechterlein, M. F. Green, R. S. Kern et al., "The MATRICS consensus cognitive battery, part 1: test selection, reliability, and validity," *American Journal of Psychiatry*, vol. 165, no. 2, pp. 203–213, 2008.

[14] S. M. August, J. N. Kiwanuka, R. P. McMahon, and J. M. Gold, "The MATRICS Consensus Cognitive Battery (MCCB): clinical and cognitive correlates," *Schizophrenia Research*, vol. 134, no. 1, pp. 76–82, 2012.

[15] S. M. Eack, C. G. Greeno, M. F. Pogue-Geile, C. E. Newhill, G. E. Hogarty, and M. S. Keshavan, "Assessing social-cognitive deficits in schizophrenia with the mayer-salovey-caruso emotional intelligence test," *Schizophrenia Bulletin*, vol. 36, no. 2, pp. 370–380, 2010.

[16] K. S. Kee, W. P. Horan, P. Salovey et al., "Emotional intelligence in schizophrenia," *Schizophrenia Research*, vol. 107, no. 1, pp. 61–68, 2009.

[17] J. van Os and S. Kapur, "Schizophrenia," *The Lancet*, vol. 374, no. 9690, pp. 635–645, 2009.

[18] S. Shamsi, A. Lau, T. Lencz et al., "Cognitive and symptomatic predictors of functional disability in schizophrenia," *Schizophrenia Research*, vol. 126, no. 1–3, pp. 257–264, 2011.

[19] M. Brüne, M. Abdel-Hamid, C. Lehmkämper, and C. Sonntag, "Mental state attribution, neurocognitive functioning, and psychopathology: what predicts poor social competence in schizophrenia best?" *Schizophrenia Research*, vol. 92, no. 1–3, pp. 151–159, 2007.

[20] A. K. J. Fett, W. Viechtbauer, M. D. G. Dominguez, D. L. Penn, J. van Os, and L. Krabbendam, "The relationship between neurocognition and social cognition with functional outcomes in schizophrenia: a meta-analysis," *Neuroscience and Biobehavioral Reviews*, vol. 35, no. 3, pp. 573–588, 2011.

[21] S. M. Eack, M. F. Pogue-Geile, D. P. Greenwald, S. S. Hogarty, and M. S. Keshavan, "Mechanisms of functional improvement in a 2-year trial of cognitive enhancement therapy for early schizophrenia," *Psychological Medicine*, vol. 41, no. 6, pp. 1253–1261, 2011.

[22] American Psychiatric Association, *Diagnostic and Statistical Manual of Mental Disorders*, American Psychiatric Association, Washington, DC, USA, 4th edition, 2000.

[23] D. V. Sheehan, Y. Lecrubier, K. H. Sheehan et al., "The Mini-International Neuropsychiatric Interview (M.I.N.I.): the development and validation of a structured diagnostic psychiatric interview for DSM-IV and ICD-10," *Journal of Clinical Psychiatry*, vol. 59, no. 20, pp. 22–33, 1998.

[24] P. Salovey and D. A. Pizarro, "The value of emotional intelligence," in *Models of Intelligence*, American Psychological Association, Washington, DC, USA, 2004.

[25] J. D. Mayer, P. Salovey, and D. R. Caruso, "Emotional intelligence: theory, findings, and implications," *Psychological Inquiry*, vol. 15, no. 3, pp. 197–215, 2004.

[26] H. Nelson and J. Willson, *National Adult Reading Test (NART): Test Manual*, Nelson Publishing, Windsor, UK, 2nd edition, 1991.

[27] R. S. E. Keefe, P. D. Harvey, T. E. Goldberg et al., "Norms and standardization of the Brief Assessment of Cognition in Schizophrenia (BACS)," *Schizophrenia Research*, vol. 102, no. 1–3, pp. 108–115, 2008.

[28] R. S. E. Keefe, T. E. Goldberg, P. D. Harvey, J. M. Gold, M. P. Poe, and L. Coughenour, "The Brief Assessment of Cognition in Schizophrenia: reliability, sensitivity, and comparison with

a standard neurocognitive battery," *Schizophrenia Research*, vol. 68, no. 2-3, pp. 283–297, 2004.

[29] M. Birchwood, J. Smith, R. Cochrane, S. Wetton, and S. Copestake, "The Social Functioning Scale. The development and validation of a new scale of social adjustment for use in family intervention programmes with schizophrenic patients," *British Journal of Psychiatry*, vol. 157, pp. 853–859, 1990.

[30] G. G. Pijnenborg, J. M. Spikman, B. F. Jeronimus, and A. Aleman, "Insight in schizophrenia: associationswith empathy," *European Archives of Psychiatry and Clinical Neuroscience*. In press.

[31] S. K. Chan, K. K. Chan, M. M. Lam et al., "Clinical and cognitive correlates of insight in first-episode schizophrenia," *Schizophrenia Research*, vol. 135, no. 1–3, pp. 40–45, 2012.

[32] M. Erickson, N. Jaafari, and P. Lysaker, "Insight and negative symptoms as predictors of functioning in a work setting in patients with schizophrenia," *Psychiatry Research*, vol. 189, no. 2, pp. 161–165, 2011.

12

Schizophrenia and Suicide Attempts: Findings from a Representative Community-Based Canadian Sample

Esme Fuller-Thomson and Bailey Hollister

Factor-Inwentash Faculty of Social Work, University of Toronto, Toronto, ON, Canada M5S 1V4

Correspondence should be addressed to Esme Fuller-Thomson; esme.fuller.thomson@utoronto.ca

Academic Editor: L. Citrome

This study examined factors associated with suicide attempts among those with schizophrenia (n = 101) versus those without (n = 21,643) in a representative sample of noninstitutionalized Canadians. The lifetime prevalence of suicide attempts among persons with schizophrenia was 39.2% versus 2.8% of nonafflicted individuals. After adjusting for sociodemographics, childhood adversities, substance abuse/dependence, depression/anxiety, and chronic pain, those with schizophrenia had 6 times the odds (OR = 6.47) of attempting suicide. Among persons with schizophrenia, suicide attempts were associated with female gender (OR = 4.59), substance abuse/dependence (OR = 6.31), depression (OR = 4.93), and childhood physical abuse (OR = 5.75). Community-dwelling persons with schizophrenia appear to be at high risk for suicide attempts.

1. Introduction

In conjunction with the complexities and difficulties of the symptoms of schizophrenia, individuals with schizophrenia are more likely to attempt suicide than those without schizophrenia [1]. The prevalence of lifetime suicide attempts in those with schizophrenia ranges from 20% to 40% [2–6]. A meta-analysis estimated that one in every 20 individuals with schizophrenia will commit suicide [7]. The average age at suicide is younger among those with schizophrenia than those without the disorder [8]. It is unclear whether men or women with schizophrenia are more likely to attempt suicide with some sources stating that men and women are equally likely [9] while others indicate that women with schizophrenia are more likely to attempt suicide as compared to men with schizophrenia [10]. As will be elaborated below, the direct relationship between schizophrenia and suicide attempts may be attenuated when adjusting for several factors including socioeconomic status, pain, substance use, depression, anxiety, and early adversities.

The evidence concerning the relationship between schizophrenia and socioeconomic status (SES) is mixed [11]. Some studies have demonstrated that growing up in a low income home is associated with increased rates of schizophrenia [12, 13]. In contrast, other studies report an association between growing up in a higher income home and increased rates of schizophrenia [11, 14]. Higher levels of education have been associated with a greater likelihood of suicide completion among those with schizophrenia [15]. The association between social class and suicide completion amongst those with schizophrenia is inconclusive with some studies indicating high social class as a risk factor, while others find homelessness as a risk factor [15].

It is well documented that individuals with schizophrenia experience pain differently compared to the general population [16, 17]. A systematic review found that when there is a clear medical cause for pain, individuals with schizophrenia report a lower prevalence and intensity of pain as compared to the general population [17]. Other studies, both experimental and population-based, support the idea that individuals with schizophrenia experience a decrease in pain sensitivity [16, 18].

A strong association between substance abuse disorders and schizophrenia has been documented [19, 20]. Almost half of Americans with schizophrenia have had some form of substance abuse disorder [21]. A systematic review indicated that for individuals with schizophrenia, alcohol and drug misuse increased the risk of suicide [15].

Symptoms of depression and anxiety are common among individuals with schizophrenia [15, 22, 23]. It is estimated that approximately 50% of individuals with schizophrenia also experience comorbid depression [24]. As in the general population, individuals with schizophrenia who experience depressive symptoms have an increased risk of suicide [5, 15]. A recent systematic review estimated that one in ten (9.8%) of those with schizophrenia had Generalized Anxiety Disorder (GAD) [23]. In the schizophrenia population, individuals with a concurrent social anxiety disorder are more likely to have attempted suicide and to have a greater lethality of suicide attempts than those with schizophrenia without an anxiety disorder [25]. In addition, suicide among those with schizophrenia seems to be less likely a reaction to life events as compared to those without schizophrenia [26].

Early physical, emotional, and sexual abuse, as well as neglect, have been associated with the development of adult onset psychosis and schizophrenia [27–29]. In a systematic review, childhood adversity was indicated as a risk factor for the development of schizophrenia as compared to nonpsychiatric populations [28]. Physical and emotional abuse in childhood are also significantly associated with the development of disassociation symptoms in patients with schizophrenia and psychotic disorders [29]. Patients with schizophrenia who have a history of child maltreatment can experience worse peer relationships, difficulties in school, and more hospital visits at younger ages than those with schizophrenia without a history of child maltreatment [30]. Possibly because of these issues, those with schizophrenia who were maltreated in childhood are more likely than individuals without a history of maltreatment to express intentions of suicide and report depressive symptoms [30]. Childhood trauma in individuals with schizophrenia is associated with an increase in suicide attempts [31, 32], which is similar to findings of studies of the general population [33].

There are several gaps in the current literature. Most studies attempt to understand the relationship between suicidal behaviors and schizophrenia using clinical samples [4, 31, 34, 35]. Studies using representative samples of community dwellers are important too because they can provide information about individuals with schizophrenia who are relatively high functioning, rather than focusing only on those who are institutionalized and tend to be at the more extreme end of the illness continuum. However, the few population-based studies that do exist often use data from outside of North America [36, 37]. One Canadian population-based study found that schizophrenia is associated with an increased risk of suicide, particularly within the first 90 days of diagnosis [38]. An increased risk of suicide in those with schizophrenia has also been demonstrated immediately after discharge from hospitals [39].

A few population-based studies have been conducted with those diagnosed with schizophrenia outside of North America. For example, a Danish cohort study found that low birth weight, low IQ, and low socioeconomic status are associated with the development of psychiatric illnesses as well as drug and alcohol abuse in men later in life [40]. This drug and alcohol abuse was related to poorer survival rates [40]. A population-based study in Denmark found that younger people (<35) were most at risk for suicide as compared to other age categories [41]. This was true for both genders [41]. A Swedish population-based study concerning violent behavior and suicide indicated that, for men, alcohol use, drug use, previous self-harm, and previous violent offenses all increased suicide risk [42]. For women, self-harm was found to be associated with an increased suicide risk [42].

Another gap in the literature is that most studies analyze suicide risk, suicidal ideation, or suicide in general [1, 15, 43] and, thus, there is less known about suicide attempts, which are strongly associated with both future attempts and completed suicides [1, 3, 34]. To our knowledge, no studies have examined the role of witnessing parental domestic violence and its relationship to schizophrenia and suicide attempts. As witnessing domestic violence has been associated with several negative outcomes in adults, research to better understand its role and relationship to schizophrenia and suicide attempts is needed [44]. Our hypotheses are as follows: (1) noninstitutionalized people with schizophrenia will have higher odds of suicide attempts than those without the disorder, and this association will be partially attenuated when adverse childhood experiences, sociodemographics, and mental health and substance abuse are accounted for in the analysis and (2) among community-dwellers with schizophrenia the odds of suicide attempts will be associated with each of the three types of childhood adversity (childhood physical abuse, childhood sexual abuse, and witnessing parental domestic violence), substance abuse, depression, and anxiety disorders.

2. Methods

Data from the 2012 Canadian Community Health Survey-Mental Health (CCHS-MH) were analyzed in the current study. The CCHS-MH is a cross-sectional survey that collects information about the factors, influences, and processes that contribute to mental health through a multidisciplinary approach focusing on health, social, and economic determinants [45]. While the survey covers the population of individuals at age of 15 and older living in the 10 provinces, residents of the three territories, those living on reserves or other aboriginal settlements, full-time members of the armed forces, and the institutionalized population were excluded. The latter groups represent less than 3% of the target population [45].

2.1. Sample. Respondents for the CCHS-MH were sampled using a three-stage design, which began with selecting individuals from geographical areas and then households within each geographical area. Out of all eligible respondents, one individual within each household was randomly selected according to varying selection probabilities [45]. Based on the selected units, 36,443 were in-scope for the survey and, of these, 29,088 households agreed to participate in the survey, resulting in an overall household-level response rate of 79.8%. From responding households, 29,088 persons were selected to participate and 25,113 provided a valid questionnaire, which yielded an overall person-level response rate of 86.3%. At the national level, these figures result in a combined response rate of 68.9%.

The analysis for the current study is based on two subsamples of the full CCHS-MH. More specifically, the first analysis was restricted to those with complete data on each of the measures in the analyses ($n = 21{,}744$). It only contains respondents at age of 20 and older because younger respondents were not asked questions about adverse childhood experiences. The second analysis was a subsample of the first analysis restricted to respondents who reported that they had been diagnosed with schizophrenia ($n = 101$).

2.2. Measures. *Schizophrenia* was assessed based upon a list of "conditions diagnosed by a health professional that are expected to last or have already lasted 6 months or more." Those with a positive response to the question "do you have schizophrenia?" were coded as such.

Suicide attempt was ascertained by a positive response to the question: Have you ever "attempted suicide or tried to take your own life?" The questions were found in a section of the CCHS-MH that focuses specifically on suicide and beginning with a statement that "the questions may be sensitive to some people, but we have to ask the same questions of everyone."

Sociodemographic variables include gender, self-identified race (nonaboriginal White versus visible minority and/or aboriginal), age (in decades), and *Socioeconomic Position* (SEP) measured by the highest level of achieved education (less than high school, high school graduate, some postsecondary school, postsecondary diploma, or university degree). Statistics Canada's measure of household income as a ratio related to the national low-income cut-off, divided into deciles, was also used to assess SEP. This variable takes into account the number of people in the household and the size of the community.

Adverse Childhood Experiences (ACEs) included the following.

(i) Witnessing Parental Domestic Violence (PDV). Individuals were determined as having been exposed to intimate partner violence if they reported they had seen or heard 11 or more times one of their "parents, step-parents, or guardians hit each other or another adult" aged 18 or over in their home.

(ii) Childhood Sexual Abuse (CSA). Childhood sexual abuse was measured by the question "How many times did an adult force you or attempt to force you into any unwanted sexual activity, by threatening you, holding you down, or hurting you in some way?" This variable was coded never versus ever.

(iii) Childhood Physical Abuse (CPA). Individuals were ascertained as having been physically abused if they reported that, before they reached the age of 16, an adult had at least once kicked, bit, punch, choked, burned, or physically attacked them.

Mental health factors include lifetime anxiety and depression. Individuals were coded as having an anxiety disorder if they met the WHO-CIDI lifetime criteria for Generalized Anxiety Disorder. Similarly, respondents were ascertained as a depressive disorder if they met the WHO-CIDI lifetime criteria for Major Depressive Episode. For more details please see [45].

Chronic pain was assessed in a section of the survey focusing on pain and discomfort that began with the following statement: the next set of questions asks about the level of pain or discomfort you usually experience. They are not about illnesses like colds that affect people for short periods of time. Respondents were determined to be regularly in pain if they responded no to the question "Are you usually free of pain or discomfort?"

Substance abuse was measured based on the WHO-CIDI using a combination of the derived variables created by Statistics Canada "Drug Abuse or Dependence (including Cannabis)" and "Alcohol Abuse or Dependence." Both were derived using the lifetime algorithm. For more information, please see the Canadian Community Health Survey (CCHS) mental health derived variable specifications [45].

2.3. Statistical Analyses. The lifetime prevalence of suicide attempts among those with schizophrenia was calculated in SPSS 22. Chi-square analysis was conducted to examine gender difference in the lifetime prevalence of suicide attempts among those with and without schizophrenia. Two series of logistic regression analyses were conducted. In the first series of analyses, the outcome was lifetime suicide attempt and the key exposure variable was schizophrenia status. The goals of the analyses were to document the odds of suicide attempts among those with schizophrenia in comparison to those without and to calculate the degree to which inclusion of the potentially confounding factors attenuated the relationship. Age, race, income, and education were controlled for in the first model and each subsequent model. The second and third model adjusted for three early adversities (witnessing parental domestic violence, being physically abused, and being sexually abused as a child) and chronic pain, respectively. The fourth model controlled for drug and alcohol abuse. The fifth model accounted for lifetime depression and anxiety disorders. The sixth and final model controlled for all the above-named factors simultaneously.

A second series of logistic regression analyses was completed using the subsample of those diagnosed with schizophrenia ($n = 101$). The first model controlled for childhood adversities only, the next adjusted for gender and substance abuse/dependence, and a third accounted for mental health factors. A final model controlled for all the above-named variables simultaneously. Data from all the analyses were weighted to adjust for the probability of selection and nonresponse. Sample sizes are reported in their unweighted form. Odds ratios and 95% confidence intervals are reported.

3. Results

In our population-based sample of noninstitutionalized Canadians, the lifetime prevalence of suicide attempts among those with schizophrenia was 39.2% compared to 2.8% of individuals without schizophrenia. One-third of males (33%) with schizophrenia had attempted suicide in contrast to 2.2%

of males without schizophrenia ($p < 0.001$). Almost half of women (47.3%) with schizophrenia had attempted suicide in comparison to 3.5% of women without schizophrenia ($p < 0.001$).

When the data were adjusted for age, race, income, and education, noninstitutionalized individuals with schizophrenia had 15 times the odds of attempting suicide (OR: 15.74, 95% CI = 9.84, 25.2) in comparison to those without schizophrenia (please see Table 1). We conducted a series of logistic regression analyses all of which included the above variables in addition to several different clusters of risk factors that we anticipated would attenuate the association between schizophrenia and suicide attempts. When three early adversities (witnessing parental domestic violence, being physically abused, and being sexually abused as a child) were added to the equation, the odds of suicide attempts among those with schizophrenia declined to 12.92 (OR: 12.92, 95% CI = 7.96, 21.753). When drug and alcohol abuse were included, people with schizophrenia still had 13 times the odds (OR: 13.06) of attempting suicide as compared to individuals without schizophrenia. When pain was added to the sociodemographic variables, people with schizophrenia had 14.5 times the odds of attempting suicide (OR: 14.5, CI = 8.91, 23.74). The greatest attenuation in the schizophrenia-suicide attempt association was due to the inclusion of lifetime depression and anxiety disorders. Inclusion of these mental health characteristics reduced the odds of suicide attempts among those with schizophrenia to 7.22 (95% CI = 4.22–12.36). After adjusting for all of the factors discussed above, individuals with schizophrenia had 6 times the odds (OR: 6.47) of attempting to suicide as compared to individuals who did not have schizophrenia. Among the variables controlled for, mental health factors explained the largest share of the relationship between schizophrenia and suicide attempts at 58%, followed by childhood adversities at 20% and substance use at 18%. All the factors together accounted for 63% of the association.

In order to identify the key factors associated with suicide attempts among those with schizophrenia, we conducted additional analyses restricted to the 101 respondents in the CCHS-MH data set who reported that they had been diagnosed with schizophrenia by a medical professional (please see Table 2). In a model adjusting for all variables simultaneously, we found that suicide attempts were associated with female gender (OR = 4.59), substance dependence (OR = 6.31), depression (OR = 4.93), and a history of physical abuse in childhood (OR = 5.75). When only early adversities were included, exposure to chronic parental domestic violence was associated with almost 7 times the odds of suicide attempts (OR = 6.95). After adjustments for gender, substance abuse, and depression and anxiety, this number decreased to nonsignificance (OR: 2.58, 95% CI = 0.65, 10.30). Among those with schizophrenia, early adversity accounted for 24% of the variability in suicide attempts (Nagelkerke $R^2 = 0.24$). When gender, drug and alcohol abuse, and lifetime anxiety and depressive disorders were added to the analysis, 38% of the variability in suicide attempts was accounted for (Nagelkerke $R^2 = 0.38$).

4. Discussion

The purpose of this study was to examine the relationship between suicide attempts and schizophrenia using representative community-based data. In individuals with schizophrenia, 39.2% had attempted suicide as compared to 2.8% of individuals without schizophrenia. Previous studies have estimated the prevalence of suicide attempts in individuals with schizophrenia to range from 20 to 40% [2–6]. Although the percentage of individuals with schizophrenia who attempted suicide fell between previously estimated rates, it was theorized that, with population-based data of noninstitutionalized individuals, these numbers would be lower than in studies using clinical samples. The data suggest, however, that rates of suicide attempts in those with schizophrenia living within the community may be similar to those found in clinical settings.

We found that the odds of suicide attempt were over 6 times higher among those with schizophrenia compared to those without, even when accounting for lifetime depression and anxiety disorders, substance use, childhood adversities, pain, and sociodemographics. Among the latter factors, depression and anxiety explained the largest share of the relationship between schizophrenia and suicide attempts, which is consistent with research showing that as much as half of individuals with schizophrenia suffer from depressive symptoms and that these symptoms are associated with an increase in suicide attempts [5, 15, 24]. Among those with schizophrenia, we found that depression was associated with 7 times the odds of a suicide attempt and that depression and anxiety together explained 17.5% of the variability in suicide attempts. These findings suggest that it is important for health care professionals working in the community to be aware of the need to assess for the presence of other mental health problems alongside the symptoms of schizophrenia. Developing best practices to support individuals who are experiencing schizophrenia comorbid with other mental health conditions could help decrease the prevalence of suicide attempts among those living in the community.

Interestingly, in the fully adjusted model, those with an anxiety disorder were 69% less likely to attempt suicide. Rapp et al. [46] found that individuals with schizophrenia who also had anxiety demonstrated higher verbal IQ, better problem solving, attention, and verbal fluency. Possessing these qualities might indicate that individuals with both schizophrenia and anxiety may be more likely to have the necessary skills to express themselves verbally and communicate with those around them should they be experiencing suicidal ideation, increasing the chances of a successful intervention. More research is required to understand the differences in characteristics between those with schizophrenia with an anxiety disorder and those with schizophrenia without an anxiety disorder.

In the general population, women are more likely to attempt suicide than men [47]. Some research has also identified this trend for women with schizophrenia [10], which is in keeping with what we found in our data. When only sociodemographics and substance abuse history were included in the analysis, women's odds of suicide attempts were elevated

Table 1: Odds ratios and 95% confidence interval of lifetime suicide attempts among those with schizophrenia versus those without in a representative community-based sample ($n = 21744$).

	Model 1 Demographics + SES	Model 2 Demographics + SES + ACEs	Model 3 Demographics + SES + substance abuse	Model 4 Demographics + SES + mental health	Model 5 Demographics + SES + pain	Model 6 Fully adjusted
Has schizophrenia						
Yes	15.74 (9.84, 25.18)	12.92 (7.68, 21.75)	13.06 (7.95, 21.47)	7.23 (4.22, 12.36)	14.54 (8.91, 23.74)	6.47 (3.73, 11.20)
No (Ref)	1.00	1.00	1.00	1.00	1.00	1.00
Adverse childhood experiences						
Witnessed parental domestic violence						
>10 times	—	2.40 (1.88, 3.06)	—	—	—	2.21 (1.71, 2.86)
≤10 times (Ref)	—	1.00	—	—	—	1.00
Physical abuse						
Abused	—	3.35 (2.72, 4.13)	—	—	—	2.28 (1.84, 2.83)
None (Ref)	—	1.00	—	—	—	1.00
Sexual abuse						
Abused	—	4.21 (3.41, 5.21)	—	—	—	2.85 (2.28, 3.56)
None (Ref)	—	1.00	—	—	—	1.00
Demographics						
Sex						
Female	1.57 (1.33, 1.85)	1.44 (1.21, 1.72)	2.33 (1.95, 2.77)	1.25 (1.05, 1.48)	1.50 (1.27, 1.77)	1.49 (1.23, 1.80)
Male (Ref)	1.00	1.00	1.00	1.00	1.00	1.00
Race						
White only	1.33 (1.09, 1.61)	1.31 (1.07, 1.61)	0.97 (0.79, 1.19)	0.99 (0.81, 1.22)	1.22 (1.01, 1.49)	0.94 (0.76, 1.17)
Visible minority or aboriginal (Ref)	1.00	1.00	1.00	1.00	1.00	1.00
Age						
Age by decade	0.82 (0.78, 0.86)	0.80 (0.76, 0.84)	0.88 (0.84, 0.93)	0.84 (0.79, 0.88)	0.77 (0.73, 0.81)	0.82 (0.77, 0.87)
Socioeconomic status						
Education						
No high school graduation (Ref)	1.00	1.00	1.00	1.00	1.00	1.00
High school graduate	0.64 (0.50, 0.83)	0.73 (0.56, 0.96)	0.64 (0.50, 0.83)	0.58 (0.45, 0.76)	0.69 (0.54, 0.90)	0.64 (0.48, 0.85)
Postsecondary graduate	0.79 (0.64, 0.99)	0.93 (0.74, 1.18)	0.87 (0.70, 1.09)	0.73 (0.58, 0.91)	0.87 (0.70, 1.09)	0.93 (0.73, 1.19)
Household income (decile)	0.84 (0.81, 0.87)	0.87 (0.85, 0.90)	0.83 (0.80, 0.86)	0.86 (0.84, 0.89)	0.86 (0.83, 0.89)	0.89 (0.86, 0.92)
Drug or alcohol abuse						
Yes	—	—	5.57 (4.68, 6.64)	—	—	2.77 (2.29, 3.34)
No (Ref)	—	—	1.00	—	—	1.00

Table 1: Continued.

	Model 1 Demographics + SES	Model 2 Demographics + SES + ACEs	Model 3 Demographics + SES + substance abuse	Model 4 Demographics + SES + mental health	Model 5 Demographics + SES + pain	Model 6 Fully adjusted
Mental health						
Lifetime generalized anxiety disorder						
Yes	—	—	—	3.23 (2.66, 3.93)	—	2.13 (1.73, 2.63)
No (Ref)	—	—	—	1.00	—	1.00
Lifetime depression						
Yes	—	—	—	5.43 (4.51, 6.55)	—	3.85 (3.17, 4.68)
No (Ref)	—	—	—	1.00	—	1.00
Chronic pain						
Pain						
Moderate or severe	—	—	—	—	4.13 (3.46, 4.93)	1.82 (1.49, 2.22)
Less than moderate (Ref)	—	—	—	—	1.00	1.00
Nagelkerke R square value	0.070	0.193	0.140	0.201	0.112	0.303
−2 Log likelihood	5431.6	4787.3	5068.4	4747.6	5213.9	4194.1

SES = socioeconomic status, ACEs = adverse childhood experiences.

TABLE 2: Odds ratios and 95% confidence interval of lifetime suicide attempt among those with schizophrenia from a representative community-based sample (n = 101).

	Model 1 ACEs only	Model 2 Demographics and substance abuse	Model 3 Demographics, substance abuse, and mental health	Model 4 Fully adjusted
Adverse childhood experiences				
Witnessed parental domestic violence				
>10 times	6.95 (2.30, 20.99)	—	—	2.58 (0.64, 10.30)
≤10 times (Ref)	1.00	—	—	1.00
Physical abuse				
Abused	2.66 (0.94, 7.51)	—	—	5.75 (1.53, 21.58)
None (Ref)	1.00	—	—	1.00
Sexual abuse				
Abused	1.00 (0.33, 3.04)	—	—	0.45 (0.13, 1.61)
None (Ref)	1.00	—	—	1.00
Demographics				
Sex				
Female	—	2.13 (0.91, 4.98)	3.10 (1.19, 8.04)	4.59 (1.21, 17.35)
Male (Ref)	—	1.00	1.00	1.00
Drug or alcohol abuse				
Yes	—	2.24 (0.96, 5.22)	5.02 (1.77, 14.26)	6.31 (1.83, 21.72)
No (Ref)	—	1.00	1.00	1.00
Mental health				
Anxiety				
Lifetime anxiety disorder	—	—	0.37 (0.13, 1.02)	0.31 (0.10, 0.94)
No anxiety disorder (Ref)	—	—	1.00	1.00
Depression				
Lifetime depressive disorder	—	—	6.97 (2.37, 20.52)	4.93 (1.26, 19.28)
No depression (Ref)	—	—	1.00	1.00
Nagelkerke R square value	0.241	0.074	0.250	0.381
−2 Log likelihood	115.5	129.629	114.7	101.9

ACE: adverse childhood experience.

but failed to reach statistical significance (OR = 2.13; 95% CI = 0.91, 4.98). However, these odds increased and became statistically significant when histories of depressive disorders and anxiety disorders were included (OR = 3.10; 95% CI = 1.19, 8.04). In the final model we were surprised by the magnitude of the association in our sample: women with schizophrenia had four times the odds of suicide attempts compared to men with schizophrenia when adjustments were made for adverse childhood experiences, sociodemographics, substance abuse, depression, and anxiety disorder (OR = 4.59; 95% CI = 1.21, 17.35). It appears that women with schizophrenia are particularly at risk, even independent of these comorbid conditions. One potential factor to explain this is that females with schizophrenia tend to present with symptoms later than males [10, 47], and individuals with later onset schizophrenia have been shown to have an increased risk of suicide [48, 49].

Among those with schizophrenia, 24% of the variability in suicide attempts was explained by a history of early adversity. When only early adversities were used to predict suicide attempts among those with schizophrenia, those who had been exposed to chronic parental domestic violence had approximately seven times the odds of attempting suicide. To our knowledge, this is the first study to examine the role of exposure to parental domestic violence in those with schizophrenia and its relationship to suicide attempts. Our findings are in keeping with data from the general population which has shown that individuals who are exposed to parental domestic violence have an increased risk of suicide attempts [50]. Childhood physical abuse was associated with 2.66 higher odds of suicide in those with schizophrenia; however, it only reached borderline significance (model 1: $p < 0.065$). After adjustments for demographics, substance abuse, and history of depression and anxiety disorders, the relationship between parental domestic violence and suicide attempts decreased to nonsignificance but childhood physical abuse reached statistical signficance. Our findings are in contrast to a recent clinical study of suicide attempts before and after first episode of schizophrenia which found no association between childhood traumas and suicide attempts [51]. There were numerous design differences between Togay et al.'s study [51] and this study which may have led to the different findings including source of sample (clinical sample of first episode clients versus representative population-based study), study location (Turkey versus Canada), period of suicide attempts (average of 5 years after first episode versus lifetime), and different measures of early adversities (combined measure of 5 types of abuse using a standardized scale versus separate inclusion of 3 specific types of childhood adversities). Physical, emotional, and sexual abuse, neglect, and witnessing parental domestic violence have been associated with an increased risk in suicide attempts in the general population [31, 32]. In our Canadian study, early childhood adversities explained a large portion of the variability in suicide attempts among those with schizophrenia. These findings reinforce the need to develop targeted programs for individuals with schizophrenia who have experienced early childhood abuse [31, 32].

In the fully adjusted model, substance abuse/dependence was associated with 6 times the odds of suicide attempts among those with schizophrenia. Both in the general population and in the schizophrenia literature drug abuse and addictions have been associated with increased risk of suicide attempts [19, 20, 52, 53]. Interestingly, substance abuse/dependence explained just 7% of the variation in suicide attempts. A potential explanation for the finding rests in exploring the self-medication hypothesis [54]. It is theorized that part of the reason individuals with schizophrenia have such high rates of substance abuse is that they try to alleviate the pain and suffering they feel as a result of the symptoms of schizophrenia by using substances [54, 55]. It is possible that, due to our use of population-based data of noninstitutionalized individuals, our sample may not be experiencing the same level of intensity of symptoms as one would see in a clinical sample and, thus, is less likely to be using substances to cope and, subsequently, turn to attempting suicide.

There are a several limitations present in this study. It is possible that recall bias may have occurred considering the retrospective nature of reporting suicide attempts as well as early adversities. There has been a lack of research aimed at establishing the validity and reliability of self-report measures related to suicide attempts [56]. In the general population, the evidence concerning the validity and reliability of retrospective reporting of child maltreatment is mixed, with some studies finding the self-reports an accurate way of assessing child maltreatment [57], while others are finding significant instability in retrospective reports of child maltreatment [58]. In individuals with schizophrenia, concerns about memory and cognition could be cited as a potential challenge to relying on self-report data [59]. Although slower recall and deficits in recalling emotion laden memories have been reported in individuals with schizophrenia, most of these studies have relied on clinical samples, thus potentially skewing the understanding of memory deficits in those with schizophrenia [60–62]. Other research has found good validity in self-report measures of childhood abuse among patients with mental disorders [63]. There are some potential risk factors for suicide attempts in individuals with schizophrenia that were not included in our analysis. These include insight into disease, poor adherence to treatment, schizophrenia symptom profile, housing conditions, marital status, and living alone. The absence of these important potential confounds could have biased our findings.

Questions have also been raised as to whether self-report of a medical diagnosis of schizophrenia is a reasonable method to assess the presence or absence of this condition. Self-reports of a medical diagnosis of schizophrenia are a prominent technique used in large, population-based data sets [64]. The prevalence of schizophrenia based on self-report of a medical diagnosis in the current sample was in keeping with the systematic review by Saha and colleagues [65] which estimated that the lifetime prevalence of schizophrenia was approximately 0.44%. However, alternative techniques for assessing schizophrenia status, such as screening tools and self-report measures, also carry the risk of missing cases of psychiatric illnesses [66]. There is particularly the potential for missing those with negative symptoms [66, 67]. In a previous study using an earlier wave of the CCHS, self-report of a clinical diagnosis of schizophrenia was found to be a reasonable way to assess the existence of schizophrenia [64]. There have been few studies examining this phenomenon, and it has been suggested that more research is to be conducted using diagnostic interviewing as a comparison to produce better, more reliable data [64]. Although the overall response rate of 68.9% was quite good for a large population-based survey, it is possible that those with schizophrenia, particularly those with more severe symptoms, may be less likely to participate in a survey such as this. If the most severe cases are most likely to have had suicide attempts, it is likely that such an underrepresentation of these individuals would result in our analyses underestimating the magnitude of the relationship between schizophrenia and suicide attempts. Additionally, it is possible that the question *"How many times did an adult force you or attempt to force you into any unwanted sexual activity, by threatening you, holding you down, or hurting you in some way?"* does not adequately capture all types of sexual abuse, specifically forms that would be subtler in nature. Consequently, our study might underestimate the history of sexual abuse.

Our nationally representative sample suggests noninstitutionalized individuals with schizophrenia are 6 times more likely than individuals without schizophrenia to attempt suicide. The presence of depressive symptoms, as well as early childhood adversities, played significant roles in explaining the high rates of suicide within the schizophrenia population. With this information, it is important to recognize that individuals who are experiencing psychosis are also vulnerable to other serious mental health issues, which are related to suicide attempts. This, alongside targeted programs for those with schizophrenia who have experienced early adversity, could help reduce the suicide attempts by individuals with schizophrenia living in the community.

Disclaimer

The views expressed in this paper do not necessarily represent the CRDCN's or that of its partners.

Conflict of Interests

The authors declare that there is no conflict of interests regarding the publication of this paper.

Acknowledgment

The authors would like to thank Rafael Riviere for assistance with paper preparation. Esme Fuller-Thomson would like to gratefully acknowledge support received from the Sandra Rotman Endowed Chair in Social Work at the University of Toronto. The analysis presented in this paper was conducted at the Toronto RDC, which is part of the Canadian Research Data Centre Network (CRDCN). The services and activities provided by the Toronto RDC are made possible by the financial or in-kind support of the SSHRC, the CIHR, the CFI, Statistics Canada, and University of Toronto. The opinions expressed do not represent the views of Statistics Canada.

References

[1] K. Hawton, L. Sutton, C. Haw, J. Sinclair, and J. J. Deeks, "Schizophrenia and suicide: a systematic review of risk factors," *The British Journal of Psychiatry*, vol. 187, no. 1, pp. 9–20, 2005.

[2] M. Pompili, X. F. Amador, P. Girardi et al., "Suicide risk in schizophrenia: learning from the past to change the future," *Annals of General Psychiatry*, vol. 6, article 10, 2007.

[3] S. G. Siris, "Suicide and schizophrenia," *Journal of Psychopharmacology*, vol. 15, no. 2, pp. 127–135, 2001.

[4] A. C. Altamura, R. Bassetti, S. Bignotti, R. Pioli, and E. Mundo, "Clinical variables related to suicide attempts in schizophrenic patients: a retrospective study," *Schizophrenia Research*, vol. 60, no. 1, pp. 47–55, 2003.

[5] J. T. Suokas, J. Perälä, K. Suominen, S. Saarni, J. Lönnqvist, and J. M. Suvisaari, "Epidemiology of suicide attempts among persons with psychotic disorder in the general population," *Schizophrenia Research*, vol. 124, no. 1-3, pp. 22–28, 2010.

[6] M. Yildiz, A. Yazici, and O. Böke, "Demographic and clinical characteristics in schizophrenia: a multi center cross-sectional case record study," *Turkish Journal of Psychiatry*, vol. 21, no. 3, pp. 213–224, 2010.

[7] B. A. Palmer, V. S. Pankratz, and J. M. Bostwick, "The lifetime risk of suicide in schizophrenia. A reexamination," *Archives of General Psychiatry*, vol. 62, no. 3, pp. 247–253, 2005.

[8] F. Limosin, J.-Y. Loze, A. Philippe, F. Casadebaig, and F. Rouillon, "Ten-year prospective follow-up study of the mortality by suicide in schizophrenic patients," *Schizophrenia Research*, vol. 94, no. 1-3, pp. 23–28, 2007.

[9] J. M. Harkavy-Friedman, E. A. Nelson, and D. F. Venarde, "Suicidal behavior in schizophrenia and schizoaffective disorder," *Clinical Neuroscience Research*, vol. 1, no. 5, pp. 345–350, 2001.

[10] C. M. Canuso and G. Pandina, "Gender and schizophrenia," *Psychopharmacology Bulletin*, vol. 40, no. 4, pp. 178–190, 2007.

[11] S. Goldberg, E. Fruchter, M. Davidson, A. Reichenberg, R. Yoffe, and M. Weiser, "The relationship between risk of hospitalization for schizophrenia, SES, and cognitive functioning," *Schizophrenia Bulletin*, vol. 37, no. 4, pp. 664–670, 2011.

[12] C. Corcoran, M. Perrin, S. Harlap et al., "Effect of socioeconomic status and parents' education at birth on risk of schizophrenia in offspring," *Social Psychiatry and Psychiatric Epidemiology*, vol. 44, no. 4, pp. 265–271, 2009.

[13] B. Saraceno, I. Levev, and R. Kohn, "The public mental health significance of research on socio-economic factors in schizophrenia and major depression," *World Psychiatry*, vol. 4, no. 3, pp. 181–185, 2005.

[14] F. Mulvany, E. O'Callaghan, N. Takei, M. Byrne, P. Fearon, and C. Larkin, "Effect of social class at birth on risk and presentation of schizophrenia: case-control study," *British Medical Journal*, vol. 323, no. 7326, pp. 1398–1401, 2001.

[15] K. Hor and M. Taylor, "Suicide and schizophrenia: a systematic review of rates and risk factors," *Journal of Psychopharmacology*, vol. 24, no. 4, pp. 81–90, 2010.

[16] M. K. Singh, L. L. Giles, and H. A. Nasrallah, "Pain insensitivity in schizophrenia: trait or state marker?" *Journal of Psychiatric Practice*, vol. 12, no. 2, pp. 90–102, 2006.

[17] G. Engels, A. L. Francke, B. van Meijel et al., "Clinical pain in schizophrenia: a systematic review," *The Journal of Pain*, vol. 15, no. 5, pp. 457–467, 2014.

[18] T. Jochum, A. Letzsch, W. Greiner, G. Wagner, H. Sauer, and K.-J. Bär, "Influence of antipsychotic medication on pain perception in schizophrenia," *Psychiatry Research*, vol. 142, no. 2-3, pp. 151–156, 2006.

[19] G. Carrà and S. Johnson, "Variations in rates of comorbid substance use in psychosis between mental health settings and geographical areas in the UK. A systematic review," *Social Psychiatry and Psychiatric Epidemiology*, vol. 44, no. 6, pp. 429–447, 2009.

[20] I. L. Fowler, V. J. Carr, N. T. Carter, and T. J. Lewin, "Patterns of current and lifetime substance use in schizophrenia," *Schizophrenia Bulletin*, vol. 24, no. 3, pp. 443–455, 1998.

[21] D. A. Reiger, M. E. Farmer, D. S. Rae et al., "Comorbidity of mental disorders with alcohol and other drug abuse," *The Journal of the American Medical Association*, vol. 264, no. 19, pp. 2511–2518, 1990.

[22] C. Mulholland and S. Cooper, "The symptom of depression in schizophrenia and its management," *Advances in Psychiatric Treatment*, vol. 6, no. 3, pp. 169–177, 2000.

[23] A. M. Achim, M. Maziade, É. Raymond, D. Olivier, C. Mérette, and M.-A. Roy, "How prevalent are anxiety disorders in schizophrenia? A meta-analysis and critical review on a significant association," *Schizophrenia Bulletin*, vol. 37, no. 4, pp. 811–821, 2011.

[24] P. F. Buckley, B. J. Miller, D. S. Lehrer, and D. J. Castle, "Psychiatric comorbidities and schizophrenia," *Schizophrenia Bulletin*, vol. 35, no. 2, pp. 383–402, 2009.

[25] S. Pallanti, L. Quercioli, and E. Hollander, "Social anxiety in outpatients with schizophrenia: a relevant cause of disability," *The American Journal of Psychiatry*, vol. 161, no. 1, pp. 53–58, 2004.

[26] H. Heilä, M. E. Heikkinen, E. T. Isometsä, M. M. Henriksson, M. J. Marttunen, and J. K. Lönnqvist, "Life events and completed suicide in schizophrenia: a comparison of suicide victims with and without schizophrenia," *Schizophrenia Bulletin*, vol. 25, no. 3, pp. 519–531, 1999.

[27] F. Varese, F. Smeets, M. Drukker et al., "Childhood adversities increase the risk of psychosis: a meta-analysis of patient-control, prospective-and cross sectional cohort studies," *Schizophrenia Bulletin*, vol. 38, no. 4, pp. 661–671, 2012.

[28] S. L. Matheson, A. M. Shepherd, R. M. Pinchbeck, K. R. Laurens, and V. J. Carr, "Childhood adversity in schizophrenia: a systematic meta-analysis," *Psychological Medicine*, vol. 43, no. 2, pp. 225–238, 2013.

[29] D. W. Holowka, S. King, D. Saheb, M. Pukall, and A. Brunet, "Childhood abuse and dissociative symptoms in adult schizophrenia," *Schizophrenia Research*, vol. 60, no. 1, pp. 87–90, 2003.

[30] L. S. Schenkel, W. D. Spaulding, D. DiLillo, and S. M. Silverstein, "Histories of childhood maltreatment in schizophrenia: relationships with premorbid functioning, symptomatology, and cognitive deficits," *Schizophrenia Research*, vol. 76, no. 2-3, pp. 273–286, 2005.

[31] A. Roy, "Reported childhood trauma and suicide attempts in schizophrenic patients," *Suicide & Life-Threatening Behavior*, vol. 35, no. 6, pp. 690–693, 2005.

[32] J. Read, K. Agar, N. Argyle, and V. Aderhold, "Sexual and physical abuse during childhood and adulthood as predictors of hallucinations, delusions and thought disorder," *Psychology and Psychotherapy: Theory, Research and Practice*, vol. 76, no. 1, pp. 1–22, 2003.

[33] R. Gilbert, C. S. Widom, K. Browne, D. Fergusson, E. Webb, and S. Janson, "Burden and consequences of child maltreatment in high-income countries," *The Lancet*, vol. 373, no. 9657, pp. 68–81, 2009.

[34] Y. Barak, Y. Baruch, A. Achiron, and D. Aizenberg, "Suicide attempts of schizophrenia patients: a case-controlled study in tertiary care," *Journal of Psychiatric Research*, vol. 42, no. 10, pp. 822–826, 2008.

[35] A. Gut-Fayand, A. Dervaux, J.-P. Olié, H. Lôo, M.-F. Poirier, and M.-O. Krebs, "Substance abuse and suicidality in schizophrenia: a common risk factor linked to impulsivity," *Psychiatry Research*, vol. 102, no. 1, pp. 65–72, 2001.

[36] J. Tiihonen, J. Lönnqvist, K. Wahlbeck et al., "11-year follow-up of mortality in patients with schizophrenia: a population-based cohort study (FIN11 study)," *The Lancet*, vol. 374, no. 9690, pp. 620–627, 2009.

[37] J. Suokas, K. Suominen, E. Isometsä, A. Ostamo, and J. Lönnqvist, "Long-term risk factors for suicide mortality after attempted suicide—findings of a 14-year follow-up study," *Acta Psychiatrica Scandinavica*, vol. 104, no. 2, pp. 117–121, 2001.

[38] J. R. Randall, R. Walld, G. Finlayson, J. Sareen, P. J. Martens, and J. M. Bolton, "Acute risk of suicide and suicide attempts associated with recent diagnosis of mental disorders: a population-based, propensity score-matched analysis," *Canadian Journal of Psychiatry*, vol. 59, no. 10, p. 531, 2014.

[39] P. Qin and M. Nordentoft, "Suicide risk in relation to psychiatric hospitalization: evidence based on longitudinal registers," *Archives of General Psychiatry*, vol. 62, no. 4, pp. 427–432, 2005.

[40] M. Osler, E. Rostrup, M. Nordentoft, E. L. Mortensen, H. Bruunsgaard, and B. Fagerlund, "Influence of early life characteristics on psychiatric admissions and impact of psychiatric disease on inflammatory biomarkers and survival: a Danish cohort study," *World Psychiatry*, vol. 14, no. 3, pp. 364–365, 2015.

[41] P. Qin, "The impact of psychiatric illness on suicide: differences by diagnosis of disorders and by sex and age of subjects," *Journal of Psychiatric Research*, vol. 45, no. 11, pp. 1445–1452, 2011.

[42] S. Fazel, A. Wolf, C. Palm, and P. Lichtenstein, "Violent crime, suicide, and premature mortality in patients with schizophrenia and related disorders: a 38-year total population study in Sweden," *The Lancet Psychiatry*, vol. 1, no. 1, pp. 44–54, 2014.

[43] Y. P. S. Balhara and R. Verma, "Schizophrenia and suicide," *East Asian Archives of Psychiatry*, vol. 22, no. 3, pp. 126–133, 2012.

[44] J. L. Edleson, "Children's witnessing of adult domestic violence," *Journal of Interpersonal Violence*, vol. 14, no. 8, pp. 839–870, 1999.

[45] Statistics Canada, *Canadian Community Health Survey—Mental Health (CCHS)*, 2013, http://www23.statcan.gc.ca/imdb/p2SV.pl?Function=getSurvey&SDDS=5015.

[46] E. K. Rapp, M. L. White-Ajmani, D. Antonius et al., "Schizophrenia comorbid with panic disorder: evidence for distinct cognitive profiles," *Psychiatry Research*, vol. 197, no. 3, pp. 206–211, 2012.

[47] R. Lewine, "At issue: sex and gender in schizophrenia," *Schizophrenia Bulletin*, vol. 30, no. 4, pp. 755–762, 2004.

[48] J. Reutfors, L. Brandt, E. G. Jönsson, A. Ekbom, P. Sparén, and U. Ösby, "Risk factors for suicide in schizophrenia: findings from a Swedish population-based case-control study," *Schizophrenia Research*, vol. 108, no. 1–3, pp. 231–237, 2009.

[49] C.-J. Kuo, S.-Y. Tsai, C.-H. Lo, Y.-P. Wang, and C.-C. Chen, "Risk factors for completed suicide in schizophrenia," *Journal of Clinical Psychiatry*, vol. 66, no. 5, pp. 579–585, 2005.

[50] T. I. Herrenkohl, C. Sousa, E. A. Tajima, R. C. Herrenkohl, and C. A. Moylan, "Intersection of child abuse and children's exposure to domestic violence," *Trauma, Violence, & Abuse*, vol. 9, no. 2, pp. 84–99, 2008.

[51] B. Togay, H. Noyan, R. Tasdelen, and A. Ucok, "Clinical variables associated with suicide attempts in schizophrenia before and after the first episode," *Psychiatry Research*, vol. 229, no. 1-2, pp. 252–256, 2015.

[52] M. Backmund, K. Meyer, C. Schütz, and J. Reimer, "Factors associated with suicide attempts among injection drug users," *Substance Use & Misuse*, vol. 46, no. 12, pp. 1553–1559, 2011.

[53] A. Roy, "Characteristics of drug addicts who attempt suicide," *Psychiatry Research*, vol. 121, no. 1, pp. 99–103, 2003.

[54] E. J. Khantzian, "The self-medication hypothesis revisited: the dually diagnosed patient," *Primary Psychiatry*, vol. 10, no. 9, pp. 47–54, 2003.

[55] K. T. Mueser and S. R. McGurk, "Schizophrenia," *The Lancet*, vol. 363, no. 9426, pp. 2063–2072, 2004.

[56] N. D. Brener, J. O. G. Billy, and W. R. Grady, "Assessment of factors affecting the validity of self-reported health-risk behavior among adolescents. Evidence from the scientific literature," *Journal of Adolescent Health*, vol. 33, no. 6, pp. 436–457, 2003.

[57] R. Pinto, L. Correia, and Â. Maia, "Assessing the reliability of retrospective reports of adverse childhood experiences among adolescents with documented childhood maltreatment," *Journal of Family Violence*, vol. 29, no. 4, pp. 431–438, 2014.

[58] D. M. Fergusson, L. J. Horwood, and L. J. Woodward, "The stability of child abuse reports: a longitudinal study of the reporting behaviour of young adults," *Psychological Medicine*, vol. 30, no. 3, pp. 529–544, 2000.

[59] E. Stefanopoulou, A. Manoharan, S. Landau, J. R. Geddes, G. Goodwin, and S. Frangou, "Cognitive functioning in patients with affective disorders and schizophrenia: a meta-analysis,"

International Review of Psychiatry, vol. 21, no. 4, pp. 336–356, 2009.

[60] S. Raffard, A. D'Argembeau, C. Lardi, S. Bayard, J.-P. Boulenger, and M. Van Der Linden, "Exploring self-defining memories in schizophrenia," *Memory*, vol. 17, no. 1, pp. 26–38, 2009.

[61] A. D'Argembeau, S. Raffard, and M. Van der Linden, "Remembering the past and imagining the future in schizophrenia," *Journal of Abnormal Psychology*, vol. 117, no. 1, pp. 247–251, 2008.

[62] A. Aleman, R. Hijman, E. H. F. de Haan, and R. S. Kahn, "Memory impairment in schizophrenia: a meta-analysis," *American Journal of Psychiatry*, vol. 156, no. 9, pp. 1358–1366, 1999.

[63] H. L. Fisher, T. K. Craig, P. Fearon et al., "Reliability and comparability of psychosis patients' retrospective reports of childhood abuse," *Schizophrenia Bulletin*, vol. 37, no. 3, pp. 546–553, 2011.

[64] A. L. Supina and S. B. Patten, "Self-reported diagnoses of schizophrenia and psychotic disorders may be valuable for monitoring and surveillance," *Canadian Journal of Psychiatry*, vol. 51, no. 4, pp. 256–259, 2006.

[65] S. Saha, D. Chant, J. Welham, and J. McGrath, "A systematic review of the prevalence of schizophrenia," *PLoS Medicine*, vol. 2, no. 5, pp. 413–433, 2005.

[66] O. Nielssen and S. Misrachi, "Prevalence of psychoses on reception to male prisons in New South Wales," *Australian and New Zealand Journal of Psychiatry*, vol. 39, no. 6, pp. 453–459, 2005.

[67] S. Rosenman, A. Korten, J. Medway, and M. Evans, "Characterising psychosis in the Australian National Survey of Mental Health and Wellbeing study on low prevalence (psychotic) disorders," *Australian and New Zealand Journal of Psychiatry*, vol. 34, no. 5, pp. 792–800, 2000.

13

Schizophrenia as a Disorder of Social Communication

Cynthia Gayle Wible

Laboratory of Neuroscience, Department of Psychiatry VA Boston Healthcare System, Harvard Medical School, Psychiatry 116A, 940 Belmont Street, Brockton, MA 02301, USA

Correspondence should be addressed to Cynthia Gayle Wible, cindy@bwh.harvard.edu

Academic Editor: Margaret A. Niznikiewicz

Evidence is reviewed for the existence of a core system for moment-to-moment social communication that is based on the perception of dynamic gestures and other social perceptual processes in the temporal-parietal occipital junction (TPJ), including the posterior superior temporal sulcus (PSTS) and surrounding regions. Overactivation of these regions may produce the schizophrenic syndrome. The TPJ plays a key role in the perception and production of dynamic social, emotional, and attentional gestures for the self and others. These include dynamic gestures of the body, face, and eyes as well as audiovisual speech and prosody. Many negative symptoms are characterized by deficits in responding within these domains. Several properties of this system have been discovered through single neuron recording, brain stimulation, neuroimaging, and the study of neurological impairment. These properties map onto the schizophrenic syndrome. The representation of dynamic gestures is multimodal (auditory, visual, and tactile), matching the predominant hallucinatory categories in schizophrenia. Inherent in the perceptual signal of gesture representation is a computation of intention, agency, and anticipation or expectancy (for the self and others). The neurons are also tuned or biased to rapidly detect threat-related emotions. I review preliminary evidence that overactivation of this system can result in schizophrenia.

1. Introduction

Is there a system for dynamic moment to moment social communication in the brain? Social perception has now been extensively studied in humans and nonhuman primates and is defined as follows: "...the initial states of evaluating the social communicative intentions of others by analysis of eye-gaze direction, facial expressions, body movements, and other types of biological motion." [1]. Recent evidence suggests that such a system does exist and that abnormal activity in this system may produce the symptoms and cognitive deficits that comprise the syndrome of schizophrenia. A posterior system will be described whose activity may correspond to or underlie the perceptual experience of conversing and interacting with others. Until recently, communication has primarily been studied through language research. This line of research has focused mainly on the structure of the representation and the neural basis of language input (graphemes, phonemes), the internal lexical/semantic representation, and language output (writing and speech production) and has made significant progress in understanding language.

2. Communication Involves Not Only Language Processing but Also Social Cognitive Functions

Communication with another individual involves a set of representations or processes that are outside the scope of traditional language research. Many of these representational systems are studied under the rubric of social cognition. Social communication (in humans) necessitates the dynamic perception of speech, social-emotional cues, and the production of the communicative message (narrative, intonation, and gestures).

The speech signal that is used to communicate is (primarily) both auditory and visual in nature. In naturalistic settings, the perception of speech occurs simultaneously with the dynamic visual perception of gestures, especially of the face. The audiovisual speech signal not only conveys meaning through words but also contains information about emotion (facial expressions and prosody). Perception during conversation also necessitates a host of other functions that are crucial for communication. During the rapid interplay of conversation, the ability to anticipate other's thoughts and actions is also essential. Theory of mind is used; this is the ability to "think about thoughts" and to represent other's point of view. The representation of agency (who is doing what) and intention, both in other's and in one's self, are important. The correct deployment of attention and working memory are needed as well as the ability to follow or track other's behavior and speech. A narrative of the conversation must be built up and maintained; this is an understanding of the context and the story or message that is being conveyed by the individual words and sentences. During conversation, meaning is built up not only from words but also from body and facial gestures as well as intonation (prosody). Recent evidence suggests that there may be a set of brain areas whose functionality matches the representations and processes needed during moment to moment social communication [2–6]. The temporal parietal occipital junction or TPJ (especially in the right hemisphere) is referred to as the "social brain area" [7] because it has been implicated in numerous neuroimaging studies of social cognitive functions such as theory of mind, empathy, social attention, and other functions [2, 3]. Figures 1 and 2 show the functional architecture of the TPJ. It has been hypothesized that the TPJ is involved in lower-level processes associated with empathy, theory of mind, agency, and attentional orienting to salient stimuli and that these processes are crucial to higher-level social function [2] (see Figure 2). The TPJ includes the inferior parietal region as well as the posterior superior temporal sulcus (PSTS) and gyrus (note that only the right hemisphere is shown, but the left TPJ region is also involved in these functions). The functional territory for the PSTS is often thought to extend inferiorly to at least the posterior middle temporal gyrus. The notion that the TPJ is crucial for social interaction/communication has now been tested directly in human subjects. A recent naturalistic functional magnetic resonance imaging (FMRI) study of live face-to-face interaction within an MRI scanner showed strong evidence that the TPJ is a core region for moment to moment social interaction [4]. Medial prefrontal regions have also been hypothesized to play a role in social functioning and data on this point will be reviewed (predominately in the later section of the paper).

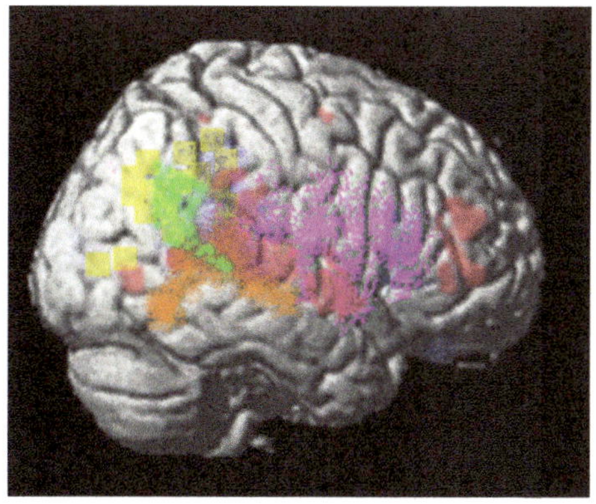

Figure 1: Summary figure of the overlap of functional regions in the TPJ (inferior parietal and PSTS); this region is involved in eye gaze (red); audiovisual speech (orange); self-representation (yellow); theory of mind (green); emotional perception of faces and prosody (dark blue and purple). Rerepresentation of data is, respectively, from [37–40, 47].

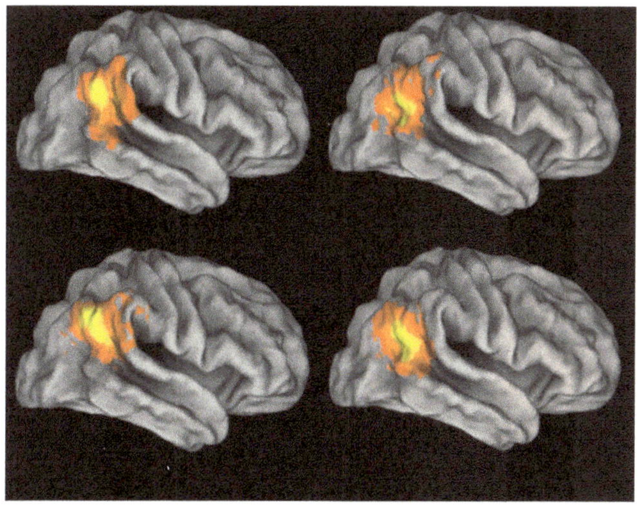

Figure 2: Results of a quantitative meta-analysis of 70 functional neuroimaging studies. Activation likelihood estimation maps in the right temporoparietal junction are shown. Colors code the probability of activation with brighter yellow indicating the highest activation (reprinted with permission from [2]).

3. General Characteristics and Anatomical Connections of the TPJ

The PSTS has a major role in the perception of dynamic gestures. A basic function of the inferior parietal region is in the formation of intentions for action and this region (as well as the intraparietal sulcus) contains mirror representations that are active during either the perception or production of an action [8]. The intraparietal sulcus separates the inferior and superior parietal lobe. Portions of the intraparietal sulcus such as the lateral intraparietal region or LIP are thought to contain a dynamically constructed saliency map that is used to guide gestures such as saccades [8–10]. The TPJ and surrounding regions project to the inferior frontal region and are closely anatomically associated with hippocampal and insular regions [5, 6, 11]. Interoceptive and homeostatic body signals activate the insula (including thirst, sensual touch, sexual arousal, warmth, heartbeat, and bladder distension) [12]. Subjective ratings of these body signals correlate most strongly with activation in the anterior insula and this region has been hypothesized to underlie emotional awareness [12]. Craig describes the anterior insula for "feeling emotion and homeostatic and body feelings" relative to the anterior cingulate's limbic motor function or role in initiating or motivating behavior.

4. Social Cognition Is Abnormal in Schizophrenia

It is well known that social cognitive deficits form a major part of the schizophrenic syndrome. Social cognitive deficits are considered to be a major determinant of functional outcome for schizophrenic individuals [13]. Social responsiveness is affected in schizophrenia; the negative symptoms include asociality as well as a lack of facial movement, facial expression, eye contact, and vocal inflection (prosody). In fact the four most prevalent so-called negative symptoms of schizophrenia are a lack of expressive gestures, a lack of vocal inflection and social inattention, as well as a general impairment in attention. Schizophrenic individuals also present with theory of mind deficits and these deficits are related to a lack of expressiveness [14, 15]. It is also important to note that internal experiences of emotion and related sensations (perhaps related to insular function) do not seem to be as abnormal in schizophrenia as emotional responsiveness [16, 17].

5. Building Links between the Syndrome of Schizophrenia and Brain Dysfunction: a Parsimonious Account of Positive and Negative Symptoms as Stemming from the Same, Similar, and/or Adjacent Social Cognitive Modules within the TPJ

These negative symptoms and social cognitive deficits could clearly be described as problems with social communicative representations or systems. However, I will argue that most, if not all, of the schizophrenic syndrome can be understood under the rubric of social communication. Recent advances in understanding this system will be described and used to reframe the symptoms of schizophrenia and to then link them to brain function. It is proposed that the overactivation of the functional modules in the TPJ that subserve social communication produces the syndrome of schizophrenia. Direct evidence for TPJ involvement in schizophrenia will be presented near the end of the paper. The formulation presented here is new and remains to be systematically tested. However there are many lines of evidence that will be described below here in after. For example, schizophrenic symptoms are evoked by stimulation to the TPJ [18–21], electrical brain activity within the TPJ coincides with the presence and absence of symptoms [22], and the disruption of TPJ activity alleviates symptoms [23–28].

6. Reframing the Schizophrenic Syndrome and Evaluating the Evidence for the Involvement of the TPJ in Social Processing

Understanding aspects of this system at the neural (single cell) and systems neuroscience levels may provide a basis for the understanding the disparate symptoms and cognitive deficits found in the schizophrenic syndrome. Several principles were used to guide the construction of the current framework. Neuroimaging alone cannot provide evidence for a region's involvement in a particular function and taken alone constitutes relatively weak evidence for a link between a function and a brain region. Lesion studies must also show that the function is impaired when the region is damaged. In evaluating human lesion data it is important to analyze each case individually [29]. The extent of involvement of other damaged regions should be taken into account. Data from patients with brain trauma from head injury or with epilepsy should be viewed with caution as these patients often have diffuse damage that may be missed in a radiologic examination. Converging evidence from several sources provides the strongest basis for positing a relationship between brain and function. For example, in interpreting functional imaging data, it is also important that other sources show convergence with the theory, including brain stimulation, transcranial magnetic stimulation (TMS), and data from neuronal recordings in humans or animals. Data from single case studies with circumscribed brain lesions that contradict a specific theoretical position must be accounted for and are a serious indictment of the theoretical position [29]. For each functional domain discussed here in after, I will cite neuroimaging and lesion data to show that the TPJ is a core substrate for the function (as well as data from the other techniques as discussed previously). When single neuron data are described, I will cite evidence showing similar findings from human studies in order to provide explicit links between cellular properties and systems level function (a detailed description of all the studies cited here can be found in [5, 6]).

7. The Phenomenology of the Schizophrenic Syndrome Reframed

For brevity, this paper will describe the most prominent symptoms and their relationship to brain function; a detailed account for the other symptoms can be found in [6]. Auditory hallucinations of voices are the most prevalent symptom [30]. Patients have the feeling that someone is actually there and speaking. Auditory hallucinations can also take the form of hearing conversations between voices. Patients will sometimes report that it seems like there is actually another person or persons in their head. Some types of auditory hallucinations may be due to a misattribution of the patient's thoughts to an outside source (abnormal agency attribution for the voice). Visual hallucinations of people in action are the next most prominent category of hallucination [31]. The most common delusions, delusions of persecution and delusions of reference, are characterized by the feeling of being followed, watched, or that people are secretly communicating using gestures or clothes [32]. The prominent positive symptoms of schizophrenia revolve around *the perception or feeling of an entity* that is speaking, communicating, watching, following, observing, or spying. Schizophrenia is also characterized *by abnormal agency judgments*; patients can feel as though their actions and thoughts are controlled by an outside force or entity (e.g., delusions of control, thought insertion, thought broadcasting). Therefore, the prominent hallucinations and delusions may be reframed as the misperception of a social entity or entities or overactivation of representations in the TPJ that subserve many aspects of dynamic social processing. Throughout the paper I will review properties of dynamic social perception and interaction that may be important for understanding the schizophrenic syndrome. For example, recent advances in cognitive neuroscience show that the perception of a social entity is accompanied by an intrinsic and automatic perception of agency, intention, and social prediction [33–36]. These functions are intrinsic to the representation of dynamic action at the single neuron level [33, 34, 36]. It has also been shown that self and other processing overlap and the feeling of a presence can also stem from abnormal activation of the self-representation [19–21, 37]. The prominent negative symptoms are related to abnormal social responding and a lack of social expression or response primarily in the face and voice. The regions that are used to perceive dynamic social interaction are also used in the formation of intentions for the production of social, emotional, and attentional gestures as well as for theory of mind [2, 7, 38–42]. This reframing of the syndrome is parsimonious in that it postulates that the symptoms can be understood as the integrated action of one region (as opposed to widespread abnormalities or complex interactions between anterior and posterior regions).

In the following sections, I will describe the functional architecture (the arrangement or juxtaposition of functional regions) as well as properties of the neuronal representation of dynamic social action that can be used to understand the schizophrenic syndrome. The functional contributions of the TPJ have been described in several disparate subfields of neuroscience and cognitive neuroscience that are conceptually overlapping but motivated by the investigation of different psychological functions [2, 5, 6]. In describing these findings, I will also show how individual schizophrenic symptoms can be reframed and organized under the rubric of TPJ function.

8. The Communicative Signal Is Based on TPJ Function, Is Multimodal (Especially Auditory and Visual), and Carries an Automatic Computation of Agency, Intention, and Social Prediction

The neural code used by the TPJ reflects the fact that communication occurs not only through auditory language comprehension but also through gestures that can occur simultaneously with the speech signal. A basic and prominent function of the TPJ is to represent dynamic gestures, especially in lateral temporal and inferior parietal regions centered on the PSTS in humans [42]. Lesions and repetitive transcranial magnetic stimulation (rTMS) to these regions impair biological motion perception [43, 44]. The homologous regions in the monkey have neurons that are multimodal and respond to the sight, sound, and somatosensory aspects of biological motion [41, 45]. Single-cell recordings in monkeys show that audiovisual representation is the most predominant type of representation followed by visual-tactile representation [45]. The PSTS combines information about biological motion, social/biographical information and speech [41, 46]. In humans, the representation of audiovisual speech occupies a large portion of the TPJ territory (see Figure 1 [47]). These relative proportions match the fact that hallucinations of voices and the feeling that someone is speaking predominate in schizophrenia followed by visual hallucinations of people and then by tactile hallucinations. Hearing voices also activates the TPJ [48].

Multimodal gesture representations have properties that allow the neurons to participate in more conceptual functions such as the computation of agency, the ability to keep track of other's behavior, and the ability to predict the actions of others (social prediction) [33, 34, 49–51]. For example, repetition suppression in the monkey STS creates a situation in which neurons that are tuned to sequences of dynamic gestures are maximally responsive to gestures that are about to occur [33]. Single-cell recordings in monkeys have shown that these functions are automatically computed and are an inherent part of the gesture representation at the single neuron level. Neuroimaging has confirmed that activity in the PSTS in humans is also modulated by the perceived intentionality of the gesture or movement [35]. In addition, the human STS was found to be a region in which interactions occur between observed action and the reafferent motor-related copy of that action [52].

Hence, overactivation of this dynamic gesture system could produce the erroneous perception of speech, visual human action (visual hallucinations of people), or tactile hallucinations. Direct evidence for this supposition comes from the fact that cortical stimulation of the TPJ (in nonpsychotic individuals) and lateral posterior temporal lobe can result in visual hallucinations of action scenes involving people [18]. Cortical stimulation of the TPJ can also cause feelings of limbs or body parts changing shape in nonpsychotic individuals (e.g., somatosensory hallucinations and delusions [19]). The overactivation of gesture representations could be graded so that some patients might experience frank hallucinations and others might experience a feeling that there are persons acting, watching, or communicating with them. In addition, this overactivation would be predicted to produce a feeling of agency or of an agent with intentions and would be expected to interfere with social prediction and social interaction.

Activity in these PSTS/TPJ multimodal neurons that encode gestures (especially audiovisual gestures) has been shown in monkeys and humans to provide rapid feedback excitation (within 30 msec) to unimodal regions and to result in gamma synchronization [53]. This phenomenon has been documented in several studies (reviewed in [5, 6]). Hence, erroneously activated audiovisual speech representations may cause the aberrant activation of auditory cortex and the gamma synchronization of TPJ and primary auditory regions. This would result in increased attention and activity in auditory channels.

9. The TPJ Is a Core Substrate for Theory of Mind

The TPJ is a core neural substrate for theory of mind or the ability to understand and represent another's point of view or thoughts [39, 54, 55]. Neuroimaging studies of theory of mind have shown several foci including the TPJ, the orbital frontal cortex, amygdala, anterior insula, and medial frontal regions [56]. The medial prefrontal cortex or the anterior paracingulate cortex—approximately corresponding to Brodmann area (BA) 9/32—had been thought to be a key region for theory of mind function [56]. However, previous reports of an association between theory of mind, social processing, and the medial prefrontal cortex have relied on patients with traumatic brain injury or epilepsy. These types of patient often have diffuse brain damage that is difficult to detect in radiologic exams (see Bird et al. (2004) [57] for a critical discussion of these studies). There have now been several reports of circumscribed lesions to the medial prefrontal cortex where the patients *do not show theory of mind impairments* [57–60]. Bird et al. (2004) [57] present a carefully documented case of a patient whose injury is circumscribed and coincides with the region identified in several fMRI studies to be involved in theory of mind (see Figure 3). This individual did show impairments in planning and memory as well as a tendency to confabulate but did not show theory of mind deficits on any of a battery of tasks [57]. In another study, three patients with anterior cingulate damage were tested on theory of mind, social situation processing, and motivational decision making. Two of the patients had selective anterior cingulate damage (one also had temporal lobe damage). These two patients were *not impaired in theory of mind, motivational decision making, or social situation processing* [58].

TPJ lesions *do impair* theory of mind [60]. In addition, recent neuroimaging studies have shown that the (right) TPJ has a response profile that is more selective for theory of mind than other regions such as the posterior cingulate and the medial prefrontal cortex. The right TPJ was selectively involved in the attribution of mental states rather than reasoning about general socially relevant facts about a person [54]. The ability to make inferences about mental states or beliefs and intentions during moral judgments was also impaired when TMS was applied to the right TPJ [61]. Neurons in the monkey STS that respond to dynamic action or biological motion are tuned to respond to physical or vocal actions that are about to occur or to anticipate action [33, 49]. Aberrant activity in the TPJ would interfere with theory of mind computations resulting in abnormal or slowed social behavior. This abnormal activity would also interfere with dynamic social response and the tracking and hence understanding of other's social behavior. These impairments are core components of the schizophrenic syndrome which includes symptoms such as asociality and social inattention as well as theory of mind deficits as described previously [13–15, 62, 63].

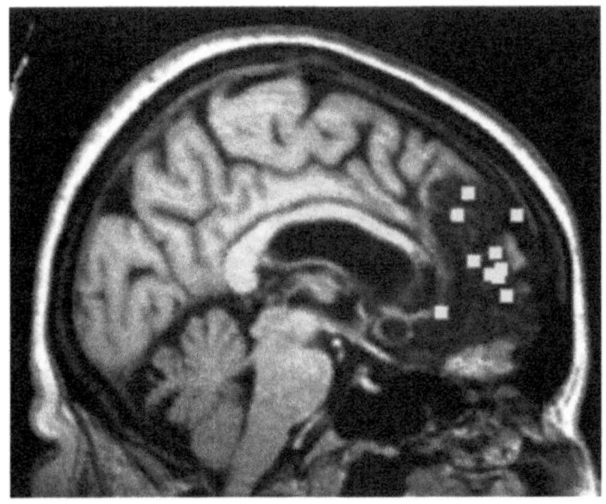

Figure 3: Figure from Bird et al., 2004, showing the lesion site of a patient with anterior cingulate damage who did not show theory of mind impairments. Peak activation foci related to theory of mind from ten different neuroimaging studies are shown (boxes) superimposed onto the lesion site. The figure shows that a lesion in the region of the anterior cingulate activated by theory of mind tasks does not cause impairments on these tasks (reprinted with permission from [57]).

10. Emotional Perception and Reaction

Emotional gesture perception and reaction for the face and body as well as prosody perception are dependent on the TPJ, presumably because of its role in voice and gesture representation (e.g., eyes and face). Emotional perception and reaction are linked; the perception of facial expressions produces a subtle version of the expression on the viewer's face [64]. The perceptual circuits that are used to perceive other's actions are also used to represent and plan our own actions, and several regions are active during both observation and imitation of dynamic gestures [7, 64, 65]. Single neurons in the monkey PSTS respond to emotional gestures [49]. Human neuroimaging studies also show that the TPJ is involved in emotional gesture and prosody perception [66, 67]. Lesions within the primary/secondary somatosensory cortex, supramarginal gyrus (part of inferior parietal cortex/TPJ), and insula (adjacent and medial to the TPJ) result in a deficit in the ability to perceive facial emotion and prosody [40]. The supramarginal gyrus may be especially important for the creation of the intentions or plans for emotional and prosodic reaction. Hence, the overexcitation of emotional gesture perceptual circuits could interfere with reaction or with the formation of intentions for facial emotional reaction. This would result in social unreactivity or asociality as well as a lack of facial movement, eye contact, vocal inflection, and facial expression; these are all prominent negative symptoms of schizophrenia.

11. Eye Gestures, Social Attention, and Agency

Movements of the eyes are especially important in social cognition and communication; they not only convey emotion but also convey the focus of attention. Dynamic representations of emotional gesture and attention are used in the perception of more conceptual aspects of social cognition [35, 68]. The TPJ and especially the posterior STS and superior temporal regions are core components of a system for the representation and perception of eye gaze [38, 69, 70]. The TPJ was shown to be selectively involved in representing joint or social attention in a neuroimaging investigation of live social interaction [39]. The perception of gaze direction and the control of attention via gaze are impaired with TPJ damage [70, 71]. Aberrant activity in this system could produce a deficit in the tracking of others eye gestures resulting in abnormal social attention and hence social reaction and understanding.

As discussed previously, the perception of intentionality and agency are an inherent component of the perception of dynamic gestures, including eye gaze [35, 72–74]. For example, in the monkey, neurons in the STS combine information about gestures of the arm (e.g., reaching) with information about the direction of gaze (the focus of attention) to compute agency or intentionality [34]. Overactivation of gaze and other gesture representations would produce the qualia not only of a presence (of being watched) but also of a presence with intentions. This assumption is corroborated with data; direct cortical stimulation of the TPJ can cause the feeling of a "shadowy presence" [20].

12. Gesture Neurons Are Tuned to Rapidly Detect Threat

Another property of gesture representation in the TPJ is that the neurons in this neural circuit are tuned to rapidly detect emotionally negative or socially threating gestures. The amygdala is most often cited with regard to this function. However, amygdala damage does not cause a deficit in the detection of dynamic body expressions of fear [75, 76]. This means that there is another brain region that is the core substrate for this function. Single neuron recording in the monkey STS showed that the neurons are tuned or biased to detect potentially threatening biological motion [41]. Event-related potential (ERP) and neuroimaging studies in humans have confirmed that the TPJ is used to perceive threating or emotionally negative gestures [41, 77]. Hence, although this region is generally used to perceive dynamic gestures, there is a neural tuning for the detection of social threat. Hence, overactivation of these gesture representations might produce the feeling of being in a socially threating situation. This feeling could be a component of delusions of persecution and other symptoms.

13. Self-Representation, Embodiment, and Agency

The perception of self-made gestures from our own visuospatial perspective and the corresponding auditory, visual, tactile, and vestibular information resulting from actions may provide the concrete scaffolding that is used to create and sustain the self-representation or the feeling of being an embodied, thinking, and acting person [37]. There are also more fixed body schemas that are presumably constructed through experience and that are used in the dynamic representation of the self (these are also located in the vicinity of the TPJ—in the intraparietal sulcus and the secondary somatosensory cortex; see [6] for a summary). Our sense of self is so evident and constant that it may be surprising to learn that it is actually a perceptual construct. However, this construct can break down and be demonstrably associated with certain neural circuits in the same way as other psychological functions such as memory and language. Changes in the feeling of embodiment can be affected by manipulating visual-somatosensory percepts that are represented within the TPJ, by stimulation of the TPJ, or by lesions in the TPJ [37, 78]. For example, the experimental manipulation of visuospatial perspective and simultaneous tactile stimulation can cause the feeling of inhabiting a different body or body swapping [79]. Stimulation or lesion in the TPJ region can cause out-of-body experiences and other changes in the feeling of embodiment [19]. For example, a patient (Susan) with right temporoparietal damage was reported who had a "Capgras syndrome for her mirror image" [80] (see pages 73–75). This patient used sign language and was observed communicating with the person in the mirror (her own reflection). She believed that there was this other "Susan" in the mirror who had the same background, appearance, and age and went to the same school as she did (but she did not know her in school). The other Susan was judged to be a bit slower and not as good at sign language as the real Susan.

The regions and representations that are used to represent the self overlap with those that are used to represent others (see detailed discussion in [6, 37, 81]). The regions that are thought to compute the self-representation are also activated by the perception of dynamic visual (gesture), auditory, or somatosensory stimulation from others, including the TPJ, somatosensory cortex, secondary somatosensory cortex, the extrastriate body area, the intraparietal sulcus, and ventral premotor regions [42, 82]. For example, the secondary somatosensory area responds to touch regardless of whether it was felt on one's own skin or seen on another [83]. Most of the functional components that have been identified with self-representation in the TPJ are modulated by auditory, visual, and tactile inputs and hence overactivation of these channels would be expected to disturb the self-representation [6].

Abnormal feelings of agency and of a presence could also occur as a result of a disturbance of the TPJ self-representation (reviewed in [5, 6]). The bulk of the experimental evidence shows that abnormal activity in TPJ regions and vestibular cortex (insula/inferior parietal lobe) can produce these phenomena [21]. Heautoscopy, the experience of an alternate self or Doppelganger, is associated with either abnormal activity or damage in the TPJ [21]. Visual hallucinations of people are the second most prominent type of hallucination in schizophrenia and may arise from abnormal activation of the self-representation. When the body double is seen (visual hallucination), the visual appearance may or may not mirror the person's own image, but the imitation of body gestures by the double can produce the feeling that the double contains the *real* mind. The experience of the self can be perceived to arise from the body double or can alternate between the physical body and the body double. This type of hallucination can also be experienced as a feeling of a presence or multiple presences of closely projected doubles that are not visible [21]. This feeling of a presence has been induced by electrical stimulation of the PSTS region [20]. Aberrant activation of the self-representation would be expected to interfere with feelings of embodiment and agency for one's thoughts and actions as is seen in symptoms such as delusions of control and could also produce the qualia (feeling of a presence) associated with delusions of persecution, delusions of jealousy, and delusions of reference or visual hallucinations.

Several neuroimaging studies of schizophrenia have shown that abnormal agency processing in patients is related to overactivation in (especially the right) IP or TPJ (reviewed in [5, 84]). For example, one study of agency processing found abnormal activity in the right inferior parietal region in schizophrenic subjects and this overactivation was also positively correlated with the Schneiderian score [85].

14. The Medial and Orbital Frontal Regions, Social Cognition, and Self-Representation

Impairments in self-awareness related to abnormal activity in midline structures have been hypothesized to play a role in the social processing problems that have been identified in schizophrenia [86]. Several central and medial regions of the brain, including those in the frontal lobe (medial orbital, the ventromedial prefrontal cortex, the anterior cingulate cortex, dorsomedial prefrontal cortex), have been theorized to be involved in self-referential processing and self-reflection [87, 88]. The evidence for this supposition comes mainly from neuroimaging studies where central midline regions have been found to show activity in tasks such as the recall of personal information, the assessment of self-personality traits, appearance, attitudes, or feelings [87, 88]. Gillihan and Farah (2005) [89], in a critical review of this literature, noted that confounding factors were not adequately controlled in many of these studies. A recent study used TMS to disrupt processing and to probe the brain response to self-related stimuli with non-self-related stimuli. Superior performance on self-related items (the self-reference effect) was found. TMS to left and right parietal cortex suppressed the self reference effect, but no effects on the self-reference effect were found with TMS to the medial prefrontal lobe [90]. It was discussed previously how patients with circumscribed and well-documented medial frontal lesions do not present with a deficit in social situation processing nor have deficits in self-related processing been reported [57, 58, 91]. Confabulation is known to occur with frontal lobe damage [80]. The current framework assumes that delusions are not confabulations but rather explanations of bizarre sensory phenomena as suggested by Brendan Maher (2006) [92].

The dorsal anterior cingulate has previously been associated with action monitoring or the monitoring of response conflict and in cognitive control (see review in [93]). This function is thought to be used in social situations [87, 93, 94]. However, there are now several reports of individuals with circumscribed lesions of this area. These individuals have not been found to have deficits in tasks used to measure response conflict such as the Stroop nor in behavioral measures of cognitive control; see for example, [91]. In fact, recent evidence suggests that the dorsal anterior cingulate response to errors may be more related to levels of negative affect during task performance than to response conflict [95]. These results are consistent with the view that the dorsal anterior cingulate plays a role in the control of autonomic responses that accompany cognitive effort (see review in [91]). The dorsal anterior cingulate may be involved in response selection based on reward contingencies; data from single unit studies in monkeys and in humans and further lesion data from humans undergoing cingulotomy support this hypothesis (see review in [91]). The dorsomedial aspect of the prefrontal cortex may have a role in empathy, in representing emotional pain in others, and/or in the ability to use emotional pain or negative consequences to constrain behavior [96]. Although empathy and theory of mind scores are correlated, the precise relationship between them is unclear [57]. A recent FMRI study found that the anterior middle cingulate cortex responded to both emotionally and physically painful events, while the dorsomedial prefrontal cortex responded selectively to emotional pain [96]. A lack of empathy does not seem to be central to schizophrenia, although it is a symptom of the manic phase of bipolar disorder.

Orbital and ventral medial frontal lesions also do not cause theory of mind deficits [97] but rather result in an acquired sociopathy [98]. Orbital and ventral medial frontal lobe damage has generally been reported to result in a lack of empathy, euphoria, irresponsibility, a lack of concern for the future, and a lack of concern for social rules [97–99]. When tested explicitly on measures of social judgment and responding, individuals with orbital and inferior medial frontal lesions present with an intact knowledge of social rules and the ability to judge the outcomes [98]. However, their autonomic responses to socially meaningful stimuli may be abnormal and it is has been hypothesized that these patients fail to activate somatic (body emotional) states in response to social stimuli [99]. Another report surmised that orbital damage results in a reduced ability to use the expectation of negative emotional reactions (anger) to constrain behavior [97]. Recently it has been reported that orbitofrontal lesions cause a diminished sensitivity to varying reward magnitudes [100]. These data are consistent with single unit recordings in monkeys showing neuronal responses that were associated with various aspects of reward computed from experience with behavioral choices [101]. It is claimed that damage to the orbital and ventral medial prefrontal cortex leads to an inability to "develop a coherent model of one's own self" and hence emotional liability and aberrant social functioning [87]. However, the function of orbital and ventral medial frontal cortices has been repeatedly shown to be related to an inability to use negative emotions to constrain behavior or to competently compute and use reward or punishment outcomes. This syndrome seems more closely aligned with mania where decision making is impaired and individuals often do risky things without regard to the emotions of others (manic symptoms include euphoria, lack of empathy, impulsiveness, lack of concern for consequences of behavior and for social rules) and manic patients sometimes confabulate as is seen in patients with frontal lobe lesions [80].

In summary, medial prefrontal regions have been shown to be activated during tasks assessing theory of mind and self related processing; this presupposes a role for these regions in social processing. Anterior cingulate regions show coactivation with the TPJ in many neuroimaging studies and hence abnormal activity in the TPJ could be expected to affect activity in this region. However, as yet there are many competing theories concerning the role of this part of the system and hence it is unclear what the functional consequences of abnormal activity would be and what form they would take (overactivation, lack of activation).

15. Direct Evidence for TPJ Involvement in Schizophrenia

It is hypothesized that the TPJ (and primary efferent areas) should show slightly elevated baseline activity interposed with epochs of hyperactivation that correspond to the abnormal qualia (hallucinations and delusions) and responsive deficiencies (negative symptoms) seen in schizophrenia [5, 6, 102]. Although it is not often acknowledged (perhaps because of the almost axiomatic belief in frontal lobe abnormalities), there is strong evidence for TPJ involvement in psychosis and schizophrenia. Activity has been recorded in the TPJ that corresponds to the experience of symptoms, activity has been found that is correlated with symptoms, and recent large-scale morphometric studies show volume reductions in the TPJ in schizophrenia. Torrey [103] wrote an extensive review of the evidence for inferior parietal involvement in schizophrenia that includes an account of the relationship between prodromal symptoms and parietal function (we will not reiterate that evidence here). The TPJ region is a relatively anatomically variable region and hence volume abnormalities could be relatively difficult to detect; the inferior parietal region is one of the last regions in the brain to be myelinated and develops into late adolescence [104]. However, recently two large-scale morphometric studies of schizophrenic volume reductions have been published. Both of these studies show core reductions in TPJ volumes [105, 106]. Direct evidence for abnormal activity in the TPJ during psychosis comes from brain recordings; right inferior parietal activity was related a delusional state in a magnetoencephalography (MEG) study [22]. When the abnormal activity subsided, the delusions subsided. Correspondingly, interference with TPJ activity alleviates schizophrenic symptoms. At first TMS was applied to the TPJ to treat auditory hallucinations; at least 6 published studies have now shown that TMS applied to the TPJ alleviates auditory hallucinations and some reports show reductions in other symptoms as well [23–28]. For example, in one study schizophrenic subjects with treatment-resistant auditory hallucinations were given daily rTMS treatments for 10 days and showed a reduction in the frequency of auditory hallucinations and an improvement in many other symptoms [23].

Data from our previously published studies have consistently supported TPJ involvement; schizophrenic symptoms such as auditory hallucinations and thought disorder were correlated with levels of FMRI activity in the inferior parietal and superior temporal sulcus in several studies [107–109]. One of the most systematic FMRI symptom capture studies of schizophrenia was one of a single schizophrenic subject who heard voices for approximately 26 seconds and then no voices for approximately 26 seconds; this periodicity is relatively optimal for an FMRI design [110]. FMRI activation was detected surrounding the PSTS approximately 3 seconds prior to the conscious detection of the auditory hallucination. Activation of the inferior parietal and inferior frontal regions followed. The PSTS activation (which extended into the superior and middle temporal regions) was persistent through the entire experience. This coincides with the unusual extended neural responses (e.g., 7 seconds) recorded in monkey STS neurons that are activated by dynamic multimodal gestures [49].

TPJ over-activation could stem from a number of causes, but it is hypothesized that in schizophrenia the source is most often from over-activation of the hippocampal system [111]. The activity of the hippocampus shows a high association or correlation with activity in the TPJ (so-called default mode or cortical hub activity) and evidence from epileptic individuals shows that abnormal hippocampal activity underlies active psychosis and that the TPJ region is also involved [6]. Note that resting state abnormalities have been repeatedly found in schizophrenia and that a seed placed within the hippocampus will produce activity in most of the "default mode" regions [112–115] (see [6] for a detailed discussion of hippocampal involvement).

16. Summary

In summary, the regions that make up the TPJ form a core system for the perception and production of emotional face and body gestures as well as prosody. This region shows functional activity that indicates that it is preferentially involved in the perception of narrative (versus words or sentences) [3]. This area is a core component for the perception of social attention or of the process of joint attention (the deployment of attention according to social and communicative cues). This area is also the core region in the brain for theory of mind or understanding other's intentions and thoughts. The neural activity in this system is biased to detect or anticipate future multimodal social acts, or in other words to anticipate speech and actions. Inherent in the representation of multimodal gestures is a coding of intention and agency. Even though this system is used for the perception and production of biological motion or gestures, there is a neural bias or tuning for the rapid identification of social threat and parts of the TPJ are core components of fear perception (reviewed in [5, 6]). The TPJ not only represents other's actions but may also be a core area for representing the self. This is the only region of the brain that produces verbal memory deficits when damaged and hence is the neural substrate for verbal working memory (reviewed in [5, 6]). Since neural activity in this region corresponds to social perception and joint attention, over-activation of this region could result in the erroneous perception of being within a dynamic social situation. Over-activation of this region would have widespread consequences for many domains including social perception, social reactivity, and attention.

When the consistency and weight of the evidence is considered, the characteristics of TPJ function more closely match the symptoms of schizophrenia. Hippocampal activity has been consistently shown to be abnormal in schizophrenia which is highly correlated with both TPJ and anterior cingulate/paracingulate activity [113–115]. The characteristics of medial prefrontal function (especially from the lesion data) may match those of bipolar disorder more closely than those of schizophrenia.

Conflict of Interests

The authors declare that this paper was conducted in the absence of any commercial or financial relationships that could be construed as a potential conflict of interests (6, 2950-2967).

Acknowledgments

This work was supported by an NIMH Grant 1 R01 MH067080-01A2 and by the Harvard Neuro-Discovery Center (formally HCNR). It was funded also by the Biomedical Informatics Research Network (U24RR021992), National Institute of Mental Health. The author would like to thank Israel Molina for help with the paper.

References

[1] T. Allison, A. Puce, and G. McCarthy, "Social perception from visual cues: role of the STS region," *Trends in Cognitive Sciences*, vol. 4, no. 7, pp. 267–278, 2000.

[2] J. Decety and C. Lamm, "The role of the right temporoparietal junction in social interaction: how low-level computational processes contribute to meta-cognition," *Neuroscientist*, vol. 13, no. 6, pp. 580–593, 2007.

[3] E. Redcay, "The superior temporal sulcus performs a common function for social and speech perception: implications for the emergence of autism," *Neuroscience and Biobehavioral Reviews*, vol. 32, no. 1, pp. 123–142, 2008.

[4] E. Redcay, D. Dodell-Feder, M. J. Pearrow et al., "Live face-to-face interaction during fMRI: a new tool for social cognitive neuroscience," *NeuroImage*, vol. 50, no. 4, pp. 1639–1647, 2010.

[5] C. G. Wible, A. P. Preus, and R. Hashimoto, "A cognitive neuroscience view of schizophrenic symptoms: abnormal activation of a system for social perception and communication," *Brain Imaging and Behavior*, vol. 3, no. 1, pp. 85–110, 2009.

[6] C. G. Wible, "Hippocampaltemporal-parietal junction interaction in the production of psychotic symptoms: a framework for understanding the schizophrenic syndrome," In press.

[7] J. Decety and J. Grezes, "The power of simulation: imagining one's own and other's behavior," *Brain Research*, vol. 1079, no. 1, pp. 4–14, 2006.

[8] J. Gottlieb, "From thought to action: the parietal cortex as a bridge between perception, action, and cognition," *Neuron*, vol. 53, no. 1, pp. 9–16, 2007.

[9] J. T. Klein, R. O. Deaner, and M. L. Platt, "Neural correlates of social target value in macaque parietal cortex," *Current Biology*, vol. 18, no. 6, pp. 419–424, 2008.

[10] K. G. Thompson and N. P. Bichot, "A visual salience map in the primate frontal eye field," *Progress in Brain Research*, vol. 147, pp. 251–262, 2005.

[11] T. Brandt, P. Bartenstein, A. Janek, and M. Dieterich, "Reciprocal inhibitory visual-vestibular interaction. Visual motion stimulation deactivates the parieto-insular vestibular cortex," *Brain*, vol. 121, no. 9, pp. 1749–1758, 1998.

[12] A. D. Craig, "How do you feel—now? The anterior insula and human awareness," *Nature Reviews Neuroscience*, vol. 10, no. 1, pp. 59–70, 2009.

[13] D. C. Javitt, "When doors of perception close: bottom-up models of disrupted cognition in schizophrenia," *Annual Review of Clinical Psychology*, vol. 5, pp. 249–275, 2009.

[14] M. Brune, M. Abdel-Hamid, C. Sonntag, C. Lehmkamper, and R. Langdon, "Linking social cognition with social interaction: non-verbal expressivity, social competence and "mentalising" in patients with schizophrenia spectrum disorders," *Behavioral and Brain Functions*, vol. 5, article 6, 2009.

[15] N. C. Andreasen, C. A. Calarge, and D. S. O'Leary, "Theory of mind and schizophrenia: a positron emission tomography study of medication-free patients," *Schizophrenia Bulletin*, vol. 35, no. 5, p. 1030, 2009.

[16] A. M. Kring, S. L. Kerr, D. A. Smith, and J. M. Neale, "Flat affect in schizophrenia does not reflect diminished subjective experience of emotion," *Journal of Abnormal Psychology*, vol. 102, no. 4, pp. 507–517, 1993.

[17] A. M. Kring and E. K. Moran, "Emotional response deficits in schizophrenia: insights from affective science," *Schizophrenia Bulletin*, vol. 34, no. 5, pp. 819–834, 2008.

[18] W. Penfield and P. Perot, "The brain's record of auditory and visual experience: a final summary and discussion," *Brain*, vol. 86, no. 4, pp. 595–696, 1963.

[19] O. Blanke, S. Ortigue, T. Landis, and M. Seeck, "Stimulating illusory own-body perceptions," *Nature*, vol. 419, no. 6904, pp. 269–270, 2002.

[20] S. Arzy, M. Seeck, S. Ortigue, L. Spinelli, and O. Blanke, "Induction of an illusory shadow person," *Nature*, vol. 443, no. 7109, article 287, 2006.

[21] P. Brugger, O. Blanke, M. Regard, D. T. Bradford, and T. Landis, "Polyopic heautoscopy: case report and review of the literature," *Cortex*, vol. 42, no. 5, pp. 666–674, 2006.

[22] R. Ishii, L. Canuet, M. Iwase et al., "Right parietal activation during delusional state in episodic interictal psychosis of epilepsy: a report of two cases," *Epilepsy and Behavior*, vol. 9, no. 2, pp. 367–372, 2006.

[23] S. H. Lee, W. Kim, Y. C. Chung et al., "A double blind study showing that two weeks of daily repetitive TMS over the left or right temporoparietal cortex reduces symptoms in patients with schizophrenia who are having treatment-refractory auditory hallucinations," *Neuroscience Letters*, vol. 376, no. 3, pp. 177–181, 2005.

[24] E. Poulet, J. Brunelin, B. Bediou et al., "Slow transcranial magnetic stimulation can rapidly reduce resistant auditory hallucinations in schizophrenia," *Biological Psychiatry*, vol. 57, no. 2, pp. 188–191, 2005.
[25] R. E. Hoffman, R. Gueorguieva, K. A. Hawkins et al., "Temporoparietal transcranial magnetic stimulation for auditory hallucinations: safety, efficacy and moderators in a fifty patient sample," *Biological Psychiatry*, vol. 58, no. 2, pp. 97–104, 2005.
[26] A. Vercammen, H. Knegtering, R. Bruggeman et al., "Effects of bilateral repetitive transcranial magnetic stimulation on treatment resistant auditory-verbal hallucinations in schizophrenia: a randomized controlled trial," *Schizophrenia Research*, vol. 114, no. 1–3, pp. 172–179, 2009.
[27] O. Rosenberg, Y. Roth, M. Kotler, A. Zangen, and P. Dannon, "Deep transcranial magnetic stimulation for the treatment of auditory hallucinations: a preliminary open-label study," *Annals of General Psychiatry*, vol. 10, no. 1, article 3, 2011.
[28] R. Jardri, B. Lucas, Y. Delevoye-Turrell et al., "An 11-year-old boy with drug-resistant schizophrenia treated with temporo-parietal rTMS," *Molecular Psychiatry*, vol. 12, no. 4, article 320, 2007.
[29] A. Caramazza, "On drawing inferences about the structure of normal cognitive systems from the analysis of patterns of impaired performance: the case for single-patient studies," *Brain and Cognition*, vol. 5, no. 1, pp. 41–66, 1986.
[30] D. Silbersweig and E. Stern, "Functional neuroimaging of hallucinations in schizophrenia: toward an integration of bottom-up and top-down approaches," *Molecular Psychiatry*, vol. 1, no. 5, pp. 367–375, 1996.
[31] J. Gauntlett-Gilbert and E. Kuipers, "Phenomenology of visual hallucinations in psychiatric conditions," *Journal of Nervous and Mental Disease*, vol. 191, no. 3, pp. 203–205, 2003.
[32] M. Startup and S. Startup, "On two kinds of delusion of reference," *Psychiatry Research*, vol. 137, no. 1-2, pp. 87–92, 2005.
[33] D. I. Perrett, D. Xiao, N. E. Barraclough, C. Keysers, and M. W. Oram, "Seeing the future: natural image sequences produce anticipatory neuronal activity and bias perceptual report," *Quarterly Journal of Experimental Psychology*, vol. 62, no. 11, pp. 2081–2104, 2009.
[34] T. Jellema, C. I. Baker, B. Wicker, and D. I. Perrett, "Neural representation for the perception of the intentionality of actions," *Brain and Cognition*, vol. 44, no. 2, pp. 280–302, 2000.
[35] J. P. Morris, K. A. Pelphrey, and G. McCarthy, "Perceived causality influences brain activity evoked by biological motion," *Social Neuroscience*, vol. 3, no. 1, pp. 16–25, 2008.
[36] D. I. Perrett, P. A. Smith, D. D. Potter et al., "Visual cells in the temporal cortex sensitive to face view and gaze direction," *Proceedings of the Royal Society B*, vol. 223, pp. 293–317, 1985.
[37] O. Blanke and S. Arzy, "The out-of-body experience: disturbed self-processing at the temporo-parietal junction," *Neuroscientist*, vol. 11, no. 1, pp. 16–24, 2005.
[38] L. Nummenmaa, L. Passamonti, J. Rowe, A. D. Engell, and A. J. Calder, "Connectivity analysis reveals a cortical network for eye gaze perception," *Cerebral Cortex*, vol. 20, no. 8, pp. 1780–1787, 2010.
[39] L. Young, D. Dodell-Feder, and R. Saxe, "What gets the attention of the temporo-parietal junction? An fMRI investigation of attention and theory of mind," *Neuropsychologia*, vol. 48, no. 9, pp. 2658–2664, 2010.
[40] R. Adolphs, H. Damasio, and D. Tranel, "Neural systems for recognition of emotional prosody. A 3-D lesion study," *Emotion*, vol. 2, no. 1, pp. 23–51, 2002.
[41] A. Puce and D. Perrett, "Electrophysiology and brain imaging of biological motion," *Philosophical Transactions of the Royal Society B*, vol. 358, no. 1431, pp. 435–445, 2003.
[42] K. A. Pelphrey, J. P. Morris, C. R. Michelich, T. Allison, and G. McCarthy, "Functional anatomy of biological motion perception in posterior temporal cortex: an fMRI study of eye, mouth and hand movements," *Cerebral Cortex*, vol. 15, no. 12, pp. 1866–1876, 2005.
[43] J. Billino, D. I. Braun, K. D. Bohm, F. Bremmer, and K. R. Gegenfurtner, "Cortical networks for motion processing: effects of focal brain lesions on perception of different motion types," *Neuropsychologia*, vol. 47, no. 10, pp. 2133–2144, 2009.
[44] E. D. Grossman, L. Battelli, and A. Pascual-Leone, "Repetitive TMS over posterior STS disrupts perception of biological motion," *Vision Research*, vol. 45, no. 22, pp. 2847–2853, 2005.
[45] C. Bruce, R. Desimone, and C. G. Gross, "Visual properties of neurons in a polysensory area in superior temporal sulcus of the macaque," *Journal of Neurophysiology*, vol. 46, no. 2, pp. 369–384, 1981.
[46] M. I. Gobbini and J. V. Haxby, "Neural systems for recognition of familiar faces," *Neuropsychologia*, vol. 45, no. 1, pp. 32–41, 2007.
[47] T. M. Wright, K. A. Pelphrey, T. Allison, M. J. McKeown, and G. McCarthy, "Polysensory interactions along lateral temporal regions evoked by audiovisual speech," *Cerebral Cortex*, vol. 13, no. 10, pp. 1034–1043, 2003.
[48] K. V. Kriegstein and A.-L. Giraud, "Distinct functional substrates along the right superior temporal sulcus for the processing of voices," *NeuroImage*, vol. 22, no. 2, pp. 948–955, 2004.
[49] N. E. Barraclough, D. Xiao, C. I. Baker, M. W. Oram, and D. I. Perrett, "Integration of visual and auditory information by superior temporal sulcus neurons responsive to the sight of actions," *Journal of Cognitive Neuroscience*, vol. 17, no. 3, pp. 377–391, 2005.
[50] M. S. Beauchamp, "Statistical criteria in fMRI studies of multisensory integration," *Neuroinformatics*, vol. 3, no. 2, pp. 93–113, 2005.
[51] M. S. Beauchamp, B. D. Argall, J. Bodurka, J. H. Duyn, and A. Martin, "Unraveling multisensory integration: patchy organization within human STS multisensory cortex," *Nature Neuroscience*, vol. 7, no. 11, pp. 1190–1192, 2004.
[52] M. Iacoboni, L. M. Koski, M. Brass et al., "Reafferent copies of imitated actions in the right superior temporal cortex," *Proceedings of the National Academy of Sciences of the United States of America*, vol. 98, no. 24, pp. 13995–13999, 2001.
[53] A. A. Ghazanfar, C. Chandrasekaran, and N. K. Logothetis, "Interactions between the superior temporal sulcus and auditory cortex mediate dynamic face/voice integration in rhesus monkeys," *Journal of Neuroscience*, vol. 28, pp. 4457–4469, 2008.
[54] R. Saxe and A. Wexler, "Making sense of another mind: the role of the right temporo-parietal junction," *Neuropsychologia*, vol. 43, no. 10, pp. 1391–1399, 2005.
[55] J. Scholz, C. Triantafyllou, S. Whitfield-Gabrieli, E. N. Brown, and R. Saxe, "Distinct regions of right temporo-parietal junction are selective for theory of mind and exogenous attention," *PLoS ONE*, vol. 4, no. 3, Article ID e4869, 2009.

[56] C. D. Frith and U. Frith, "How we predict what other people are going to do," *Brain Research*, vol. 1079, no. 1, pp. 36–46, 2006.

[57] C. M. Bird, F. Castelli, O. Malik, U. Frith, and M. Husain, "The impact of extensive medial frontal lobe damage on "Theory of Mind" and cognition," *Brain*, vol. 127, no. 4, pp. 914–928, 2004.

[58] A. Baird, B. K. Dewar, H. Critchley, S. J. Gilbert, R. J. Dolan, and L. Cipolotti, "Cognitive functioning after medial frontal lobe damage including the anterior cingulate cortex: a preliminary investigation," *Brain and Cognition*, vol. 60, no. 2, pp. 166–175, 2006.

[59] L. J. Bach, F. Happe, S. Fleminger, and J. Powell, "Theory of mind: independence of executive function and the role of the frontal cortex in acquired brain injury," *Cognitive Neuropsychiatry*, vol. 5, no. 3, pp. 175–192, 2000.

[60] D. Samson, I. A. Apperly, C. Chiavarino, and G. W. Humphreys, "Left temporoparietal junction is necessary for representing someone else's belief," *Nature Neuroscience*, vol. 7, no. 5, pp. 499–500, 2004.

[61] L. Young, F. Cushman, M. Hauser, and R. Saxe, "The neural basis of the interaction between theory of mind and moral judgment," *Proceedings of the National Academy of Sciences United States*, vol. 104, no. 20, pp. 8235–8240, 2007.

[62] Y. Sarfati, M. C. Hardy-Bayle, C. Besche, and D. Widlocher, "Attribution of intentions to others in people with schizophrenia: a non- verbal exploration with comic strips," *Schizophrenia Research*, vol. 25, no. 3, pp. 199–209, 1997.

[63] Y. Sarfati, M. C. Hardy-Bayle, E. Brunet, and D. Widlocher, "Investigating theory of mind in schizophrenia: influence of verbalization in disorganized and non-disorganized patients," *Schizophrenia Research*, vol. 37, no. 2, pp. 183–190, 1999.

[64] U. Dimberg, M. Thunberg, and K. Elmehed, "Unconscious facial reactions to emotional facial expressions," *Psychological Science*, vol. 11, no. 1, pp. 86–89, 2000.

[65] L. Carr, M. Iacoboni, M. C. Dubeaut, J. C. Mazziotta, and G. L. Lenzi, "Neural mechanisms of empathy in humans: a relay from neural systems for imitation to limbic areas," *Proceedings of the National Academy of Sciences of the United States of America*, vol. 100, no. 9, pp. 5497–5502, 2003.

[66] J. Narumoto, T. Okada, N. Sadato, K. Fukui, and Y. Yonekura, "Attention to emotion modulates fMRI activity in human right superior temporal sulcus," *Cognitive Brain Research*, vol. 12, no. 2, pp. 225–231, 2001.

[67] D. I. Leitman, D. H. Wolf, J. D. Ragland et al., "'It's not what you say, but how you say it': a reciprocal temporo-frontal network for affective prosody," *Frontiers in Human Neuroscience*, vol. 4, article 19, 2010.

[68] S. Baron-Cohen, S. Wheelwright, and T. Jolliffe, "Is there a "language of the eyes"? Evidence from normal adults, and adults with autism or Asperger Syndrome," *Visual Cognition*, vol. 4, no. 3, pp. 311–331, 1997.

[69] M.V. Lombardo, B. Chakrabarti, E.T. Bullmore et al., "Shared neural circuits for mentalizing about the self and others," *Journal of Cognitive Neuroscience*, vol. 22, no. 7, pp. 1623–1635, 2010.

[70] T. Akiyama, M. Kato, T. Muramatsu, F. Saito, S. Umeda, and H. Kashima, "Gaze but not arrows: a dissociative impairment after right superior temporal gyrus damage," *Neuropsychologia*, vol. 44, no. 10, pp. 1804–1810, 2006.

[71] N. Boddaert, N. Chabane, H. Gervais et al., "Superior temporal sulcus anatomical abnormalities in childhood autism: a voxel-based morphometry MRI study," *NeuroImage*, vol. 23, no. 1, pp. 364–369, 2004.

[72] K. A. Pelphrey, R. J. Viola, and G. McCarthy, "When strangers pass: processing of mutual and averted social gaze in the superior temporal sulcus," *Psychological Science*, vol. 15, no. 9, pp. 598–603, 2004.

[73] R. Saxe, D. K. Xiao, G. Kovacs, D. I. Perrett, and N. Kanwisher, "A region of right posterior superior temporal sulcus responds to observed intentional actions," *Neuropsychologia*, vol. 42, no. 11, pp. 1435–1446, 2004.

[74] J. Schultz, H. Imamizu, M. Kawato, and C. D. Frith, "Activation of the human superior temporal gyrus during observation of goal attribution by intentional objects," *Journal of Cognitive Neuroscience*, vol. 16, no. 10, pp. 1695–1705, 2004.

[75] A. P. Atkinson, A. S. Heberlein, and R. Adolphs, "Spared ability to recognise fear from static and moving whole-body cues following bilateral amygdala damage," *Neuropsychologia*, vol. 45, no. 12, pp. 2772–2782, 2007.

[76] C. Cristinzio, K. N'Diaye, M. Seeck, P. Vuilleumier, and D. Sander, "Integration of gaze direction and facial expression in patients with unilateral amygdala damage," *Brain*, vol. 133, no. 1, pp. 248–261, 2010.

[77] J. Grezes, S. Pichon, and B. De Gelder, "Perceiving fear in dynamic body expressions," *NeuroImage*, vol. 35, no. 2, pp. 959–967, 2007.

[78] E. L. Altschuler and V. S. Ramachandran, "Last but not least: a simple method to stand outside oneself," *Perception*, vol. 36, no. 4, pp. 632–634, 2007.

[79] V. I. Petkova and H. H. Ehrsson, "If I were you: perceptual illusion of body swapping," *PLoS ONE*, vol. 3, no. 12, Article ID e3832, 2008.

[80] T. E. Feinberg, *Altered Egos: How the Brain Creates the Self*, Oxford University Press, 2001.

[81] M. Tsakiris, "My body in the brain: a neurocognitive model of body-ownership," *Neuropsychologia*, vol. 48, no. 3, pp. 703–712, 2010.

[82] K. J. Wheaton, J. C. Thompson, A. Syngeniotis, D. F. Abbott, and A. Puce, "Viewing the motion of human body parts activates different regions of premotor, temporal, and parietal cortex," *NeuroImage*, vol. 22, no. 1, pp. 277–288, 2004.

[83] C. Keysers, B. Wicker, V. Gazzola, J. L. Anton, L. Fogassi, and V. Gallese, "A touching sight: SII/PV activation during the observation and experience of touch," *Neuron*, vol. 42, no. 2, pp. 335–346, 2004.

[84] S. A. Spence, D. J. Brooks, S. R. Hirsch, P. F. Liddle, J. Meehan, and P. M. Grasby, "A PET study of voluntary movement in schizophrenic patients experiencing passivity phenomena (delusions of alien control)," *Brain*, vol. 120, no. 11, pp. 1997–2011, 1997.

[85] C. Farrer, N. Franck, C. D. Frith et al., "Neural correlates of action attribution in schizophrenia," *Psychiatry Research*, vol. 131, no. 1, pp. 31–44, 2004.

[86] D. J. Holt, B. S. Cassidy, J. R. Andrews-Hanna et al., "An anterior-to-posterior shift in midline cortical activity inschizophrenia during self-reflection," *Biological Psychiatry*, vol. 69, no. 5, pp. 415–423, 2011.

[87] G. Northoff, A. Heinzel, M. de Greck, F. Bermpohl, H. Dobrowolny, and J. Panksepp, "Self-referential processing in our brain—a meta-analysis of imaging studies on the self," *NeuroImage*, vol. 31, no. 1, pp. 440–457, 2006.

[88] L. T. Rameson, A. B. Satpute, and M. D. Lieberman, "The neural correlates of implicit and explicit self-relevant processing," *NeuroImage*, vol. 50, no. 2, pp. 701–708, 2010.

[89] S. J. Gillihan and M. J. Farah, "Is self special? A critical review of evidence from experimental psychology and cognitive neuroscience," *Psychological Bulletin*, vol. 131, no. 1, pp. 76–97, 2005.

[90] H. C. Lou, B. Luber, A. Stanford, and S. H. Lisanby, "Self-specific processing in the default network: a single-pulse TMS study," *Experimental Brain Research*, vol. 207, no. 1-2, pp. 27–38, 2010.

[91] L. K. Fellows and M. J. Farah, "Is anterior cingulate cortex necessary for cognitive control?" *Brain*, vol. 128, no. 4, pp. 788–796, 2005.

[92] B. A. Maher, "The relationship between delusions and hallucinations," *Current Psychiatry Reports*, vol. 8, no. 3, pp. 179–183, 2006.

[93] D. M. Amodio and C. D. Frith, "Meeting of minds: the medial frontal cortex and social cognition," *Nature Reviews Neuroscience*, vol. 7, no. 4, pp. 268–277, 2006.

[94] G. Northoff, "Self and brain: what is self-related processing?" *Trends Cognitive Science*, vol. 15, no. 5, pp. 186–187, 2011, Author reply 187–188.

[95] R. P. Spunt and M. D. Lieberman, "An integrative model of the neural systems supporting the comprehension of observed emotional behavior," *NeuroImage*, vol. 59, no. 3, pp. 3050–3059, 2012.

[96] E. G. Bruneau, A. Pluta, and R. Saxe, "Distinct roles of the "Shared Pain" and "Theory of Mind" networks in processing others' emotional suffering," *Neuropsychologia*, vol. 50, no. 2, pp. 219–231, 2012.

[97] R. J. Blair and L. Cipolotti, "Impaired social response reversal. A case of 'acquired sociopathy'," *Brain*, vol. 123, no. 6, pp. 1122–1141, 2000.

[98] J. L. Saver and A. R. Damasio, "Preserved access and processing of social knowledge in a patient with acquired sociopathy due to ventromedial frontal damage," *Neuropsychologia*, vol. 29, no. 12, pp. 1241–1249, 1991.

[99] A. R. Damasio, D. Tranel, and H. Damasio, "Individuals with sociopathic behavior caused by frontal damage fail to respond autonomically to social stimuli," *Behavioural Brain Research*, vol. 41, no. 2, pp. 81–94, 1990.

[100] J. Kim, E. Yang, L. Overhalser et al., "Orbitofrontal cortex lesions disrupt adaptation of choice-behavior to varying affective context in economic decision-making," In press.

[101] J. W. Kable and P. W. Glimcher, "The neurobiology of decision: consensus and controversy," *Neuron*, vol. 63, no. 6, pp. 733–745, 2009.

[102] D. H. Ffytche, R. J. Howard, M. J. Brammer, A. David, P. Woodruff, and S. Williams, "The anatomy of conscious vision: an fMRI study of visual hallucinations," *Nature Neuroscience*, vol. 1, no. 8, pp. 738–742, 1998.

[103] E. F. Torrey, "Schizophrenia and the inferior parietal lobule," *Schizophrenia Research*, vol. 97, no. 1–3, pp. 215–225, 2007.

[104] N. Geschwind, "Disconnexion syndromes in animals and man," *Brain*, vol. 88, no. 2, pp. 237–294, 1965.

[105] R. A. Honea, A. Meyer-Lindenberg, K. B. Hobbs et al., "Is gray matter volume an intermediate phenotype for schizophrenia? A voxel-based morphometry study of patients with schizophrenia and their healthy siblings," *Biological Psychiatry*, vol. 63, no. 5, pp. 465–474, 2008.

[106] J. M. Segall, J. A. Turner, T. G. Van Erp et al., "Voxel-based morphometric multisite collaborative study on schizophrenia," *Schizophrenia Bulletin*, vol. 35, no. 1, pp. 82–95, 2009.

[107] S. D. Han, P. G. Nestor, M. Hale-Spencer et al., "Functional neuroimaging of word priming in males with chronic schizophrenia," *NeuroImage*, vol. 35, no. 1, pp. 273–282, 2007.

[108] C. G. Wible, K. Lee, I. Molina et al., "FMRI activity correlated with auditory hallucinations during performance of a working memory task: data from the FBIRN consortium study," *Schizophrenia Bulletin*, vol. 35, no. 1, pp. 47–57, 2009.

[109] R. I. Hashimoto, K. Lee, A. Preus, R. W. McCarley, and C. G. Wible, "An fMRI study of functional abnormalities in the verbal working memory system and the relationship to clinical symptoms in chronic schizophrenia," *Cerebral Cortex*, vol. 20, no. 1, pp. 46–60, 2010.

[110] B. R. Lennox, S. Bert, G. Park, P. B. Jones, and P. G. Morris, "Spatial and temporal mapping of neural activity associated with auditory hallucinations," *The Lancet*, vol. 353, no. 9153, p. 644, 1999.

[111] S. A. Schobel, N. M. Lewandowski, C. M. Corcoran et al., "Differential targeting of the CA1 subfield of the hippocampal formation by schizophrenia and related psychotic disorders," *Archives of General Psychiatry*, vol. 66, no. 9, pp. 938–946, 2009.

[112] A. G. Garrity, G. D. Pearlson, K. McKiernan, D. Lloyd, K. A. Kiehl, and V. D. Calhoun, "Aberrant "default mode" functional connectivity in schizophrenia," *American Journal of Psychiatry*, vol. 164, no. 3, pp. 450–457, 2007.

[113] J. L. Vincent, A. Z. Snyder, M. D. Fox et al., "Coherent spontaneous activity identifies a hippocampal-parietal memory network," *Journal of Neurophysiology*, vol. 96, no. 6, pp. 3517–3531, 2006.

[114] R. L. Buckner, J. Sepulcre, T. Talukdar et al., "Cortical hubs revealed by intrinsic functional connectivity: mapping, assessment of stability, and relation to Alzheimer's disease," *Journal of Neuroscience*, vol. 29, no. 6, pp. 1860–1873, 2009.

[115] M. Föcking, P. Dicker, J. A. English, K. O. Schubert, M. J. Dunn, and D. R. Cotter, "Commonproteomic changes in the hippocampus in schizophrenia and bipolar disorder and particular evidence for involvement of cornu ammonis regions 2 and 3," *Archives of General Psychiatry*, vol. 68, no. 5, pp. 477–488, 2011.

14

The Psychotomimetic Nature of Dreams: An Experimental Study

Oliver Mason and Dominic Wakerley

Research Department of Clinical, Educational and Health Psychology, 1-19 Torrington Place, University College London, London WC1N 6BT, UK

Correspondence should be addressed to Oliver Mason, o.mason@ucl.ac.uk

Academic Editor: Anil K. Malhotra

Several theories promote the similarities between dreaming and psychosis, but this has rarely been tested empirically. We assessed dreaming and waking reality using the Psychotomimetic States Inventory, a measure of psychotic-like experience originally designed for drug studies. Twenty participants completed the measure in each of two dream conditions and one waking condition. Dreams were assessed upon waking naturally and also using a movement-activated (actigraph) alarm during the night. Overall, participants reported more quasipsychotic characteristics during dreams (in both conditions) than when awake. This was most marked for paranoia and delusional thinking, but differences were also seen for perceptual abnormalities, mania, and anhedonia. The quality of dream experience seems particularly similar to psychosis in sometimes being highly self-referential and having a paranoid content. Subjective changes to cognition and affect are consistent with alterations in prefrontal cortical activity during REM sleep that mirror those of schizophrenia.

1. Introduction and Methods

The phenomenological similarity between the dream state and psychosis has been often remarked upon but rarely empirically tested. Kant declared "the lunatic is a wakeful dreamer," while Schopenhauer said "a dream is a short-lasting psychosis, and a psychosis is a long-lasting dream." Perhaps the most developed neurobiological account, Hobson [1] has advanced a recent hypothesis of the dreaming brain as a model of psychosis, suggesting dreams mimic the distortion of reality seen in the positive symptoms of schizophrenia, though he prefers the term "delirium." "In dreams, as in delirium, consciousness is clouded, attention is distractible, intellectual functions are dull, perceptions are hallucinatory, cognition is illogical, emotion is unstable and uncontrolled, memory is poor, and thought processes are at a concrete, not a symbolic, level" [2, page 23]. Although in some ways adversaries of Hobson's wider model (see [3]), Sohms and Turnbull also advocate that "the functional anatomy of dreaming is almost identical to that of schizophrenic psychosis" [4, page 213]. Pushing the analogy to the furthest by describing psychosis itself as a dream state with the neurobiology of REM stage sleep, Gottesmann [5] outlines the best delineated areas of neurobiological overlap in terms of "common intracerebral disconnections, disturbed responsiveness and sensory deafferentation processes (and) dorsolateral prefrontal deactivation" (page 1105).

The commonest metric for assessing and asserting this commonality has been that of dream bizarreness, though the frequency of bizarre elements seems to vary depending on what is included, and may well be overclaimed by some theorists [3]. One large study of dream recall [6] found 36% to have more than one bizarre element, while another found bizarreness in 14% of dream characters [7]. If small distortions are included, figures rise to 40–60% (e.g., [8]). As Domhoff (page 4, [3]) notes "it is not obvious that [...] unusual events in dreams are inherently bizarre if they are compared with either the stories people are familiar with in waking life or waking thought flow." Interestingly, schizophrenia patients' waking fantasies may be more like dreams at least as measured by the Thematic Apperception Test rated for cognitive bizarreness [9].

Whether dreams take the form and content of types of delusional and hallucinatory experiences reported by patients is an interesting aspect of the question: two recent studies by Yu [10, 11] have attempted to characterize typical dreams in order to elucidate a typology of what is recalled of these. Paranoia and grandiosity were repeated factors that shared much with common delusional themes, while other more ego-ideal contents did not.

1.1. Aims and Hypotheses. A naturalistic setting is crucial to any study of dream content, as it has been repeatedly found that in dream laboratories the sleeper dreams of dream laboratories: thus we aimed to capture REM-sleep dreaming by the least intrusive means possible. In addition to testing upon waking naturally, the study used an activity-monitoring wristwatch set to wake the participant when movement (potentially REM-related) was detected. As major body movements occur predominantly before and after REM sleep periods [12], we hypothesized that use of the actigraphically triggered alarm would maximize dream recall. Actigraph-based methods have a good degree of correspondence with the gold standard of polysomnography for sleep recording in good sleepers at least [13, 14]. To measure the psychotic qualities of dreams, we used the Psychotomimetic State Inventory (PSI, [15]), a measure developed for recreational drug studies and other analogous settings (e.g., sensory deprivation [16]). This is not a symptomatic measure; rather it assesses schizotypal experiences that are thought to be analogous to psychosis. We hypothesized that dreams would be characterized by greater PSI scores that the natural awake state. In particular, we hypothesized greater paranoia and delusional content based on the earlier work of Yu [10, 11].

1.2. Method. 20 participants (13 male and 7 female) with an average age of 20.5 took part. All were undergraduate students with no history of psychiatric or neurological disorder. In this within-subject repeated measures design, all were asked to complete the PSI on three occasions: upon waking naturally; following artificial waking using actigraph recording; in the normal waking state during the day. Participants recorded their responses in their own homes following thorough briefing on the use of the questionnaires and the actigraph watch (Sleep Tracker Pro, Innovative Sleep Solutions Inc., Atlanta, GA, USA). As REM sleep stages last longer towards the end of the sleep cycle, the watch alarm was set to respond to movement within a two-hour period around an hour prior to natural waking for each participant. Participants were asked to refrain from use of alcohol or recreational drugs on the day prior to testing. As use of the actigraph watch necessarily required curtailing sleep this was only performed on a single night; however, participants were able to report on a dream upon natural waking should this occur while in the study over a one week period. Waking state data was obtained by sending a text message reminder at time of day, 6 hours after the individual's usual stated waking time (most usually in the early afternoon). University College London ethical approval was obtained.

1.2.1. Psychotomimetic State Inventory [13]. Participants rate statements that describe their experience from 0 (not at all) to 3 (strongly) across 48 items: the instructions state

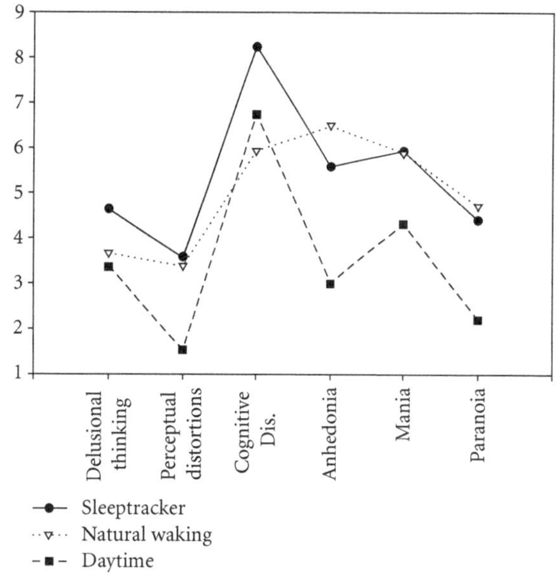

Figure 1: PSI results across the three conditions.

"Please complete the following questions by circling the number that best describes your experience *in the past few hours.*" The PSI yields six subscales: "delusional thinking," "perceptual distortion," "anhedonia," "mania," "paranoia," and "cognitive disorganization." The scale has a test-retest reliability of 0.84 and a Cronbach's alpha overall of 0.94.

2. Results

One participant failed to recall a dream by either method, one more after waking naturally over the course of the week and two further participants did not recall a dream using the actigraph.

Results using the PSI in the three conditions (awake, dream-natural waking, and dream-sleeptracker waking) are given in Table 1 and illustrated in Figure 1. Repeated measure analyses of variance were conducted to test the hypotheses (see Table 1 for planned comparisons). Overall, both dream conditions produced greater overall PSI scores than those reported during the day. Dreams were rated as having greater psychotomimetic qualities than the daytime-awake state, with no difference between those reported when waking naturally and those using the sleeptracker device, though there were slightly greater ratings for the device. Dream/awake differences were seen for almost all subscales except for cognitive disorganization. Although some dream/awake differences failed to reach significance, in every case the pattern was the same with, both dream conditions tending to have higher means than that of the daytime-awake condition. In line with the hypotheses, this was most marked for delusional thinking and paranoia. However, significant differences were also seen for anhedonia and mania suggesting changes in affect are also important aspects of dream experience that parallel psychotic experience.

TABLE 1: Means and standard deviations of PSI and subscales.

	Dream-natural waking (NW)	Dream-sleeptracker (ST)	Awake-daytime (AD)	Pairwise comparisons
*PSI Total***	27.3 (16.9)	33.1 (21.8)	18.5 (14.2)	NW = ST > AD
Delusional thinking**	3.2 (2.9)	5.9 (5.4)	2.1 (2.3)	ST > AD
Perceptual distortions*	3.4 (4.1)	3.6 (4.3)	1.5 (2.1)	NW = ST > AD
Cognitive Disorganization	5.9 (5.1)	8.2 (6.4)	6.7 (5.3)	—
Anhedonia*	6.5 (3.2)	6.0 (3.8)	3.0 (3.0)	NW > AD
Mania*	5.9 (3.8)	5.9 (2.9)	4.3 (3.1)	NW = ST > AD
Paranoia**	4.7 (4.4)	4.4 (4.7)	1.4 (1.8)	NW = ST>AD

* $P < .05$, ** $P < .01$ RM-ANOVA, and pairwise comparisons $P < .05$ Bonferroni corrected.

3. Discussion

The study attempted to measure dream experience as soon as possible after it occurred in addition to test completion upon waking. The use of an actigraphic approach, waking participants during periods of greater movement during sleep did successfully elicit dream material for seventeen of the twenty participants. We would, therefore, tentatively suggest the utility of actigraphy in obtaining dream reports, though their sleep staging cannot be directly ascertained.

The hypothesis that dreams would be characterized by greater PSI scores than the "daytime-awake" state was confirmed both for the dreams recalled using actigraphy and upon natural morning wakening. Dreams were characterized by significantly greater delusional thinking, perceptual distortions, anhedonia, mania, and paranoia. Thus, the results are consistent with those of Yu [10, 11] on delusional content and paranoid ideation. In the present study, many of the items concern ideas of reference or special/magical powers; the scores suggest a high degree of self-referential dream content. Paranoia was the largest effect of all and suggests common experiences of being watched, plotted against, or harmed with associated fear. This is consistent with one evolutionary theory that dreams are specialized to simulate threatening events [8].

Differences in mania and anhedonia were perhaps more surprising and suggest cognitive-affective experience is altered in additional ways that resemble psychotic experience. Perusal of the anhedonia questions, many of which tap feeling distant, uninvolved or uncomfortable with people, suggest that in dreams, one's experience of self in relation to others is in some ways altered, or experienced at one stage removed. Whether this is a true parallel to anhedonia in the psychotic sense is an intriguing idea as many neurocognitive accounts of negative symptoms focus on failures to construct and sustain accurate representations of oneself and others—itself a fair description of some dreams.

Mania taps a sense of increased subjective speed of thought and action, mood swings, and greater impulsivity. A weakened sense of cognitive control is a clear parallel between the dream and psychotic states. The organization of cognitive control within the lateral prefrontal cortex (LFFC) in both normals and schizophrenia patients is only now being delineated by fMRI ([17]). Schizophrenic patients exhibited *hypoactivation* in caudal LPFC regions suggesting a weakening of contextual influence and thus inappropriate behavioural representation (and hence bizarre behaviour). They interpreted *hyperactivation* in rostral LPFC regions as an attempt to compensate by drawing excessively on temporal episodic information. While the caudal LPFC may or may not be deactivated in NREM sleep, it certainly is in REM, and other areas of PFC are activated including orbital frontal areas that serve temporal and emotional processing (see [18] for review). However, complex patterns of specific landscapes of activation are associated with different sleep stages, and it is difficult to allocate specific changes to dreaming or individual aspects of dream experience: as a recent review [19, page 1004] states "no study to date has been able to directly relate, in the same individuals, brain activation during sleep with emotions experienced in dreams." We are simply drawing the analogy between the heightened sense of emotion reported in some dreams and clinical states of mania or paranoia. Of course a wide range of emotions occur in dreams with fear and anxiety prominent among these: Schwartz and Maquet [20, page 25] highlight the role of the amygdala in organizing emotional processing during sleep in a way that "might favor fearful experience in dreams." Even amongst a range of structural and functional alternations seen in limbic structures in schizophrenia, grey matter loss in the left amygdale appears particularly marked and extends to patients' relatives [21].

It is important to note several limitations. The study does not compare dreaming with schizotypal experiences occurring when awake, and indeed there may be bias introduced by the methods of obtaining dream experience ratings as compared to waking state ratings. In retrospect, averaging across a large set of data points would help provide a richer picture of whether dreams differ from schizotypal mentation when awake. As a measure derived from psychotic phenomena was used, assessment of visual hallucinosis formed a very small aspect of the measurement (two items of 48). As a consequence, the study was very definitely *not* a test of the "dream-as-psychosis" versus "dream-as-delirium" hypotheses. The final limitation is that sleep-staging was not directly assessed, and no neurobiological correlates of dream experiences obtained.

References

[1] A. Hobson, "A model for madness?" *Nature*, vol. 430, no. 6995, p. 21, 2004.

[2] J. A. Hobson, *Dreaming: An Introduction to the Science of Sleep*, Oxford University Press, New York, NY, USA, 2002.
[3] G. William Domhoff, "Refocusing the neurocognitive approach to dreams: a critique of the hobson versus solms debate," *Dreaming*, vol. 15, no. 1, pp. 3–20, 2005.
[4] M. Sohms and O. Turnbull, *The Brain and the Inner World*, Other Press, New York, NY, USA, 2002.
[5] C. Gottesmann, "The dreaming sleep stage: a new neurobiological model of schizophrenia?" *Neuroscience*, vol. 140, no. 4, pp. 1105–1115, 2006.
[6] I. Strauch and B. Meier, *In Search of Dreams: Results of Experimental Dream Research*, SUNY Press, Albany, NY, USA, 1996.
[7] D. Kahn, R. Stickgold, E. F. Pace-Schott, and J. A. Hobson, "Dreaming and waking consciousness: a character recognition study," *Journal of Sleep Research*, vol. 9, no. 4, pp. 317–325, 2000.
[8] A. Revonsuo and C. Salmivalli, "A content analysis of bizarre elements in dreams," *Dreaming*, vol. 5, pp. 169–187, 1995.
[9] S. Scarone, M. L. Manzone, O. Gambini et al., "The dream as a model for psychosis: an experimental approach using bizarreness as a cognitive marker," *Schizophrenia Bulletin*, vol. 34, no. 3, pp. 515–522, 2008.
[10] C. K. C. Yu, "Paranoia in dreams and the classification of typical dreams," *Dreaming*, vol. 19, no. 4, pp. 255–272, 2009.
[11] C. K. C. Yu, "Delusions and the factor structure of typical dreams," *Dreaming*, vol. 19, no. 1, pp. 42–54, 2009.
[12] J. A. Hobson, T. Spagna, and R. Malenka, "Ethology of sleep studied with time-lapse photography: postural immobility and sleep-cycle phase in humans," *Science*, vol. 201, no. 4362, pp. 1251–1253, 1978.
[13] S. Ancoli-Israel, R. Cole, C. Alessi, M. Chambers, W. Moorcroft, and C. P. Pollak, "The role of actigraphy in the study of sleep and circadian rhythms," *Sleep*, vol. 26, no. 3, pp. 342–392, 2003.
[14] T. Blackwell, S. Redline, S. Ancoli-Israel et al., "Comparison of sleep parameters from actigraphy and polysomnography in older women: the SOF study," *Sleep*, vol. 31, no. 2, pp. 283–291, 2008.
[15] O. J. Mason, C. J. M. Morgan, A. Stefanovic, and H. V. Curran, "The Psychotomimetic States Inventory (PSI): measuring psychotic-type experiences from ketamine and cannabis," *Schizophrenia Research*, vol. 103, no. 1–3, pp. 138–142, 2008.
[16] O. J. Mason and F. Brady, "The psychotomimetic effects of short-term sensory deprivation," *Journal of Nervous and Mental Disease*, vol. 197, no. 10, pp. 783–785, 2009.
[17] G. Barbalat, V. Chambon, N. Franck, E. Koechlin, and C. Farrer, "Organization of cognitive control within the lateral prefrontal cortex in schizophrenia," *Archives of General Psychiatry*, vol. 66, no. 4, pp. 377–386, 2009.
[18] A. Muzur, E. F. Pace-Schott, and J. A. Hobson, "The prefrontal cortex in sleep," *Trends in Cognitive Sciences*, vol. 6, no. 11, pp. 475–481, 2002.
[19] M. Desseilles, T. T. Dang-Vu, V. Sterpenich, and S. Schwartz, "Cognitive and emotional processes during dreaming: a neuroimaging view," *Consciousness and Cognition*, vol. 20, pp. 998–1008, 2011.
[20] S. Schwartz and P. Maquet, "Sleep imaging and the neuropsychological assessment of dreams," *Trends in Cognitive Sciences*, vol. 6, no. 1, pp. 23–30, 2002.
[21] L. Tian, C. Meng, H. Yan et al., "Convergent evidence from multimodal imaging reveals amygdala abnormalities in schizophrenic patients and their first-degree relatives," *PLoS One*, vol. 6, no. 12, article e28794, 2011.

15

Evaluation of Factors Affecting Continuous Performance Test Identical Pairs Version Score of Schizophrenic Patients in a Japanese Clinical Sample

Takayoshi Koide,[1] Branko Aleksic,[1] Tsutomu Kikuchi,[1,2] Masahiro Banno,[1] Kunihiro Kohmura,[1] Yasunori Adachi,[1] Naoko Kawano,[1] Tetsuya Iidaka,[1] and Norio Ozaki[1]

[1] *Department of Psychiatry, Nagoya University Graduate School of Medicine, 65 Tsurumai-cho, Showa-ku, Nagoya 466-8550, Japan*
[2] *Department of Psychiatry, Matsuzaki Hospital, 67 Azamotosanbongi, Sanbongi-cho, Aichi, Toyohashi 441-8152, Japan*

Correspondence should be addressed to Branko Aleksic, branko@med.nagoya-u.ac.jp

Academic Editor: Nakao Iwata

Aim. Cognitive impairment in schizophrenia strongly relates to social outcome and is a good candidate for endophenotypes. When we accurately measure drug efficacy or effects of genes or variants relevant to schizophrenia on cognitive impairment, clinical factors that can affect scores on cognitive tests, such as age and severity of symptoms, should be considered. To elucidate the effect of clinical factors, we conducted multiple regression analysis using scores of the Continuous Performance Test Identical Pairs Version (CPT-IP), which is often used to measure attention/vigilance in schizophrenia. *Methods.* We conducted the CPT-IP (4-4 digit) and examined clinical information (sex, age, education years, onset age, duration of illness, chlorpromazine-equivalent dose, and Positive and Negative Symptom Scale (PANSS) scores) in 126 schizophrenia patients in Japanese population. Multiple regression analysis was used to evaluate the effect of clinical factors. *Results.* Age, chlorpromazine-equivalent dose, and PANSS-negative symptom score were associated with mean d′ score in patients. These three clinical factors explained about 28% of the variance in mean d′ score. *Conclusions.* As conclusion, CPT-IP score in schizophrenia patients is influenced by age, chlorpromazine-equivalent dose and PANSS negative symptom score.

1. Introduction

Schizophrenia is a complex, heritable psychiatric disorder, affecting approximately 1% of the general population. The heritability of schizophrenia is estimated to be 64% [1]. Genes relevant to schizophrenia or variants that may modulate risk for the disease have been identified using both linkage and candidate-based or whole-genome association studies [2–5]. A complementary approach examines the genetics of schizophrenia from the neurobiological perspective with neurocognitive endophenotypic markers of putative brain function. The underlying brain dysfunctions (and related endophenotypes) are more stable, trait-like markers that can be used to refine the psychiatric diagnosis. This approach is further motivated by the need to elucidate pathophysiological pathways after candidate variants are established [6].

The Consortium on the Genetics of Schizophrenia is a 7-site collaboration that examines the genetic architecture of quantitative endophenotypes in families with schizophrenia. The authors suggested that the Continuous Performance Test Identical Pairs Version (CPT-IP), Degraded Stimulus Continuous Performance Test (DS-CPT), Verbal Declarative Memory Test, Working Memory Test, and Penn Computerized Neurocognitive Battery are the most appropriate tests to evaluate endophenotypes relevant to schizophrenia. Furthermore, the heritability of attention/vigilance using sample comprised of 30 healthy families was estimated to be 0.39 and 0.49 based on verbal and spatial CPT-IP scores, respectively

[7]. The effect size was 1.18 when schizophrenia patients and controls were compared. Accordingly, the comparison between the first-degree relatives of schizophrenic patients and controls resulted in smaller effect size (0.54) [6].

CPT-IP is included as a core test in major psychological batteries used to evaluate cognitive functioning of psychiatric patients, such as the Measurement and Treatment Research to Improve Cognition in Schizophrenia and the Consensus Cognitive Battery (MCCB) for schizophrenia. Cognitive impairment is one of the core symptoms of schizophrenia and is associated with impaired quality of life and poor outcome [8–10]. The CPT-IP test used to evaluate one of the cognitive endophenotypes related to schizophrenia. Specifically, CPT-IP can measure the attention/vigilance deficit that is commonly found in schizophrenic subjects and those who are at risk for the disorder [11].

Biological phenotypes (e.g., cognitive or central executive functions) are thought to more closely reflect the effects of genetic variation compared with manifested psychiatric illness; therefore, endophenotype studies have proven to be more robust and require smaller sample sizes than purely diagnosis-based studies. When genetic effects on cognitive performance are evaluated, it is important to consider measurement errors [12] as well as the effect of clinical factors that may strongly affect CPT-IP scores. In that regard, except for several reports that have evaluated the association between age and Positive and Negative Symptom Scale (PANSS) scores on cognitive performance [13], there are no comprehensive studies that looked for relevant covariates that may influence CPT-IP scores. We conducted an analysis of factors that can affect CPT-IP scores (e.g., sex, age, education years, onset age, duration of illness, chlorpromazine equivalent dose, and PANSS scores) using a Japanese population-based sample.

2. Methods

2.1. Participants. This study was approved by the Ethics Committee of each participating institute, and written informed consent was obtained from each participant. Patients were included in the study if they (1) met DSM-IV criteria for schizophrenia, (2) were physically healthy, and (3) had no mood disorders, substance abuse, neurodevelopmental disorders, epilepsy, or known mental retardation. Consensus diagnoses were made by at least two experienced psychiatrists according to DSM-IV criteria on the basis of unstructured interviews with patients and families and review of medical records. The rate of the samples excluded due to a lack of consensus was less than 5%. All subjects were unrelated to each other, living in the central area of the mainland of Japan, and self-identified as Japanese. The study included 126 unrelated Japanese patients with schizophrenia (mean age, 44.4 ± 13.3 years; 80 males and 46 females).

2.2. Measurement Settings. There are a variety of CPTs, the more commonly used being CPT-X/AX, DS-CPT, and CPT-IP [11]. CPT-IP has evolved over the course of the New York High-Risk Project [14]. In CPT-IP, the target is defined as the second stimulus in any pair of identical stimuli. The benefit of using CPT-IP instead of the other tests is due to the structure and simplicity of the examination. In other words, no number or number sequence is specified, as in the X/AX design, and the subject does not need to memorize each stimulus presented as in the DS-CPT, which can increase the information-processing load. We used CPT-IP program Release 4.0 (NewCPT.exe, Copyright 1982–2004 by Barbara A. Cornblatt, All Rights Reserved). The PC monitor was 10.4′ and letter size was at least 2.2 × 1.5 cm [7]. The distance between the subjects and the monitor was at least 50 cm.

Stimuli were flashed on the screen at a constant rate of 1 per set, with a stimulus "on" time of 50 msec and a stimulus "off" time of 950 msec. Stimuli were four-digit numbers and were presented 150 times. In each 150 trial conditions, 30 of the trials (20%) were target trials and required a response. Target trials were those on which the second of a pair of two identical stimuli appeared. Responses to target trials were scored as hits [7]. Condition also included a number of catch trials on which the stimulus presented was similar but not identical to that of the preceding trial. Responses to catch trials were considered a specific type of commission error, referred to as false alarms. There were 30 catch trials (20%) in our test. The remaining trials in both conditions were 90 randomly distributed fillers. Responses to filler trials, referred to as random errors, were also considered to be commission errors but were analysed independently of false alarms. We conducted the four-digit CPT-IP two times, with a resting time between the two examinations of 1 min. Mean d′ score was defined as the mean of first and second d′ score.

2.3. Clinical Factors. Chlorpromazine (CPZ) equivalent dose was calculated according to standard methodology based on a Japanese clinical sample [15, 16]. The PANSS was used to evaluate the severity of symptoms in patients [17].

2.4. Statistical Analysis. IBM SPSS Statistics Version 19 was used for all analyses. Intraclass correlation coefficient was calculated in d′, hits, false alarm, and random errors. Multiple regression was performed for the analysis of mean of d′ score using clinical information (sex, age, education years, onset age, duration of illness, CPZ equivalent dose of antipsychotics, and PANSS score) (positive, negative and general psychopathology). Multiple regression models were analysed using forward-backward stepwise selection. Multiple correlation coefficient adjusted for the degree of freedom (R_a^2), analysis of variance (ANOVA) P-value, and Durbin-Watson ratio were calculated to evaluate the extent of model fitting. The significance level was set at $P = 0.05$.

3. Results

Clinical profile of participants is shown in Table 1. The intraclass correlation coefficient (ICC) of the mean d′ score was 0.71 (Table 2). In multiple regression analysis, age, CPZ equivalent dose, and PANSS-negative symptom score were significantly associated with mean d′ score (Table 3). Durbin-Watson ratio indicated the absence of spurious

Table 1: Participants profile.

	Patients (n = 126)	
Sex		
Male	80	
Female	46	
	Mean	SD[a]
Age (y)	44.4	13.3
Education years (y)	12.4	2.4
Onset age (y)	26.7	10.0
Duration of illness (y)	17.6	13.0
Chlorpromazine equivalent dose (mg/day)	631.9	434.0
PANSS score		
Positive (7–49)	16.3	5.2
Negative (7–49)	19.0	5.5
General psychopathology (16–112)	36.2	9.3
Total (30–210)	71.6	17.7
Clinical diagnosis		
Paranoid type	46	
Disorganized type	3	
Catatonic type	1	
Residual type	65	
Unknown	11	
Polytherapy		
Antipsychotics		
Monotherapy	26	
Risperidone	62	
Olanzapine	16	
Aripiprazole	17	
Other atypical drug	3	
Typical drug	2	

[a]standard deviation.

Table 2: Measurement results of 4-digit CPT-IP.

P	Patients (n = 126) Mean	SD[a]	ICC[b]
d′			
1st	1.29	0.84	0.71
2nd	1.55	0.96	
mean	1.42	0.84	
Hits (0–30)			
1st	18.4	7.2	0.77
2nd	19.6	6.9	
False alarms (0–30)			
1st	6.3	4.6	0.70
2nd	5.7	4.7	
Random errors (0–90)			
1st	4.8	8.9	0.53
2nd	3.5	4.9	

[a]standard deviation
[b]intraclass correlation coefficient.

regression. Although no strong correlation (>0.8) was observed in all clinical parameters, the Pearson's correlation between age and duration of illness was high (0.72).

4. Discussion

CPT-IP is a major neurocognitive examination used to assess cognitive impairment among psychiatric patients. Included as a subtest in the MCCB, CPT-IP scores are often used to assess drug efficacy in clinical trials or endophenotypes in genetic studies. Confounding factors, such as measurement error or influence of clinical data, can hamper interpretation of results. Thus, to elucidate the effects of clinical data (age, sex, education years, duration of illness, onset age, CPZ equivalent dose, and PANSS score) on CPT-IP score in schizophrenia patients, we performed a multiple regression analysis in Japanese people suffering from schizophrenia.

4.1. Main Findings. Age and PANSS-negative symptom score were statistically associated with mean d′ score in schizophrenia patients. This finding is in concordance with a previous study [18]. Additionally, our results suggest that CPZ-equivalent dose affects CPT-IP score. Overall, using a relatively large Japanese clinical sample of schizophrenia, we showed that age, CPZ-equivalent, dose and PANSS-negative symptom score can have a major effect on the CPT-IP scores and therefore should be taken into the account when interpreting results obtained from patients with schizophrenia. Age, CPZ-equivalent dose, and PANSS negative symptom score explained about 28% of the variance in mean d′ score.

4.2. Limitations. There are several limitations that should be considered when interpreting the results of the present study. Multiple regression analysis findings in schizophrenia patients would benefit if we had been able to obtain more clinical information, such as IQ score and duration of untreated psychosis. As we could not find significant effects of sex, age at disease onset, duration of illness, and PANSS-positive and general psychopathology score in this study, weak effects of these factors might be observed when the sample size is increased.

5. Conclusion

We investigated how covariates (age, CPZ-equivalent dose, and PANSS-negative symptom score) affect mean d′ score of CPT-IP. This is the first study using a single independent large Japanese schizophrenia sample set, known as homogeneous in terms of genetic makeup. Our study suggested that those effects should be carefully considered especially when CPT-IP is performed to detect small effect size factors which are expected to be found in case of common risk variants associated with schizophrenia or cognitive-enhancing drugs. Thus, as CPT-IP is likely to be an endophenotypic measure in molecular genetic studies of schizophrenia in the post-genome-wide association study era [19, 20], our data show

TABLE 3: Multiple regression analysis of mean d′ score.

Clinical factors	Multiple regression analysis Forward-backward stepwise selection Patients (n = 126) Setting: P_{in} = 0.05, P_{out} = 0.1					
	PRC[a]	S-PRC[b]	VIF[c]	95% CI[d] Lower	95% CI[d] Upper	P value
Age (y)	−0.031	−0.45	1.04	−0.041	−0.020	**<0.001**
CPZ-equivalent dose (mg/day)	−0.00038	−0.21	1.01	−0.001	<0	**0.012**
PANSS-negative symptom score (7–49)	−0.026	−0.16	1.04	−0.052	<0	**0.017**
Intercept	3.54	—	—	2.89	4.19	<0.001
$\hat{R}^{2e}$			0.28			
ANOVA P value			**<0.001**			
Durbin-Watson ratio			1.93			

[a]partial regression coefficient
[b]standardized partial regression coefficient
[c]variance inflation factor
[d]confidence interval
[e]multiple correlation coefficient adjusted for the degrees of freedom.

that careful assessment of confounding factors is essential for interpretation of findings.

Authors' Contribution

T. Koide and B. Aleksic contributed equally to this work.

Acknowledgments

Funding for this study was provided by research grants from the Ministry of Education, Culture, Sports, Science and Technology of Japan; the Ministry of Health, Labor and Welfare of Japan; Grant-in-Aid for "Integrated research on neuropsychiatric disorders" carried out under the Strategic Research Program for Brain Sciences by the Ministry of Education, Culture, Sports, Science and Technology of Japan; Grant -in-Aid for Scientific Research on Innovative Areas (Comprehensive Brain Science Network) from the Ministry of Education, Science, Sports and Culture of Japan; The Academic Frontier Project for Private Universities, Comparative Cognitive Science Institutes, and the Core Research for Evolutional Science and Technology. The authors sincerely thank the patients and healthy volunteers for their participation in this study. They would like to express our gratitude to Ryoko Ishihara, PhD, Yoshihito Ito, MD, PhD, Hiromi Noma, Saori Yamashita, PhD and Mami Yoshida for their technical assistance, discussion, contributions to creating and managing the database, and advice about investigation of cognitive tests and their interpretation.

References

[1] P. Lichtenstein, B. H. Yip, C. Björk et al., "Common genetic determinants of schizophrenia and bipolar disorder in Swedish families: a population-based study," *The Lancet*, vol. 373, no. 9659, pp. 234–239, 2009.

[2] H. Stefansson, R. A. Ophoff, S. Steinberg et al., "Common variants conferring risk of schizophrenia," *Nature*, vol. 460, no. 7256, pp. 744–747, 2009.

[3] J. Shi, D. F. Levinson, J. Duan et al., "Common variants on chromosome 6p22.1 are associated with schizophrenia," *Nature*, vol. 460, no. 7256, pp. 753–757, 2009.

[4] S. M. Purcell, N. R. Wray, J. L. Stone et al., "Common polygenic variation contributes to risk of schizophrenia and bipolar disorder," *Nature*, vol. 460, no. 7256, pp. 748–752, 2009.

[5] M. Y. M. Ng, D. F. Levinson, S. V. Faraone et al., "Meta-analysis of 32 genome-wide linkage studies of schizophrenia," *Molecular Psychiatry*, vol. 14, no. 8, pp. 774–785, 2009.

[6] R. E. Gur, M. E. Calkins, R. C. Gur et al., "The consortium on the genetics of schizophrenia: neurocognitive endophenotypes," *Schizophrenia Bulletin*, vol. 33, no. 1, pp. 49–68, 2007.

[7] B. A. Cornblatt, N. J. Risch, G. Faris, D. Friedman, and L. Erlenmeyer-Kimling, "The continuous performance test, identical pairs version (CPT-IP): I. New findings about sustained attention in normal families," *Psychiatry Research*, vol. 26, no. 2, pp. 223–238, 1988.

[8] M. F. Green, "What are the functional consequences of neurocognitive deficits in schizophrenia?" *American Journal of Psychiatry*, vol. 153, no. 3, pp. 321–330, 1996.

[9] M. F. Green, R. S. Kern, D. L. Braff, and J. Mintz, "Neurocognitive deficits and functional outcome in schizophrenia: are we measuring the "right stuff"?" *Schizophrenia Bulletin*, vol. 26, no. 1, pp. 119–136, 2000.

[10] M. F. Green, R. S. Kern, and R. K. Heaton, "Longitudinal studies of cognition and functional outcome in schizophrenia: implications for MATRICS," *Schizophrenia Research*, vol. 72, no. 1, pp. 41–51, 2004.

[11] B. A. Cornblatt and J. G. Keilp, "Impaired attention, genetics, and the pathophysiology of schizophrenia," *Schizophrenia Bulletin*, vol. 20, no. 1, pp. 31–46, 1994.

[12] K. S. Kendler and M. C. Neale, "Endophenotype: a conceptual analysis," *Molecular Psychiatry*, vol. 15, no. 8, pp. 789–797, 2010.

[13] K. H. Nuechterlein, M. F. Green, R. S. Kern et al., "The MATRICS consensus cognitive battery, part 1: test selection, reliability, and validity," *American Journal of Psychiatry*, vol. 165, no. 2, pp. 203–213, 2008.
[14] L. Erlenmeyer-Kimling and B. A. Cornblatt, "A summary of attentional findings in the New York high-risk project," *Journal of Psychiatric Research*, vol. 26, no. 4, pp. 405–426, 1992.
[15] A. Inagaki and T. Inada, "Dose equivalence of psychotropic drugs. Part XX: dose equivalence of novel antipsychotics: blonanserin," *Japanese Journal of Clinical Psychopharmacology*, vol. 11, pp. 887–890, 2008.
[16] A. Inagaki and T. Inada, "Dose equivalence of psychotropic drugs. Part XXII: dose equivalence of depot antipsychotics III: risperidon long-acting injection," *Japanese Journal of Clinical Psychopharmacology*, vol. 13, pp. 1349–4353, 2010.
[17] S. R. Kay, A. Fiszbein, and L. A. Opler, "The positive and negative syndrome scale (PANSS) for schizophrenia," *Schizophrenia Bulletin*, vol. 13, no. 2, pp. 261–276, 1987.
[18] M. R. Nieuwenstein, A. Aleman, and E. H.F. De Haan, "Relationship between symptom dimensions and neurocognitive functioning in schizophrenia: a meta-analysis of WCST and CPT studies," *Journal of Psychiatric Research*, vol. 35, no. 2, pp. 119–125, 2001.
[19] K. E. Burdick, P. DeRosse, J. M. Kane, T. Lencz, and A. K. Malhotra, "Association of genetic variation in the MET proto-oncogene with schizophrenia and general cognitive ability," *American Journal of Psychiatry*, vol. 167, no. 4, pp. 436–443, 2010.
[20] T. D. Cannon, "Candidate gene studies in the GWAS era: the MET proto-oncogene, neurocognition, and schizophrenia," *American Journal of Psychiatry*, vol. 167, no. 4, pp. 369–372, 2010.

16

Faulty Suppression of Irrelevant Material in Patients with Thought Disorder Linked to Attenuated Frontotemporal Activation

S. M. Arcuri,[1,2] M. R. Broome,[1,3] V. Giampietro,[4] E. Amaro Jr.,[2] T. T. J. Kircher,[5] S. C. R. Williams,[4] C. M. Andrew,[4] M. Brammer,[4] R. G. Morris,[6] and P. K. McGuire[1]

[1] *Department of Psychosis Studies, Institute of Psychiatry, King's College London, London, UK*
[2] *NIF, Functional Neuroimaging, Lab/LIM 44, Instituto de Radiologia, University of Sao Paulo, Sao Paulo, Brazil*
[3] *Warwick Medical School, University of Warwick, Coventry UK and Psychosis Clinical Academic Group, Coventry, UK*
[4] *Department of Neuroimaging, Institute of Psychiatry, King's College London, London, UK*
[5] *Marburg University, Marburg, Germany*
[6] *Department of Psychology, Institute of Psychiatry, King's College London, London, UK*

Correspondence should be addressed to S. M. Arcuri, silvia.arcuri@kcl.ac.uk

Academic Editor: Christoph Mulert

Formal thought disorder is a feature schizophrenia that manifests as disorganized, incoherent speech, and is associated with a poor clinical outcome. The neurocognitive basis of this symptom is unclear but it is thought to involve an impairment in semantic processing classically described as a loosening of meaningful associations. Using a paradigm derived from the n400 event-related, potential, we examined the extent to which regional activation during semantic processing is altered in schizophrenic patients with formal thought disorder. Ten healthy control and 18 schizophrenic participants (9 with and 9 without formal thought disorder) performed a semantic decision sentence task during an event-related functional magnetic resonance imaging experiment. We employed analysis of variance to estimate the main effects of semantic congruency and groups on activation and specific effects of formal thought disorder were addressed using post-hoc comparisons. We found that the frontotemporal network, normally engaged by a semantic decision task, was underactivated in schizophrenia, particularly in patients with FTD. This network is implicated in the inhibition of automatically primed stimuli and impairment of its function interferes with language processing and contributes to the production of incoherent speech.

1. Introduction

Bleuler's work in psychosis continues to be highly influential in furthering understanding of the signs and symptoms of schizophrenia [1]. Nevertheless, one of his primary conceptual contributions in understanding schizophrenia, "disturbance of associations" [2, 3], remains to be explained in terms of underlying neural basis. In turn, Bleuler's ideas were influenced by Jung's word association task [4]. Regardless of the psychological or affective mechanisms that may influence the production of speech, Jungian word association is by nature a semantic association test. Interpretations of the broader meanings of "split mind" and "association", arising from the psychoanalytical field, are not incompatible with an inbuilt characteristic of this test, which taps into the concept of semantic priming [5], extensively investigated in schizophrenia (see Minzenberg et al. [6] for a review in single-word semantic priming in schizophrenia). However, some studies do not take into account specific symptoms proposed by Bleuler, such as formal thought disorder, as an underlying factor that would interfere with task performance (e.g., [7]), mixing up performance of patients with a range of distinct symptoms. Of note, there is a line of investigation suggesting that formal thought disorder (FTD) is associated with hyperactivation of the semantic network [8–14]. These studies mainly employ semantic tasks based on word-pair semantic priming paradigms. It is important to note that such kind of studies, although provided evidence for altered semantic processing associated with FTD, may fail to tap into the type of communication impairment clinically seen in FTD patients. The latter manifests itself in linguistic units that range from large thoughts, such as whole periods with several sentences embedded, to small utterances, such as words within the same sentence [15], or even a single word (e.g., neologism).

Bleuler also suggested that, within its symptoms, FTD is possibly the closest to the neural substrate of schizophrenia [2]. Biological evidence for a neural basis of FTD has been provided by methods employing functional measures of brain activity. EEG studies employing the n400, an event-related potential (ERP) that is a neural marker of semantic processing [16–18], demonstrated a reduction in n400 amplitudes and increased latency in schizophrenia during a sentence processing task [19–21], consistent with impairment in semantic integration, particularly associated with FTD [22–26].

Functional neuroimaging of schizophrenia suggested that FTD is associated with altered resting activity in the medial temporal cortex [27] and with altered activity (brain metabolism or Blood Oxygen Level Dependent-BOLD-activity) during tasks that engage language processing in the dorsolateral prefrontal, bilateral anterior cingulate, and lateral temporal cortices [28–32]). FTD has also been linked to reductions in grey matter volume in the inferior frontal [33, 34] and the temporo-parietal cortex [35]. Using a model of information processing, MacDonalds III and collaborators demonstrated diminished activity in the middle frontal gyrus in schizophrenic patients with disorganization symptoms (includes FTD) associated with context processing deficits [31]. Collectively, the studies particularly implicate the prefrontal, middle frontal, temporal, and anterior cingulate cortices in the pathophysiology of FTD in schizophrenia.

In summary, FTD is a symptom of schizophrenia that manifests itself as disorganized, incoherent speech. Andreasen [36] has operationalized studying this symptom by creating a scale that decomposes the concept of "loosening of meaningful associations" into measurable items. Thus, this clinical manifestation of schizophrenia, which can be objectively measured, is thought to involve impairment in semantic processing, deficits in executive functioning, and altered brain activity in the left frontal, temporal, and anterior cingulate cortices.

The objective of the present study was to use event-related fMRI to examine the extent to which regional activation during semantic processing is altered in schizophrenic patients with FTD. Methodological issues which were not tackled by some of the functional imaging studies mentioned above (small sample sizes, block design fMRI task and an overt production of speech) were carefully addressed. Particularly, we devised a task likely to engage areas associated with linguistic processes with heavier demands [37] using a paradigm derived from semantic decision procedures used in the ERP studies that originally correlated FTD with n400 abnormalities in schizophrenia. We sought to engage the top down modulation of semantic processing by requiring suppression or inhibitory mechanisms to take place, necessary to process semantic incongruent information. Activation of the left inferior frontal and left middle temporal [38, 39], right anterior cingulate [38], and bilateral precuneus [39] was found in studies that required the generation of semantically incongruent endings to complete a previously primed incomplete sentence stem. Therefore, these areas are activated in tasks requiring suppression of endings (meanings) automatically activated by sentences.

We hypothesized the following:

(1) Incongruent sentences would engage left inferior frontal, left middle temporal, right anterior cingulate, and bilateral precuneus more than congruent sentences.

(2) FTD patients with schizophrenia would show diminished activation relative to controls and patients without FTD in:

 (a) areas previously demonstrated to show aberrant activity in this group: left prefrontal (middle and inferior), left temporal, and bilateral anterior cingulate cortex and

 (b) areas associated with manipulation of incongruent material (i.e., the above and also the precuneus).

2. Methods

2.1. Subjects. Ten healthy adult volunteers and 18 patients meeting DSM-IV criteria for schizophrenia [40] took part in the study. Acutely psychotic patients with either high or low levels of positive FTD were recruited from the South London and Maudsley NHS Trust. Controls were recruited from the same geographical area through local advertisement.

All subjects were dextral [41], males with National Adult Reading Test Revised [42] IQ $\geq$ 80, and native speakers of British English. Exclusion criteria for controls were a previous history of a neurological or psychiatric disorder, substance dependence, or a medical disorder that could affect the brain. Exclusion criteria for patient were another DSM-IV axis I diagnosis and age of onset of schizophrenia prior to 18 years of age. Subjects received oral and written information about the procedures and gave written consent to participate, with £30 in return for participating. The project was approved by the Research Ethical Committee of the Institute of Psychiatry.

Psychopathology was assessed using the Scale for the Assessment of Positive Symptoms (SAPS) [36] and the Scale for the Assessment of Negative Symptoms (SANS) [43]. Positive FTD was assessed on the basis of the corresponding 8 items in the SAPS (derailment; incoherence; illogicality; circumstantiality; pressure of speech; distractible speech; tangentiality; clanging).

In each patient, the score on each FTD SAPS item (range 0–5) was summed to yield a total FTD score (range 0–40). The FTD score was then used both as a classifier to split the patients sample in two subgroups (as described below) and as a continuous measure (see Figure 2(b)), without distinctions within the patients. Thus, patients who had a FTD score 0–4 were classified as non-FTD and those with scores ranging from 5–40 were classified as FTD. The patients sample was split into two groups on this basis producing a subgroup with (FTD, $n = 9$ and a subgroup without FTD (Non-FTD, $n = 9$). There were no significant differences between these subgroup in SAPS total score, SANS total score, scale for the Assessment of Global Functioning (GAF) [40] score, antipsychotic medication dose (in chlorpromazine equivalent), duration of illness, number of psychiatric admissions, or age at first admission (Table 1). There were also no differences in the score for negative FTD, as defined by the SANS items (poverty of speech, poverty of content of speech, thought blocking, and increased latency of response).

The two patient subgroups and the healthy controls had similar demographic characteristics (Table 2).

2.2. Task

2.2.1. Sentence Stems. Eighty sentence stems (i.e., last word missing) were used with the degree of constraint previously defined in a large sample drawn from the same population as the control subjects in the present study [44]. Forty stems had a high semantic constraint (HCt) (cloze probability > 0.94) and 40 low semantic constraint (LCt) (cloze probability < 0.34). For example, "He posted the letter without a....", is a HCt stem (completed by the word "stamp" by 96% of subjects), while "She couldn't imagine anyone less..." is a LCt stem.

2.2.2. Target Words. Two types of words were presented as target stimuli, taken from completions that had originally been produced for the stems [44]. These words were either congruous with the sentence stem (i.e., semantically related) or incongruous (semantically unrelated). To avoid phonological priming [45], words with the same initial phoneme as the most frequent congruent completion (best completion) for that stem were excluded.

2.3. Experimental Paradigm

2.3.1. fMRI Stimuli. Sentence stems were presented onto a screen subtending a visual angle of approximately 1° (text height) by 7°, (stem length). Stems were presented for 2.5 sec. After an interval of 0,7 sec during which the screen was blank, the target word appeared (Figure 1). During the inter stimulus interval, subjects were instructed to fixate on an asterisk for at least 13.7 sec. Eighty trials of 20.4 seconds duration were presented, divided into 5 runs of 16 trials each. Trial type per run was pseudorandomized to control for order effects between subjects. Subjects were instructed to read the sentence stem, then decide if the target completed the stem in a sensible way or not making their choice using one of two buttons on a button box (for accuracy and response time recordings). Prior to scanning, all subjects underwent a training session to make sure they were able to understand and perform the task.

2.3.2. fMRI Data Acquisition. Gradient-echo planar MR images were acquired using a quadrature head coil in a 1.5 Tesla GE Signa System (General Electric, Milwaukee, WS, USA). Head movement was minimised by foam padding and a supporting band across the forehead. A gradient echo EPI axial acquisition (TR 1700 milliseconds-ms, TE 40 ms, FA 90°, matrix 64 × 64, FOV 24 cm, thickness 7 mm, gap 0.7 mm, 192 volumes) was used to collect 12 slices parallel to the intercommissural (AC-PC) plane. The total number of images acquired (in 5 runs) was 960 with just under five minutes between them. Structural images were acquired using gradient echo IR EPI sequence (TR 1600 ms, TE 40 ms, TI 180 ms, matrix 128 × 128, FOV 20 cm, thickness 3 mm, gap 0.3 mm, NEX 8, 43 slices). This latter image was used for normalisation to a standard template.

2.4. Analysis. This experiment is part of a larger study [46] in which a series of experiments were designed to test the semantic network and executive functions in FTD patients. The present experiment manipulated semantic constraints and congruencies. In this paper, we only addressed effects of semantic congruency.

2.5. Online Behavioral Data. Repeated Measures (SPSS, General Linear Model) analyses were performed for accuracy scores and reaction times (RT) using semantic congruency as within-subject factors. A "yes" response for a semantically incongruent word or "no" response to a congruent word was considered inaccurate. The percentage of correct responses across trials of the same condition was used as within-subject factor.

2.6. Neuroimaging Data. Imaging data were analysed with xbam v3.4, Department of Biostatistics and Computing, Institute of Psychiatry, King's College London [47]. More details about the software can be obtained at http://www.brainmap.it/.

2.6.1. Movement Estimation and Correction. The mean signal intensity over all time points (960) was averaged to create a target image (average image intensity at every voxel across all time points) and the sum of absolute differences in grey scale values between the voxels of each observed image (at each time point) and its corresponding base image was computed. A rigid body registration search algorithm was used to estimate the extent of translation and rotation (3 rotations + 3 translations), minimising the total difference between match and base images. The match images were realigned relative to the base image by tricubic spline interpolation and the realigned T2*-weighted time series were regressed on the concomitant and lagged time series of estimated movement at each voxel [48]. Residual time series resulting from the last stage of this procedure were thus uncorrelated with estimated rigid motion in 3D.

2.6.2. Data Analysis. A nonparametric procedure [49] was adopted that avoids assumptions about the distribution of statistics under the null hypothesis. First, the experimental

TABLE 1: Clinical characteristics of the Patient Groups.

Group	Non-FTD	FTD	*P* value
Positive FTD	0 (1) 0–2	17 (11) 5–20	**<0.001**[a]
Negative FTD	5 (7) 0–9	6 (6) 3–14	0.546[a]
SAPS (sum)	23 (16) 8–50	14 (10) 6–26	0.471[b]
SANS (sum)	19 (9) 1–34	27 (13) 11–52	0.588[b]
GAF	31 (13) 21–51	30 (14) 20–40	0.546[a]
Chlorpromazine equivalent in (mg/day)	700 (967) 133–1800	517 (550) 320–1200	0.772[a]
Duration of illness (in years)	6 (12) 0.5–17	11 (14) 8–28	0.190[a]
Hospital admissions			
Number	2 (4) 1–15	6 (9) 1–20	0.142[a]
Age at 1st	25 (9) 19–60	26 (11) 15–31	0.222[a]

[a] Mann-Whitney [median (interquartile range) min and max], [b] ANOVA [Mean (SD) and range], [c] Fischer Exact.

TABLE 2: Demographic Description of the Sample.

Groups	AGE Median (interquartile range); min and max	Nart IQ Mean (SD); range	Years of full-time education median (interquartile range); min and max
Controls	35 (10); 24–54	108.3 (13.5); 89–126	14.3–(5.3); 9–24
NON-TD	38 (21); 24–63	101.4 (12.7); 86–122	11.0 (1.5)*; 9–15
TD	33 (16); 23–55	99.2 (10.7); 82–115	11.0 (3)*; 9–12
Analysis results	$P = 0.222$[a]	$P = 0.267$[b]	$P = 0.029$[a]

[a] Kruskal Wallis, [b] one-way ANOVA, *no difference between TD and non-TD patients for years of education.

design was convolved with two poisson functions chosen to model the haemodynamic delays of 4 and 8 seconds (see Figure 1). The best fit (weighted sum) of these two convolutions to the observed time series at each voxel was then computed by least squares analysis. The use of the two convolutions within the experimental design allows the time delay between stimulus onset and peak bold response to vary between these limits, which encompass the normal range of haemodynamic delays. Using the parameters of the least squares model fit, the sums of squares of deviations from the mean image intensity over the whole time series due to the model and the residuals were calculated. The ratio of these sums of squares of residuals (model/residuals) was then calculated (and called SSQ ratio). The appropriate null distribution of this statistic was obtained by repeating the model fitting procedure after wavelet-based permutation of the time series [47] twenty times at each voxel and combining the data over all voxels. For any desired type I error rate, the appropriate critical threshold value of SSQ ratio could be obtained from this distribution. Any value of SSQ ratio that exceeded this threshold was deemed to indicate the presence of a voxel responding to the experimental paradigm.

In order to construct group images, the observed and "null" SSQ ratio maps for each experimental condition were then transformed into Talairach space [50]. Median activation maps for each condition were computed after smoothing with a Gaussian filter (FWHM 7.2 mm). Three maps were produced: (1) condition "b" versus "a", (2) condition "c" versus "a", and (3) condition "b" versus "c", where "a" means baseline and "b" and "c" the experimental conditions tested.

The main effect of semantic congruency was assessed by contrasting the 40 congruent trials (20 *low* congruent + 20 *high* congruent) and 40 incongruent trials (20 *low* incongruent + 20 *high* congruent) [conditions "b" and "c" maps]. In order to probe the analysis to the main cognitive process under investigation, we chose the 3rd TR in an event-related design, in which the presentation both of the sentence stem and the final word has already taken place, as shown in Figure 1.

Differences in the responses between conditions were obtained at each voxel by regression of the linear model $F = a_0 + a_1 P + e$, where the vector of responses in all subjects at a voxel, P is a dummy coding vector expressing the particular contrast between experimental conditions of interest, and e is the vector of random errors. Values of a_1^* were tested for statistical significance by randomly reallocating the data of each voxel between conditions, thus realising the null distribution under the hypothesis of no difference between responses to different experimental conditions. The analyses reported in this study were carried out using cluster-level statistics to avoid harsh multiple comparison corrections required if each voxel is tested individually [51]. Initially, maps of a_1^* were thresholded retaining only clusters with a probability of type I error = 0.0001, for main effects of the task in healthy controls. However, the patients group showed a diminished overall strength of activation relative to healthy controls. We thus decided to report results from maps thresholded at a voxel/cluster probability of type I error =

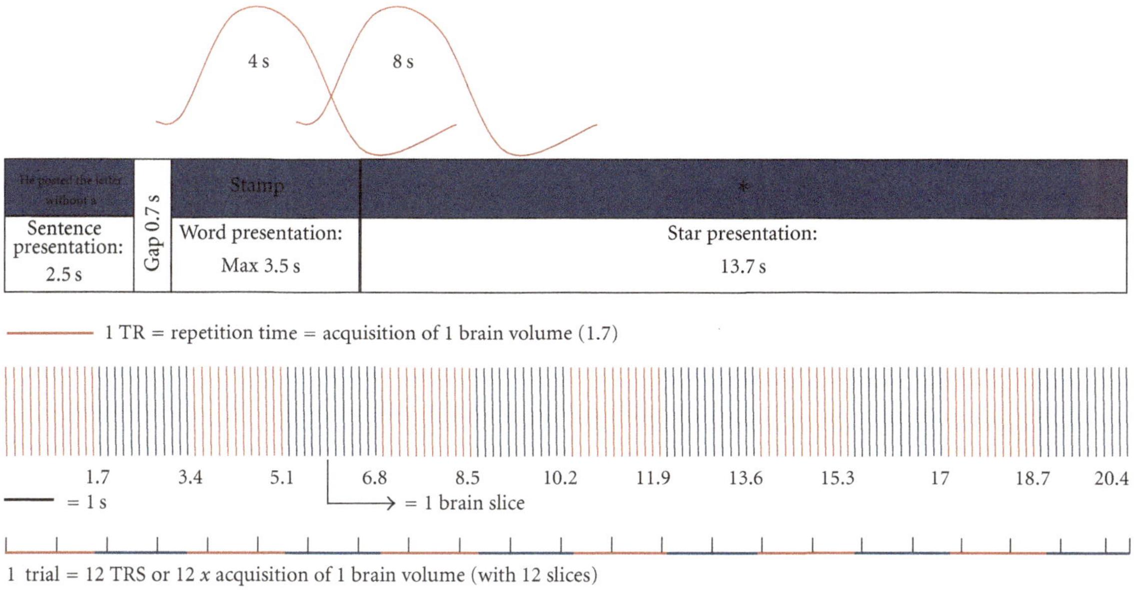

FIGURE 1: fMRI task design.

0.05/0.01, adjusted to get less than 1 false positive per map, to facilitate interpretation of the results, particularly the differences found between controls and patients and between patients themselves (FTD and Non-FTD). The integral of the SSQ ratio values for each of the resulting three-dimensional clusters was then tested against the distribution of cluster SSQ ratio integrals generated after random reallocation of data between conditions at each voxel (see above). Maps reflecting the contrast between conditions (i.e., congruent versus incongruent) in each group were analysed with ANOVAS, producing 2 maps, one showing regions more activated in the first condition and the other showing the reverse.

To minimize the potentially confounding effect of differences in task performance on brain activation, all incorrect trials were excluded from the image analysis. Thus the neuroimaging data were derived from trials in which subjects correctly decided whether the final word was or not semantically congruent with the previous sentence stem.

2.6.3. Data Analyses to Compare Groups. To investigate between group differences due to effects of semantic congruency, the images resulting from the contrast between semantic congruent versus incongruent trials were directly compared between groups, first contrasting all groups in a 3-Group ANOVA with cluster probability of type I error set at 0.01. This analysis produced a range of maps in which one group showed greater activation than the other groups and vice-versa. These maps are presented in the results section below (Figure 2 and Table 3).

Further analyses were conducted to investigate the nature of the results arising from the semantic congruency analysis: we wanted to determine whether differences in activation maps observed between controls and patients could be due to a specific pattern of activation associated with FTD or not. Therefore, separate post-hoc ANOVAS contrasting FTD with controls and FTD with Non-FTD were performed.

3. Results

3.1. Online Behavioral Responses

3.1.1. Accuracy. We did not observe an effect of semantic congruency in performance accuracy ($F = 0.65$, $P = 0.43$, $df = 1$). Equally, there was no significant interaction between congruency and group ($F = 0.46$, $P = 0.64$, $df = 1$). Post- hoc tests (Tukey) demonstrated that there was a significant contrast between FTD and controls [mean Difference = −0.128; Std error = 0.397; $P = 0.009$; CI: −0.227 to −0.029], reflecting impairment seen in incongruent trials (Figure 4) with FTD showing the worse performance (more mistakes than both other groups). Non-FTD showed an intermediate level of performance, making more mistakes than FTD and fewer relative to controls, without significant differences in both contrasts.

3.1.2. Reaction Times. In all groups, responses to congruent trials were faster than incongruent ones (see Figure 5), with an observed significant effect of semantic congruency on reaction times ($F = 14.17$, $P = 0.001$, $df = 1$) and no significant interactions between semantic congruency and group ($F = 0.84$, $P = 0.442$, $df = 2$). A robust main effect of group on RT was found ($F = 34.10$, $P < 0.001$, $df = 2$). Non-FTD patients were slower than FTD and controls in both conditions (congruent and incongruent trials). Controls were faster than FTD in both conditions. Post-hoc contrasts demonstrated significant differences in RT between all pairs contrasted, that is, controls versus FTD [mean difference = −0.442; std error = 0.800; $P < 0.001$; CI: −0.639 to −0.244], controls versus NON-FTD [mean difference = −0.672; std

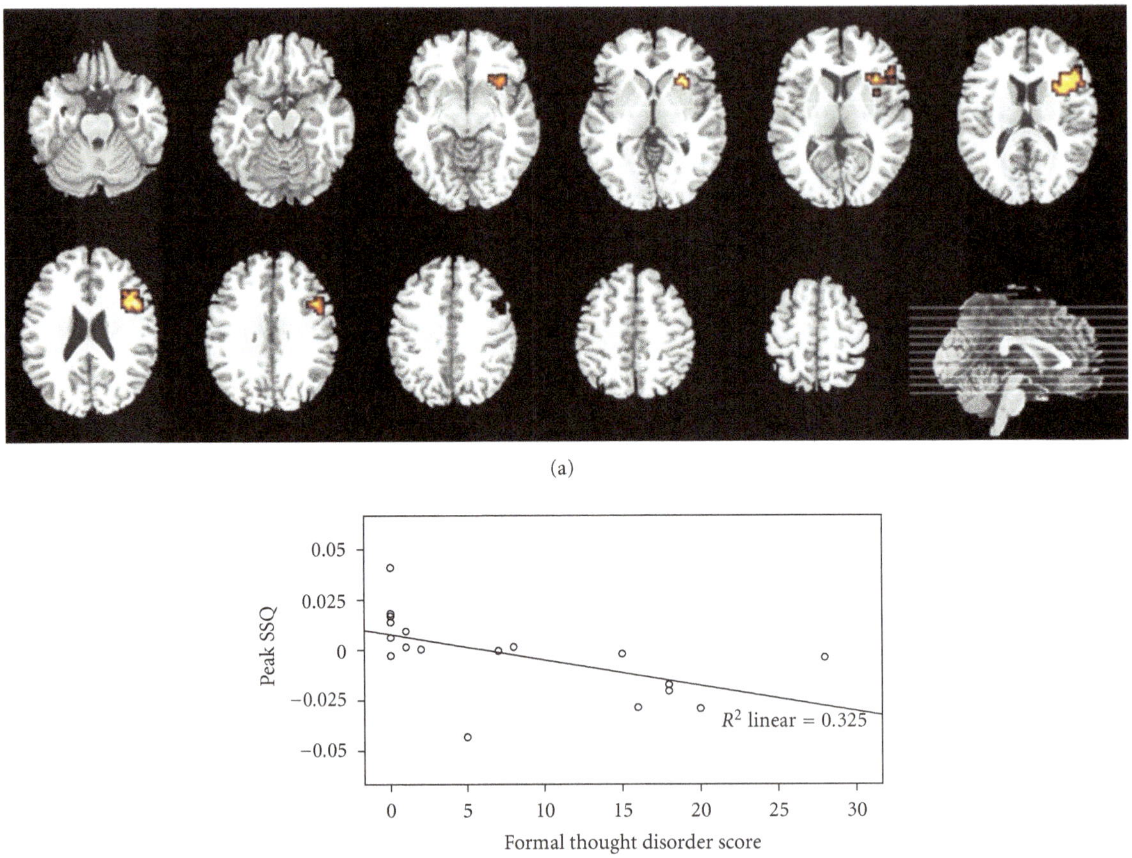

(a)

(b)

Figure 2: (a) 3-Group ANOVA: semantic congruency (congruent versus incongruent) trials. Comparison of healthy controls ($n = 10$) versus schizophrenic patients with formal thought disorder (FTD, $n = 9$) versus schizophrenic patients without formal thought disorder (Non-FTD, $n = 9$). Attenuated activation in the left inferior frontal gyrus was observed in FTD relative to Non-FTD and to controls. The latter showed greater activation in this region also relative to non-FTD. The left side of the brain images corresponds to the right side of the brain. The superior part of the brain images corresponds to the anterior brain region. (b) Scatter plot of the activity in the left inferior frontal cortex as a function of the score in formal thought disorder (FTD) within schizophrenic patients ($n = 18$). We observe that FTD higher scores in a sample of psychotic schizophrenic patients are negatively correlated with activity in the left inferior frontal cortex ($x = -43.33$, $y = 14.81$, $z = 14.85$).

error = 0.085; $P < 0.001$; CI: −0.880 to −0.463], and FTD versus NON-FTD [mean difference = −0.229; std error = 0.088; $P = 0.036$; CI: −0.446 to −0.013].

4. Neuroimaging Results

4.1. Control Subjects

4.1.1. Congruent and Incongruent Sentences (Table 3). Congruent trials were associated with increased activation relative to incongruent trials in the dorsal portion of the left inferior frontal gyrus, the orbital portion of the right inferior frontal gyrus, the anterior cingulate bilaterally, the right caudate nucleus, the left posterior middle temporal gyrus, the left parahippocampal gyrus, the right precuneus, and the right inferior frontal gyrus. Conversely, incongruent trials were associated with more activation than congruent trials in the left middle frontal gyrus, the right medial frontal gyrus, and the left superior frontal gyrus.

4.1.2. Between Group Differences: Controls versus Non-FTD versus FTD (Table 3). The contrast between congruent and incongruent sentences was associated with greater activation in the dorsal portion of the left inferior frontal cortex in controls than Non-FTD patients, which in turn had increased activation relative to FTD patients in the same region (Figure 2(a)). In this analysis, we did not find regions in which the patients groups showed more activation than controls.

4.1.3. Activation Associated with FTD. POST-HOC contrasts of FTD patients versus controls and FTD versus Non-FTD patients confirmed attenuated activation in the left inferior frontal cortex in the FTD group. Relative to controls, FTD patients showed less activation in the dorsal portion

Table 3: The semantic decision match fmri task: neuroimaging results: 3D cluster sizes, talairach coordinates (of peak voxels) and cluster P values for main effects of the semantic congruency.

(a) Within group analysis: congruent versus incongruent trials in healthy controls ($n = 10$). Displayed only clusters > or = 6 in size

Contrast	Size	Tal(x)	Tal(y)	Tal(z)	Probability	Cerebral region
Congruent > Incongruent	2189	43.33	14.81	14.85	0.000656	Left inferior frontal gyrus, dorsal portion
	312	46.94	29.63	−7.15	0.000656	Right inferior frontal gyrus, orbital portion
	181	0.00	11.11	31.35	0.000656	Bilateral anterior cingulate gyrus
	3	14.44	11.11	25.85	0.008530	Right anterior cingulate gyrus
	15	10.83	22.22	−1.65	0.000656	Right caudate
	7	−36.11	−48.15	3.85	0.001969	Left middle temporal gyrus
	6	−21.67	−29.63	−12.65	0.001969	Left parahippocampal gyrus
	6	21.67	−66.67	36.85	0.004593	Right precuneus
Incongruent > Congruent	3094	−32.50	37.04	25.85	0.000678	Left middle frontal gyrus
	15	3.61	44.44	25.85	0.004749	Right medial frontal gyrus
	14	−21.67	55.56	9.35	0.000678	Left superior frontal gyrus

(b) Between Groups Analyses:. 3-Group ANOVA: Semantic Congruency (congruent versus incongruent) trials. Comparison of healthy controls ($n = 10$) versus schizophrenic patients with Formal Thought Disorder (FTD, $n = 9$) versus schizophrenic patients without formal thought disorder (Non-FTD, $n = 9$)

Results	Size	Tal(x)	Tal(y)	Tal(z)	Probability	Cerebral Region
Controls > NTD > TD	79	−43.33	14.81	14.85	0.007784	Left inferior frontal gyrus, dorsal portion

(c) Post-hoc 2 group comparisons: semantic congruency (congruent versus incongruent trials) schizophrenic patients with formal thought disorder (FTD, $n = 9$) versus healthy controls ($n = 10$) and FTD versus schizophrenic patients without formal thought disorder (Non-FTD, $n = 9$)

Results	Size	Tal(x)	Tal(y)	Tal(z)	Probability	Cerebral Region
Controls > TD	172	−43.33	14.81	14.85	0.000284	Left inferior frontal gyrus, dorsal portion
	95	28.89	−70.37	−18.15	0.000851	Right cerebellum, posterior lobe, declive
	92	50.56	25.93	14.85	0.002553	Right inferior frontal gyrus, dorsal portion
	67	−57.78	−37.04	3.85	0.011211	Left middle temporal gyrus
	42	−25.28	−62.96	36.85	0.012766	Left Precuneus
	35	−39.72	−62.96	−18.15	0.012482	Left cerebellum, posterior lobe, declive
	25	−10.83	−92.59	−7.15	0.012482	Left lingual gyrus
NON-FTD > TD	185	−43.33	14.81	20.35	0.000256	Left middle frontal gyrus
	127	46.94	18.52	25.85	0.001282	Right middle frontal gyrus
	37	0.00	18.52	36.85	0.008720	Bilateral anterior cingulate
NON-FTD < TD	81	7.22	−55.56	20.35	0.003912	Right posterior cingulate

of the inferior frontal cortex bilaterally, the left middle temporal gyrus, precuneus, and lingual gyrus and in the cerebellum bilaterally (Figure 3(a)). No areas were relatively more activated in the FTD than the control group.

Relative to Non-FTD patients, FTD patients showed less activation in the left middle frontal gyrus and bilaterally in the anterior cingulate gyrus (Figure 3(b) and Table 3). Conversely, the FTD subgroup showed more activation than the Non-FTD subgroup in the right posterior cingulate gyrus and the left cerebellum (Figure 3(c)).

5. Discussion

5.1. Behavioral Results. Semantic congruency influenced RTs, with minimum values in trials with congruous endings, as expected (see Figure 5). Therefore, we observed an effect of inhibition (or interference) associated with processing of incongruent sentences in all groups. The patients made more errors than controls, particularly those with FTD. This was most evident on incongruent trials where patients with FTD performed much worse than both patients with no FTD and controls, showing deficiency in processes where inhibition is expected.

5.2. Neuroimaging Results

5.2.1. Semantic Processing in Healthy Controls. We found that incongruent sentences activated the left middle frontal cortex more than congruent ones, an area associated with suppression when the same type of semantic material was employed

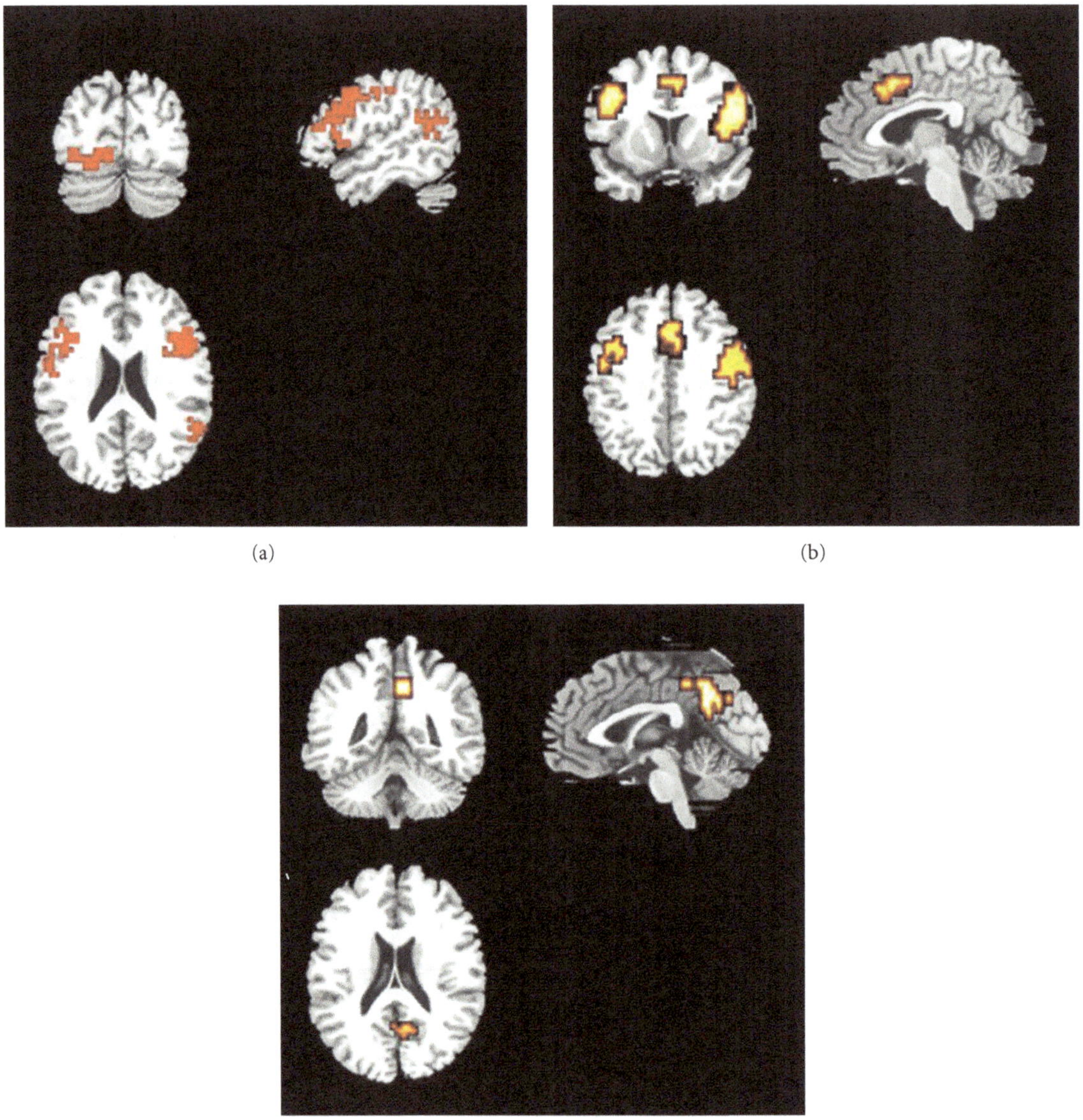

(a) (b) (c)

Figure 3: Post-hoc 2 group comparisons: semantic congruency (congruent versus incongruent trials). (a) healthy controls ($n = 10$) versus schizophrenic patients with formal thought disorder (FTD, $n = 9$) (b, c) FTD versus schizophrenic patients without formal Thought Disorder (Non-FTD, $n = 9$). (a) Controls show greater activation relative to FTD in the inferior frontal gyrus bilaterally, dorsal portions, in the left middle temporal gyrus (BA 22), in the left lingual gyrus, in the left precuneus, and in the cerebellum (posterior lobe) bilaterally. (b) Non-FTD patients showed greater activation of bilateral middle frontal gyrus and bilateral anterior cingulate, relative to FTD. (c) FTD patients show greater activation relative to Non-FTD patients in the right posterior cingulate. The left side of the brain images correspond to the right side of the brain. The superior part of the brain images correspond to the anterior brain region.

[39] and with inhibition of stereotyped responses [52]. However, in our study, we observed greater activity for *congruent* than incongruent trials in healthy controls in the right precuneus, contrary to our hypothesis. Therefore, our first hypothesis was partially confirmed. A possible explanation for these differences observed between ours and Allen et al.'s study may be the fact that their task required overt production of a final completing word for visually presented priming sentence stems, whilst ours only required making a decision upon a visually presented final word.

The general pattern of activation we found was expected because the semantic task used placed high demands on executive control, such as maintaining competing items on hold whilst checking for semantic appropriateness [53] and inhibiting unnecessary items. Thus, in healthy controls, we observed more activation for congruent than incongruent trials in the right inferior (orbital) and left inferior (dorsal) cortices, left posterior temporal cortex, bilateral anterior cingulate, and left precuneus. Our findings are in line with data supporting an important role of the left hemisphere in

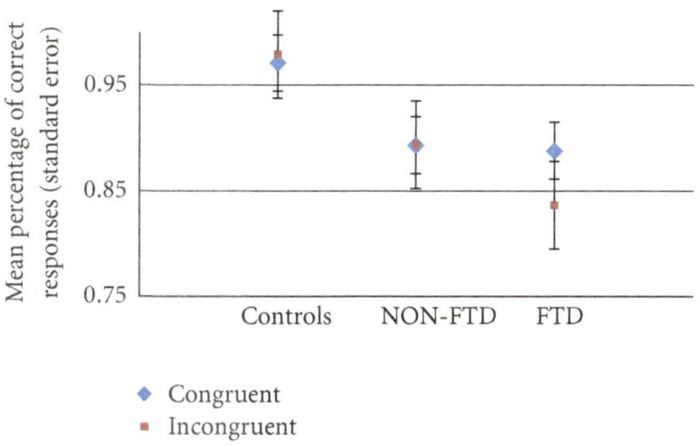

FIGURE 4: Semantic decision match fMRI task: performance accuracy in semantic congruent and incongruenet trials. Control ($n = 10$) versus NON-FTD ($n = 9$) versus FTD ($n = 9$).

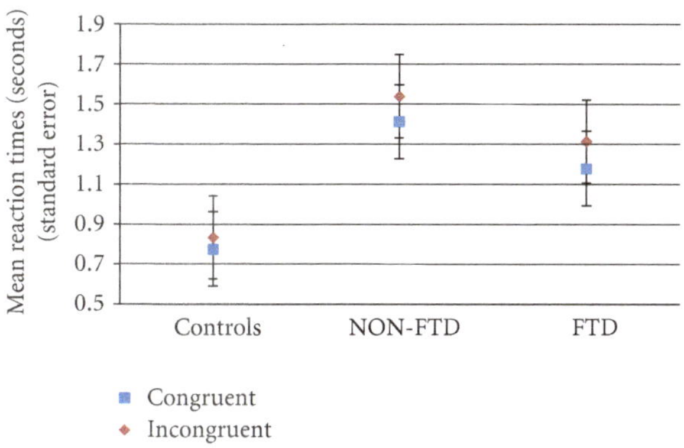

FIGURE 5: Semantic decision match fMRI task: reaction times in semantic congruent and incongruent trials. Control ($n = 10$) versus NON-FTD ($n = 9$) versus FTD ($n = 9$).

the final integration of semantic aspects present in sentences and texts [54] and recent meta-analytical studies showing activity in these regions associated with semantic processing [55–57].

5.2.2. Semantic Processing in FTD Schizophrenic Patients. We also hypothesized that FTD patients would show decreased activation in the prefrontal (middle and inferior), temporal, and cingulate cortices. Relative to controls, FTD patients showed a diminished activation in dorsal inferior frontal cortex (bilaterally) and in the left middle temporal gyrus when processing incongruent relative to congruent sentences. We predicted that these differences would also be evident when contrasting patients with and without FTD. We found that for the incongruent/congruent contrast, the FTD subgroup showed less activation than Non-FTD patients bilaterally in the left inferior/middle frontal gyri and the anterior cingulate gyri. Thus, our second hypothesis was confirmed. The differential brain activity observed in FTD patients while performing a task, without mistakes, seem to be arising from an early point of the semantic processing, since these attenuated activations were observed in areas in which controls showed increased activation for congruent trials relative to incongruent ones and *not* the other way round (contrary to our initial prediction). Although this may seem a contradictory finding, the current study confirms altered brain activity in these areas specifically associated with FTD in schizophrenia [28–32].

Manipulation of incongruent sentences requires overcoming a prepotent response, that is, suppression of automatically activated word(s) after a primed sentence stem [36]. The latter process needs to be maintained "active" for a longer period. Activity in the DLPFC has been associated with working memory and contextual information in experiments requiring heavier semantic processing demands [31, 58]. These group differences in inferior frontal and left middle temporal responses reflected less activation of these areas in patients with FTD relative to both controls and patients without FTD. This differential pattern of response is similar to that evident in their behaviour, where patients with FTD performed markedly worse than both other groups on trials involving semantically incongruent sentences, making more mistakes and also having a shorter RT than Non-FTD patients. Relative to Non-FTD, FTD also had less activation in the anterior cingulate cortices, which have been suggested by several authors to participate in demanding processes, such as monitoring conflict of response [59], engagement of cognitive control [60], top-down inhibitory modulation [61], detection of mnemonic competition, and retrieval induced forgetting [62].

A final point should be made about the activity in the precuneus. This region has been demonstrated to be involved in semantic processing [39, 57, 63, 64] episodic memory retrieval [65], retrieval-induced facilitation [66], and dopamine regulation of working memory [67]. FTD patients, but not Non-FTD patients, had less activation in the left precuneus than controls. Despite some subtle inconsistencies in hemispheric localization (not rare in fMRI studies of schizophrenia), this finding suggests a problem in episodic memory retrieval that might have contributed to the FTD group worse task performance. Thus, FTD patients showed robust diminished activation in areas implicated in the suppression of irrelevant material as well as detection and resolution of mnemonic conflict [68], selecting context-appropriate meanings in the presence of competing meanings [69], and differences between impaired and facilitated information [66]. Interestingly, Arcuri [46] found that FTD patients produced significantly more expected words than controls, when overtly producing anomalous endings for sentences of a high degree of constraint, in a modified version of the Hayling Task [70]. That study included the scanned FTD patients ($n = 9$) from the present study but had a larger sample of FTD patients ($n = 21$). Thus, FTD patients who showed diminished activation in areas implicated in aspects of executive control, when deciding whether a final target word is semantically appropriate for a previously presented sentence, also had difficulties in inhibiting automatically activated words that followed sentences of high semantic constraint, when they were asked to openly generate semantically incongruent completions for those sentences.

The differences between FTD and the Non-FTD patients are not attributable to sociodemographic or other clinical differences as they are matched in all respects other than the severity of positive FTD. Moreover, although the FTD patients performed the task more poorly than Non-FTD patients and controls, the image analysis was restricted to correct trials, indicating that the differences in activation were not simply secondary to the more impaired task performance in this subgroup. The differences in regional responses may thus be linked to the pathophysiology of incoherent speech. The prominent role of the inferior frontal cortex in language processing and particularly semantic processing is consistent with this suggestion. However, the fact that a qualitatively similar but less severe reduction in activation was evident in patients with no FTD indicates that findings in this area are also associated with the disorder of schizophrenia, independent of the presence of this particular symptom.

Liddle et al. [27] proposed that the disorganisation syndrome (disorders of the form of thought and innappropriate affect) is associated with a differential pattern of brain activity in frontal, temporal, and cingulate cortices relative to the two other syndromes (psychomotor poverty and reality distortion). In our sample, although we focused specifically on the symptom of FTD, it was significantly correlated with inappropriate affect, that is, patients with FTD had higher scores in innappropriate effect as well, pointing to the same direction of a distinct syndrome of disorganisation within schizophrenia.

5.3. Limitations. The sample was small, and larger studies should be done to confirm our results and possibly explain the limitations in the observed data, which might have contributed to a possible lack of power in our analyses.

6. Conclusion

The frontotemporal network normally engaged by a semantic decision task was underactivated in schizophrenia, particularly in patients with FTD. This network is implicated in the inhibition of automatically primed stimuli and impairment of its function interferes with language processing and contributes to the production of incoherent speech.

Acknowledgments

The authors are grateful for all the participants for their cooperation, particularly the patients. All authors contributed critically to paper writing. S. M. Arcuri designed and performed the experiment, recruited, interviewed, and tested participants (healthy controls and patients), analysed the data, and interpreted the results. M. R. Broome recruited patients and contributed to experiment performance. V.Giampietro and M. Brammer designed the fmri analysis software and contributed to fmri data analysis. E. Amaro Jr. contributed to experimental design and to event-related fmri expertise for data collection and analysis. T. T. J. Kircher contributed to recruitment and experiment performance in healthy control participants. S. C. R. Williams and C. M. Andrew provided input for the experimental design and fmri procedure. R. G. Morris contributed to the experimental design and offline data analysis and interpretation of results. P. K. McGuire provided critical input for testing a psychiatric population, data analysis, and interpretation. The authors thank Dr. Tamara Russell for helpful comments. This work is part of Dr Arcuri's Ph.D. scholarship CAPES (BEX 20–74/95-1) Brasilia, Brazil.

References

[1] V. Peralta and M. J. Cuesta, "Eugen bleuler and the schizophrenias: 100 Years after," *Schizophrenia Bulletin*, vol. 37, no. 6, pp. 1118–1120, 2011.

[2] S. Heckers, "Bleuler and the neurobiology of schizophrenia," *Schizophrenia Bulletin*, vol. 37, no. 6, pp. 1131–1135, 2011.

[3] M.-C. Hardy-Baylé, Y. Sarfati, and C. Passerieux, "The cognitive basis of disorganization symptomatology in Schizophrenia and its clinical correlates: toward a pathogenetic approach to disorganization," *Schizophrenia Bulletin*, vol. 29, no. 3, pp. 459–471, 2003.

[4] A. Moskowitz and G. Heim, "Eugen Bleuler's Dementia Praecox or the Group of Schizophrenias (1911): a centenary appreciation and reconsideration," *Schizophrenia Bulletin*, vol. 37, no. 3, pp. 471–479, 2011.

[5] M. Spitzer, "Associative networks, formal thought disorder and schizophrenia. On the experimental psychopathology of speech-dependent thought processes," *Nevernartz*, vol. 64, no. 3, pp. 147–159, 1993.

[6] M. J. Minzenberg, B. A. Ober, and S. Vinogradov, "Semantic priming in schizophrenia: a review and synthesis," *Journal of the International Neuropsychological Society*, vol. 8, no. 5, pp. 699–720, 2002.

[7] J. D. Ragland, R. C. Gur, J. Raz et al., "Effect of schizophrenia on frontotemporal activity during word encoding and recognition: a PET cerebral blood flow study," *American Journal of Psychiatry*, vol. 158, no. 7, pp. 1114–1125, 2001.

[8] M. Spitzer, U. Braun, L. Hermle, and S. Maier, "Associative semantic network dysfunction in thought-disordered schizophrenic patients: direct evidence from indirect semantic priming," *Biological Psychiatry*, vol. 34, no. 12, pp. 864–877, 1993.

[9] M. Spitzer, I. Weisker, M. Winter, S. Maier, L. Hermle, and B. A. Maher, "Semantic and phonological priming in schizophrenia," *Journal of Abnormal Psychology*, vol. 103, no. 3, pp. 485–494, 1994.

[10] M. Spitzer, "A cognitive neuroscience view of schizophrenic thought disorder," *Schizophrenia Bulletin*, vol. 23, no. 1, pp. 29–50, 1997.

[11] M. Kiefer and M. Spitzer, "Time course of conscious and unconscious semantic brain activation," *NeuroReport*, vol. 11, no. 11, pp. 2401–2407, 2000.

[12] M. Kiefer, U. Martens, M. Weisbrod, L. Hermle, and M. Spitzer, "Increased unconscious semantic activation in schizophrenia patients with formal thought disorder," *Schizophrenia Research*, vol. 114, no. 1–3, pp. 79–83, 2009.

[13] T. E. Goldberg, M. S. Aloia, M. L. Gourovitch, D. Missar, D. Pickar, and D. R. Weinberger, "Cognitive substrates of thought disorder, I: the semantic system," *American Journal of Psychiatry*, vol. 155, no. 12, pp. 1671–1676, 1998.

[14] J. G. Kerns and H. Berenbaum, "Cognitive impairments associated with formal thought disorder in people with schizophrenia," *Journal of Abnormal Psychology*, vol. 111, no. 2, pp. 211–224, 2002.

[15] T. H. McGlashan, "Eugen bleuler: centennial anniversary of his 1911 publication of dementia praecox or the group of

schizophrenias," *Schizophrenia Bulletin*, vol. 37, no. 6, pp. 1101–1103, 2011.

[16] G. McCarthy, A. C. Nobre, S. Bentin, and D. D. Spencer, "Language-related field potentials in the anterior-medial temporal lobe: I. Intracranial distribution and neural generators," *The Journal of Neuroscience*, vol. 15, no. 2, pp. 1080–1089, 1995.

[17] A. C. Nobre and G. McCarthy, "Language-related field potentials in the anterior-medial temporal lobe: II. Effects of word type and semantic priming," *The Journal of Neuroscience*, vol. 15, no. 2, pp. 1090–1098, 1995.

[18] P. J. Holcomb, "Semantic priming and stimulus degradation: implications for the role of the N400 in language processing," *Psychophysiology*, vol. 30, no. 1, pp. 47–61, 1993.

[19] P. F. Mitchell, S. Andrews, A. M. Fox, S. V. Catts, P. B. Ward, and N. McConaghy, "Active and passive attention in schizophrenia: an ERP study of information processing in a linguistic task," *Biological Psychology*, vol. 32, no. 2-3, pp. 101–124, 1991.

[20] M. A. Niznikiewicz, B. F. O'Donnell, P. G. Nestor et al., "ERP assessment of visual and auditory language processing in schizophrenia," *Journal of Abnormal Psychology*, vol. 106, no. 1, pp. 85–94, 1997.

[21] S. Andrews, A. M. Shelley, P. B. Ward, A. Fox, S. V. Catts, and N. McConaghy, "Event-related potential indices of semantic processing in schizophrenia," *Biological Psychiatry*, vol. 34, no. 7, pp. 443–458, 1993.

[22] J. Adams, S. F. Faux, P. G. Nestor et al., "ERP abnormalities during semantic processing in schizophrenia," *Schizophrenia Research*, vol. 10, no. 3, pp. 247–257, 1993.

[23] M. Kutas and S. A. Hillyard, "Brain potentials during reading reflect word expectancy and semantic association," *Nature*, vol. 307, no. 5947, pp. 161–163, 1984.

[24] D. Salisbury, "N400 to lexical ambiguity and semantic incongruity in schizophrenia," *International Journal of Psychophysiology*, vol. 75, no. 2, pp. 127–132, 2010.

[25] M. Kostova, C. Passerieux, J. P. Laurent, and M. C. Hardy-Baylé, "N400 anomalies in schizophrenia are correlated with the severity of formal thought disorder," *Schizophrenia Research*, vol. 78, no. 2-3, pp. 285–291, 2005.

[26] J. P. Laurent, M. Kostova, and C. Passerieux, "N400 and P300 modulation as functions of processing level in schizophrenia patients exhibiting formal thought disorder," *International Journal of Psychophysiology*, vol. 75, no. 2, pp. 177–182, 2010.

[27] P. F. Liddle, K. J. Friston, C. D. Frith, S. R. Hirsch, T. Jones, and R. S. J. Frackowiak, "Patterns of cerebral blood flow in schizophrenia," *British Journal of Psychiatry*, vol. 160, pp. 179–186, 1992.

[28] P. K. McGuire, D. J. Quested, S. A. Spence, R. M. Murray, C. D. Frith, and P. F. Liddle, "Pathophysiology of "positive" thought disorder in schizophrenia," *British Journal of Psychiatry*, vol. 173, pp. 231–235, 1998.

[29] T. T. J. Kircher, E. T. Bulimore, M. J. Brammer et al., "Differential activation of temporal cortex during sentence completion in schizophrenic patients with and without formal thought disorder," *Schizophrenia Research*, vol. 50, no. 1-2, pp. 27–40, 2001.

[30] T. T. J. Kircher, P. F. Liddle, M. J. Brammer, S. C. R. Williams, R. M. Murray, and P. K. McGuire, "Neural correlates of formal thought disorder in schizophrenia: preliminary findings from a functional magnetic resonance imaging study," *Archives of General Psychiatry*, vol. 58, no. 8, pp. 769–774, 2001.

[31] A. W. MacDonald III, C. S. Carter, J. G. Kerns et al., "Specificity of prefrontal dysfunction and context processing deficits to schizophrenia in never-medicated patients with first-episode psychosis," *American Journal of Psychiatry*, vol. 162, no. 3, pp. 475–484, 2005.

[32] I. H. Park, H. J. Park, J. W. Chun, E. Y. Kim, and J. J. Kim, "Prefrontal functional dissociation in the semantic network of patients with schizophrenia," *NeuroReport*, vol. 19, no. 14, pp. 1391–1395, 2008.

[33] M. Nakamura, P. G. Nestor, J. J. Levitt et al., "Orbitofrontal volume deficit in schizophrenia and thought disorder," *Brain*, vol. 131, no. 1, pp. 180–195, 2008.

[34] J. Sun, J. J. Maller, L. Guo, and P. B. Fitzgerald, "Superior temporal gyrus volume change in schizophrenia: a review on Region of Interest volumetric studies," *Brain Research Reviews*, vol. 61, no. 1, pp. 14–32, 2009.

[35] H. Horn, A. Federspiel, M. Wirth et al., "Structural and metabolic changes in language areas linked to formal thought disorder," *British Journal of Psychiatry*, vol. 194, no. 2, pp. 130–138, 2009.

[36] N. C. Andreasen, *Scale for the Assessment of Positive Symptoms (SAPS)*, The University of Iowa, Iowa City, Iowa, USA, 1984.

[37] C. Van Petten, "Words and sentences: event-related brain potential measures," *Psychophysiology*, vol. 32, no. 6, pp. 511–525, 1995.

[38] D. A. Nathaniel-James, P. Fletcher, and C. D. Frith, "The functional anatomy of verbal initiation and suppression using the Hayling Test," *Neuropsychologia*, vol. 35, no. 4, pp. 559–566, 1997.

[39] P. Allen, A. Mechelli, K. E. Stephan et al., "Fronto-temporal interactions during overt verbal initiation and suppression," *Journal of Cognitive Neuroscience*, vol. 20, no. 9, pp. 1656–1669, 2008.

[40] American Psychiatric Association, *Diagnostic and Statistical Manual of Mental Disorders*, American Psychiatric Association, Washington, DC, USA, 4th edition, 1994.

[41] M. Annett, "A classification of hand preference by association analysis," *The British journal of psychology*, vol. 61, no. 3, pp. 303–321, 1970.

[42] H. E. Nelson and J. R. Willison, *National Adult Reading Test (NART): Test Manual*, NFER-Nelson, Windsor, UK, 2nd edition, 1991.

[43] N. C. Andreasen, *Scale for the Assessment of Negative Symptoms (SANS)*, The University of Iowa, Iowa City, Iowa, USA, 1984.

[44] S. M. Arcuri, S. Rabe-Hesketh, R. G. Morris, and P. K. McGuire, "Regional variation of cloze probabilities for sentence contexts," *Behavior Research Methods, Instruments, and Computers*, vol. 33, no. 1, pp. 80–90, 2001.

[45] D. Norris, J. M. McQueen, and A. Cutler, "Bias effects in facilitatory phonological priming," *Memory and Cognition*, vol. 30, no. 3, pp. 399–411, 2002.

[46] S. M. Arcuri, *Neural and cognitive studies of thought disorder in schizophrenia*, Ph.D. thesis, King's College, University of London, London, UK, 2003.

[47] E. Bullmore, C. Long, J. Suckling et al., "Colored noise and computational inference in neurophysiological (fMRI) time series analysis: resampling methods in time and wavelet domains," *Human Brain Mapping*, vol. 12, no. 2, pp. 61–78, 2001.

[48] K. J. Friston, S. Williams, R. Howard, R. S. J. Frackowiak, and R. Turner, "Movement-related effects in fMRI time-series," *Magnetic Resonance in Medicine*, vol. 35, no. 3, pp. 346–355, 1996.

[49] E. Bullmore, M. Brammer, S. C. R. Williams et al., "Statistical methods of estimation and inference for functional MR image analysis," *Magnetic Resonance in Medicine*, vol. 35, no. 2, pp. 261–277, 1996.

[50] J. Talairach and P. Tournoux, *Co-Planar Stereotaxic Atlas of the Human Brain*, Thieme, New York, NY, USA, 1993.

[51] E. T. Bullmore, M. J. Brammer, S. Rabe-Hesketh et al., "Methods for diagnosis and treatment of stimulus-correlated motion in generic brain activation studies using fMRI," *Human Brain Mapping*, vol. 7, no. 1, pp. 38–48, 1999.

[52] H. Kadota, H. Sekiguchi, S. Takeuchi, M. Miyazaki, Y. Kohno, and Y. Nakajima, "The role of the dorsolateral prefrontal cortex in the inhibition of stereotyped responses," *Experimental Brain Research*, vol. 203, no. 3, pp. 593–600, 2010.

[53] J. M. Novick, I. P. Kan, J. C. Trueswell, and S. L. Thompson-Schill, "A case for conflict across multiple domains: memory and language impairments following damage to ventrolateral prefrontal cortex," *Cognitive Neuropsychology*, vol. 26, no. 6, pp. 527–567, 2009.

[54] F. Homae, R. Hashimoto, K. Nakajima, Y. Miyashita, and K. L. Sakai, "From perception to sentence comprehension: the convergence of auditory and visual information of language in the left inferior frontal cortex," *NeuroImage*, vol. 16, no. 4, pp. 883–900, 2002.

[55] J. R. Binder, R. H. Desai, W. W. Graves, and L. L. Conant, "Where is the semantic system? A critical review and meta-analysis of 120 functional neuroimaging studies," *Cerebral Cortex*, vol. 19, no. 12, pp. 2767–2796, 2009.

[56] M. Vigneau, V. Beaucousin, P. Y. Hervé et al., "Meta-analyzing left hemisphere language areas: phonology, semantics, and sentence processing," *NeuroImage*, vol. 30, no. 4, pp. 1414–1432, 2006.

[57] W. W. Graves, R. Desai, C. Humphries, M. S. Seidenberg, and J. R. Binder, "Neural systems for reading aloud: a multiparametric approach," *Cerebral Cortex*, vol. 20, no. 8, pp. 1799–1815, 2010.

[58] M. D'Esposito, B. R. Postle, and B. Rypma, "Prefrontal cortical contributions to working memory: evidence from event-related fMRI studies," *Experimental Brain Research*, vol. 133, no. 1, pp. 3–11, 2000.

[59] D. M. Barch, T. S. Braver, F. W. Sabb, and D. C. Noll, "Anterior cingulate and the monitoring of response conflict: evidence from an fMRI study of overt verb generation," *Journal of Cognitive Neuroscience*, vol. 12, no. 2, pp. 298–309, 2000.

[60] J. G. Kerns, J. D. Cohen, A. W. MacDonald III, R. Y. Cho, V. A. Stenger, and C. S. Carter, "Anterior cingulate conflict monitoring and adjustments in control," *Science*, vol. 303, no. 5660, pp. 1023–1026, 2004.

[61] P. H. Ghatan, J. C. Hsieh, K. M. Petersson, S. Stone-Elander, and M. Ingvar, "Coexistence of attention-based facilitation and inhibition in the human cortex," *NeuroImage*, vol. 7, no. 1, pp. 23–29, 1998.

[62] B. A. Kuhl, N. M. Dudukovic, I. Kahn, and A. D. Wagner, "Decreased demands on cognitive control reveal the neural processing benefits of forgetting," *Nature Neuroscience*, vol. 10, no. 7, pp. 908–914, 2007.

[63] T. T. J. Kircher, M. Brammer, N. T. Andreu, S. C. R. Williams, and P. K. McGuire, "Engagement of right temporal cortex during processing of linguistic context," *Neuropsychologia*, vol. 39, no. 8, pp. 798–809, 2001.

[64] G. I. de Zubicaray, F. O. Zelaya, C. Andrew, S. C. R. Williams, and E. T. Bullmore, "Cerebral regions associated with verbal response initiation, suppression and strategy use," *Neuropsychologia*, vol. 38, no. 9, pp. 1292–1304, 2000.

[65] A. E. Cavanna and M. R. Trimble, "The precuneus: a review of its functional anatomy and behavioural correlates," *Brain*, vol. 129, no. 3, pp. 564–583, 2006.

[66] M. Wimber, K. H. Bäuml, Z. Bergström, G. Markopoulos, H. J. Heinze, and A. Richardson-Klavehn, "Neural markers of inhibition in human memory retrieval," *The Journal of Neuroscience*, vol. 28, no. 50, pp. 13419–13427, 2008.

[67] P. Fusar-Poli, O. D. Howes, P. Allen et al., "Abnormal frontostriatal interactions in people with prodromal signs of psychosis: a multimodal imaging study," *Archives of General Psychiatry*, vol. 67, no. 7, pp. 683–691, 2010.

[68] B. A. Kuhl, I. Kahn, N. M. Dudukovic, and A. D. Wagner, "Overcoming suppression in order to remember: contributions from anterior cingulate and ventrolateral prefrontal cortex," *Cognitive, Affective and Behavioral Neuroscience*, vol. 8, no. 2, pp. 211–221, 2008.

[69] C. Metzler, "Effects of left frontal lesions on the selection of context-appropriate meanings," *Neuropsychology*, vol. 15, no. 3, pp. 315–328, 2001.

[70] P. W. Burgess and T. Shallice, "Response suppression, Initiation and strategy use following frontal lobe lesions," *Neuropsychologia*, vol. 34, no. 4, pp. 263–272, 1996.

17

Treatment Adherence with Early Prescription of Long-Acting Injectable Antipsychotics in Recent-Onset Schizophrenia

Annie Viala, Françoise Cornic, and Marie-Noëlle Vacheron

SM 13, Centre Hospitalier Sainte-Anne, 1 Rue Cabanis, 75014 Paris, France

Correspondence should be addressed to Annie Viala, a.viala@ch-sainte-anne.fr

Academic Editor: Robin A. Emsley

Although response to treatment for the first episode of schizophrenia is generally favourable, nonadherence with the treatment is the first cause of relapse and rehospitalisation within the next few years. Long-acting injectable antipsychotics (LAIAs) combine the advantages of the newer antipsychotics and the long-acting formulation. The evaluation concerns 25 schizophrenic patients hospitalised for the first time, treated with risperidone long-acting injectable (RLAI) associated with reintegration methods, and followed up for at least 18 months. Clinical observation was completed using Clinical Global Impression (CGI) scale and Global Assessment of Functioning (GAF). Clinical improvement was coupled with a good reintegration rate, very few relapse, or rehospitalisation. Bimonthly injection combined with psychosocial methods improved interactive followup, and therefore patients' compliance with the treatment. Treating with LAIA as early as possible, from the first episode if possible, can reduce relapse, number and duration of rehospitalisation, and cognitive symptoms and improve the quality of life and prognosis.

1. Introduction

Schizophrenia remains a chronic disease concerning about 1% of the general population in the world; although response to treatment in the early phases of evolution is generally favourable, it is estimated that rates of adherence to treatment 1 year after discharge from hospital are only about 50%, and 75% in the first two years of treatment [1, 2].

The causes are multifactorial: denial of disease, side effects of medication, cognitive impairment, comorbidity especially substance abuse [3] and also doctor-patient relationship [4].

Relapses and rehospitalisations worsen the prognosis of patients with schizophrenia, impact both patients and families'insertion and quality of life, and increase direct and indirect health costs [5, 6]. Treatment with LAIAs, which encourage adherence (fewer side-effects, stabilization of drug levels), can prevent the risk of interruption of treatment which is the main cause of relapse and rehospitalisation. This type of treatment, used as early as possible, since first-episode schizophrenia, may improve the long-term prognosis [7], particularly when associated with reintegration methods [8] and interactive followup using interest of monthly or bimonthly injection.

The aim of our study is to present the followup in "real life" of 25 patients, hospitalised for the first time, treated with RLAI associated with reintegration methods and multidisciplinary followup, for at least 18 months, in order to evaluate the impact: 1/on relapse and rehospitalisation rate; 2/on treatment adherence.

2. Materials and Methods

2.1. Study Design. The data presented here derive from a naturalistic prospective study of 120 patients treated with Risperidone Long Acting Injectable (RLAI) which was currently the only atypical long-acting injectable antipsychotic available at that time in France, associated with rehabilitation methods, and followed up for at least 18 months [9]: among them, 25 patients were hospitalised for the first time, and therefore younger in age and illness duration.

It was an epidemiological, observational, noninterventional study in usual-care settings, in which patients were treated with flexible dose of RLAI, without randomization nor controlled trial. All patients were aware of the aim of the study and had given oral informed consent.

The aim of our study was to investigate the outcome of the illness according to a better compliance with RLAI integrated in a psychosocial treatment programme, notably the number and duration of hospitalisations, and also the possibility of familial and socioprofessional reintegration.

2.2. Inclusion and Exclusion Criteria. All patients were men or women of minimally 18 years of age, recruited consecutively in the same catchman urban area corresponding to their district of psychiatric healthcare in Paris (all of them were residents of the 14th district of Paris). All of them were psychotics according to DSM IVR criteria for schizophrenia [10].

Exclusion criteria were serious medical condition, history of malignant syndrome, pregnant or breast-feeding female, history of clozapine treatment, known allergies, hypersensitivity or intolerance to risperidone, and patients who had not given informed consent.

2.3. Assessments. Patients were assessed at baseline and after 6, 12, and 18 months for adherence, efficacy, RLAI dosage, number and duration of hospitalisation, social functionality, and reintegration (work, studies, apartment).

Clinical observation was completed using Clinical Global Impression scale (CGI) [11] representative of clinical improvement, and Global Assessment of Functioning (GAF) [12] representative of functional improvement, whose results are statistically significant.

2.4. Treatment. All patients were treated with risperidone per os, with doses ranging from 4 mg to 8 mg before changing to RLAI. The first injection was given prior to discharge, and the oral treatment was continued for 3 or 4 weeks.

The following injections were given at the out-patient center, or in the hospital depending on where each patient was consulted, and on their need to maintain a more controlled therapeutic regimen. The nurses supervised administration of the treatment and could call them when they missed time of injection. The starting dose was calculated according to the patient's acute state and comorbidity, especially substance abuse (alcohol, cannabis). The initially prescribed dosage changed over time, according to the evolution, and to the physician.

2.5. Reintegration Measures. Day hospital, part-time therapy center, sheltered housing, protected employment center, and also dietetic education, physical exercise were used; each patient was cared for by two nurses and a social worker; these measures were adapted to each patient's needs, using bimonthly injection to consult their physician and/or a nurse.

2.6. Statistical Analyses. Descriptive statistics (mean standard deviation) were generated for quantitative data for all patients. For statistical analysis of the CGI and GAF data, subgroups were created with those patients who completed the survey after 18 months. Statistical analysis of hospitalisation data was performed for the subgroup of patients who had received treatment during the preceding 18 months, who completed the 18-month followup, and who had at least one hospitalisation during these two time periods. Quantitative data was first tested for normality using the Kolmogorov-Smirnov test, followed by analysis for statistical significance using either the Wilcoxon signed rank test or the paired Student's t-test, as applicable. Qualitative data was subjected to McNemar's test. Bowker's test for symmetry was used to analyse dosage change over time.

3. Results

3.1. Sociodemographic Data and Clinical Characteristics. The patient population comprised 14 men and 11 women, the mean age was 30,08 ± 7,54 years, the mean duration of illness 6,84 ± 5,45 years; all of them were hospitalised for the first time, in acute or very acute state (positive symptoms: 20 patients, negative symptoms: 5 patients); the most common diagnosis was paranoid schizophrenia (13 patients), followed by schizoaffective disorder (5 patients), disorganised schizophrenia (3 patients), undifferentiated schizophrenia (2 patients), and acute psychotic disorder (2 patients).

3.2. Previous Treatment. 17 of 25 patients (64%) were not taking any treatment before being hospitalized; only 3 of them were naïve of all treatments. 8 of 25 were treated with Olanzapine (4 patients), Haloperidol (3 patients), Pipotiazine (1 patient).

None of them had previously received Risperidone.

Reasons for prescription were lack of efficacy or compliance (16 patients), lack of tolerability (2 patients), prescriber's choice (4 patients), and comorbidity such as substance abuse.

3.3. Dosage, Tolerability, Discontinuation Rate. RLAI dosage changed over time: 24 received a starting dosage of 50 mg, according to their very acute state and coexisting alcohol dependence and substance abuse (especially cannabis use), and also our normal clinical practice; 1 received a starting dose of 37,5 mg. The dosage has been decreased during the course of the survey. Most patients (16 patients) went on 50 mg, some of them went on 37,5 mg or 25 mg, 5 of them were treated with 25 mg at M18, end of our study.

Five patients interrupted their treatment (including 3 quickly after initiation) because of illness denial, weight gain, or partial efficacy.

3.4. Socioprofessional Evolution. After RLAI instauration, 19 patients could live in their own apartment, 1 in sheltered housing; 11 could restart work or find a job (100%: 5 patients, 50%: 4 patients, professional training: 2 patients), 3 patients could restart studies. Other patients had activities in day hospital or part-time therapy center, some of them needing some more time to attend a protected employment center. All of them improved their quality of life over time, with more possibilities to meet friends and family, to live a more stable and independent life, outside the psychiatric hospital.

3.5. Clinical Efficacy CGI. Evolution of the CGI score is representative of clinical improvement: the level of severity of the illness (CGI-S) decreased from 5.44 (range 4–6, SD $\pm$ 0.58) on day 0 to 3.14 (range 1–5, SD $\pm$ 1.21) at M18. This result is statistically significant ($P < 0.0001$). CGI-I score showed that at M18, 3 patients were very greatly improved, 3 greatly improved, and 1 slightly improved.

3.6. Functional Improvement GAF. Evolution on the GAF scale is representative of functional improvement: the score increased from 36.16 (range 11–70, SD $\pm$ 13.55) on day 0 to 75.71 (range 65–85, SD $\pm$ 7.32) at M18. This result is statistically significant ($P < 0.0001$). The largest improvement was observed during the first 6 months of treatment, during which the mean GAF score increased by 20 and then more slowly until M18.

3.7. Hospitalisation Rate and Duration. Only 4 patients relapsed (16%), and only once: 3 patients between D0 and M6 (mean duration of hospitalisation: 21 days), and 1 during M6 and M12 (mean duration of hospitalisation: 7 days); no patient relapsed between M12 and M18. These results, when compared with the whole cohort's results, show that fewer patients were hospitalised after RLAI therapy, with a short duration of hospitalisation. We cannot compare with their own rate of hospitalisation, because it is their first hospitalisation, but we can notice that their rate of hospitalisation is better when compared with those who had already been treated and hospitalised in the whole cohort (37% for the whole cohort versus 16% for the 25 recent onset patients).

4. Discussion

These results compared with those of the whole cohort (120 patients) are very consistent and very close to them: marked improvements in CGI and GAF scores, reduced rates and durations of hospitalisation. They are globally better, and we think that is due to the recent onset in this population (patients younger in age and duration of illness) and they convince us to begin RLAI treatment as soon as possible (CGI improvement from 5,6 to 3,6 for the whole cohort versus 5,4 to 3,1 for 25 recent onset patients; GAF improvement from 34,1 to 67,5 for the whole cohort versus 36,1 to 75,7 for the 25 recent onset patients).

We currently used starting dosage of 50 mg, according to the very acute state and comorbidity (especially alcohol and cannabis use) of our patients, but also to our normal clinical practice in front of this "very difficult-to-treat-population," considering underdosing can contribute discontinuation when patients are severely ill [13, 14], and also lower plasma levels of Risperidone and 9OH risperidone at the beginning of the treatment [15, 16]

Clinical benefits may be linked with psychosocial programme associated with RLAI treatment from the beginning of the treatment, and multidisciplinary long-term followup (18 months in our study) in order to improve adherence with the medication.

Treatment plan including early warning signs developed for each patient, based on psychoeducation programme, family involvement in order to acquire and improve insight are regularly emphazised [1, 17–19].

Interest in functional outcome is based on subjective satisfaction with life, occupational and social functioning [18, 20], less and shorter inpatient stays, less long-term institutionalization, solitary living, and dependence on disability pension; greater frequency of outpatient visits, better information, improved access to supported employment, and rehabilitation should help the patients to agree with LAIA formulation [21, 22].

The importance of early intervention in schizophrenia treatment [23, 24] is based on acute clinical symptomatology (often positive symptoms), high risk of non- and partial adherence, risk of accruing morbidity and persistent deficits [25], and also high sensitivity to antipsychotics.

Treating as early as possible, from the first episode if possible, can reduce relapse, number and duration of hospitalisation, and also cognitive symptoms, illness worsening and suicide attempts [26], and thus improving the prognosis, and also direct and indirect cost [27–30].

Long-acting injectable antipsychotics combine the advantages of both the newer antipsychotics (efficacy, fewer extrapyramidal symptoms) and the long-acting formulation [31, 32]; they can reduce relapse through the increased medication adherence in patients with schizophrenia [33] and lower fluctuations in plasma concentrations.

Although response to treatment for the initial psychotic episode is generally favourable, most patients are unable to maintain this improvement [25, 34, 35]; poor adherence may be particularly common after a first episode of schizophrenia and may occur very early [22]: according to Coldham et al., 39% are not adherent and 20% inadequately adherent in the first year of treatment; non-adherence with medication is the first cause of relapse, it could be one of the most preventable, but it stays one of the most difficult to solve [1].

According to the neurodegenerative theory, relapse and recurrences make brain structures more neurotoxic: ventricular enlargement, cortical atrophy in brain, longer duration of illness, less effectiveness of the medication, deficient cognitive function, and prominent negative symptoms [23, 36].

Relapse predictors include medication discontinuation as a high risk [34]; relapse prevention is a major objective, and long-term treatment is indicated [37]. In recent publications concerning patients in the early phase of schizophrenia, two potentially risk factors for rehospitalisation are confirmed: short duration of first hospitalisation (shorter than two weeks) and early nonadherence to medication [38], even though periods of nonadherence are brief [35].

Long-acting injectable antipsychotics should not be considered by psychiatrists as a last resort in persistently ill patients; some recent studies show that patients, especially young patients, with a good insight, and sometimes a high study level, when informed on long-acting formulation, agree with them and prefer to receive their medication via a long-acting formulation rather than in tablet form [39, 40].

Psychiatrists' attitude towards LAIA should evolve [4, 41]. They should be recommended as a part of an integrated treatment plan, including multidisciplinary followup and treatment teams administering and supervising the medication [21], using interest of monthly or bimonthly injection in order not to forget treatment, and also to improving more frequent and regular contact between patients and healthcare professionals, interactive followup with nurse, psychiatrist, and also peers [14, 42].

A number of studies and pharmacoeconomic models have demonstrated that long-acting risperidone decreases direct healthcare costs largely by reducing the rates of relapse and hospitalisation [5, 43].

Relapse and hospitalisations are costly: direct medical costs in healthcare, indirect costs on the basis of productive activity (for the patient and family) [6, 29]. Even though adherence interventions in psychotic disorders have produced mixed results, possible cost benefits for the society and prevention of hospitalisation are necessary for patients [44] and a challenge for public health.

Limitations. No randomization, nor comparative group, the small number of patients are limitations to our study. However, results are encouraging when compared with those of the whole cohort, and the recent publications of the literature. They will need further investigations.

5. Conclusion

The treatment of schizophrenia is an ongoing challenge in psychiatry. The literature on long-acting injectable antipsychotics for early-phase schizophrenia, first episode, or recent onset, is limited, there are very few long-term data and guidelines are not yet available [38, 45, 46].

Using injectable long-acting antipsychotics as initial therapeutic treatment can reduce relapse rate and improve the prognosis and should be maintained in the long-term treatment of schizophrenia, using interactive, interdisciplinary followup, corresponding with psychosocial biological continuum, in order to progress from compliance to adherence: working with family and caregivers, information about the illness and its treatment, psychoeducation, bimonthly injection combined with nurse and psychiatrist assessment, telephone call and home visit when patient is late, and reintegration programme (housing, work, studies) may improve adherence and outcomes in these patients. An additional pertinent function is motivational enhancement fostering compliance and active participation in schizophrenia treatment plans for patients, relatives, and psychiatrists.

References

[1] E. L. Coldham, J. Addington, and D. Addington, "Medication adherence of individuals with a first episode of psychosis," *Acta Psychiatrica Scandinavica*, vol. 106, no. 4, pp. 286–290, 2002.

[2] S. J. Keith and J. M. Kane, "Partial compliance and patient consequences in schizophrenia: our patients can do better," *Journal of Clinical Psychiatry*, vol. 64, no. 11, pp. 1308–1315, 2003.

[3] D. G. Robinson, M. G. Woerner, J. M. J. Alvir, R. M. Bilder, G. A. Hinrichsen, and J. A. Lieberman, "Predictors of medication discontinuation by patients with first-episode schizophrenia and schizoaffective disorder," *Schizophrenia Research*, vol. 57, no. 2-3, pp. 209–219, 2002.

[4] S. Heres, T. Reichhart, J. Hamann, R. Mendel, S. Leucht, and W. Kissling, "Psychiatrists' attitude to antipsychotic depot treatment in patients with first-episode schizophrenia," *European Psychiatry*, vol. 26, no. 5, pp. 297–301, 2010.

[5] M. Knapp, R. Mangalore, and J. Simon, "The global costs of Schizophrenia," *Schizophrenia Bulletin*, vol. 30, no. 2, pp. 279–293, 2004.

[6] M. Knapp, "Costs of schizophrenia," *Psychiatry*, vol. 4, no. 10, pp. 33–35, 2005.

[7] R. Emsley, P. Oosthuizen, L. Koen, D. J. H. Niehaus, R. Medori, and J. Rabinowitz, "Oral versus injectable antipsychotic treatment in early psychosis: post hoc comparison of two studies," *Clinical Therapeutics*, vol. 30, no. 12, pp. 2378–2386, 2008.

[8] J. A. Lieberman, T. Scott Stroup, J. P. McEvoy et al., "Effectiveness of antipsychotic drugs in patients with chronic schizophrenia," *New England Journal of Medicine*, vol. 353, no. 12, pp. 1209–1223, 2005.

[9] A. Viala, F. Cornic, C. Benamor et al., "A descriptive, open-label, long-term follow-up survey of psychotic patients receiving risperidone long-acting injectable: preliminary results," *International Journal of Psychiatry in Clinical Practice*, vol. 13, no. 2, pp. 138–146, 2009.

[10] DSM-IVR, *Diagnostic and Statistical Manual of Mental Disorders*, American Psychiatric Association, Washington, DC, USA, 4th edition, 2000.

[11] W. Guy, *ECDEU Assessment Manual for Psychopharmacology, Revised*, US Department of Health, Education and Welfare, Washington DC, Publication ADM 76-338, 1976.

[12] J. Endicott, R. L. Spitzer, J. L. Fleiss, and J. Cohen, "The global assessment scale. A procedure for measuring overall severity of psychiatric disturbance," *Archives of General Psychiatry*, vol. 33, no. 6, pp. 766–771, 1976.

[13] C. L. Young and D. M. Taylor, "Health resource utilization associated with switching to risperidone long-acting injection," *Acta Psychiatrica Scandinavica*, vol. 114, no. 1, pp. 14–20, 2006.

[14] S. Keith, "Use of long-acting risperidone in psychiatric disorders: focus on efficacy, safety and cost-effectiveness," *Expert Review of Neurotherapeutics*, vol. 9, no. 1, pp. 9–31, 2009.

[15] R. Nesvåg, M. Hendset, H. Refsum, and L. Tanum, "Serum concentrations of risperidone and 9-OH risperidone following intramuscular injection of long-acting risperidone compared with oral risperidone medication," *Acta Psychiatrica Scandinavica*, vol. 114, no. 1, pp. 21–26, 2006.

[16] G. M. Simpson, R. A. Mahmoud, R. A. Lasser et al., "A 1-year double-blind study of 2 doses of long-acting risperidone in stable patients with schizophrenia or schizoaffective disorder," *Journal of Clinical Psychiatry*, vol. 67, no. 8, pp. 1194–1203, 2006.

[17] A. Zygmunt, M. Olfson, C. A. Boyer, and D. Mechanic, "Interventions to improve medication adherence in schizophrenia," *American Journal of Psychiatry*, vol. 159, no. 10, pp. 1653–1664, 2002.

[18] M. A. Turner, J. M. Boden, C. Smith-Hamel, and R. T. Mulder, "Outcomes for 236 patients from a 2-year early intervention

in psychosis service," *Acta Psychiatrica Scandinavica*, vol. 120, no. 2, pp. 129–137, 2009.

[19] P. J. Weiden, N. R. Schooler, J. C. Weedon, A. Elmouchtari, A. Sunakawa, and S. M. Goldfinger, "A randomized controlled trial of long-acting injectable risperidone vs continuation on oral atypical antipsychotics for first-episode schizophrenia patients: initial adherence outcome," *Journal of Clinical Psychiatry*, vol. 70, no. 10, pp. 1397–1406, 2009.

[20] R. Bodén, J. Sundström, E. Lindström, and L. Lindström, "Association between symptomatic remission and functional outcome in first-episode schizophrenia," *Schizophrenia Research*, vol. 107, no. 2-3, pp. 232–237, 2009.

[21] J. Nielsen, P. Le Quach, C. Emborg, L. Foldager, and C. U. Correll, "10-Year trends in the treatment and outcomes of patients with first-episode schizophrenia," *Acta Psychiatrica Scandinavica*, vol. 122, no. 5, pp. 356–366, 2010.

[22] J. Tiihonen, J. Haukka, M. Taylor, P. M. Haddad, M. X. Patel, and P. Korhonen, "A nationwide cohort study of oral and depot antipsychotics after first hospitalization for schizophrenia," *American Journal of Psychiatry*, vol. 168, no. 6, pp. 603–609, 2011.

[23] B. Kim, S. H. Lee, T. K. Choi et al., "Effectiveness of risperidone long-acting injection in first-episode schizophrenia: in naturalistic setting," *Progress in Neuro-Psychopharmacology and Biological Psychiatry*, vol. 32, no. 5, pp. 1231–1235, 2008.

[24] R. Emsley, R. Medori, L. Koen, P. P. Oosthuizen, D. J. H. Niehaus, and J. Rabinowitz, "Long-acting injectable risperidone in the treatment of subjects with recent-onset psychosis: a preliminary study," *Journal of Clinical Psychopharmacology*, vol. 28, no. 2, pp. 210–213, 2008.

[25] R. Emsley, P. Oosthuizen, L. Koen, D. J. H. Niehaus, R. Medori, and J. Rabinowitz, "Remission in patients with first-episode schizophrenia receiving assured antipsychotic medication: a study with risperidone long-acting injection," *International Clinical Psychopharmacology*, vol. 23, no. 6, pp. 325–331, 2008.

[26] M. Pompili, G. Serafini, M. Innamorati et al., "Suicide risk in first episode psychosis: a selective review of the current literature," *Schizophrenia Research*, vol. 129, no. 1, pp. 1–11, 2011.

[27] S. Almond, M. Knapp, C. Francois, M. Toumi, and T. Brugha, "Relapse in schizophrenia: costs, clinical outcomes and quality of life," *British Journal of Psychiatry*, vol. 184, pp. 346–351, 2004.

[28] P. M. Llorca, H. Miadi-Fargier, C. Lançon et al., "Cost-effectiveness analysis of schizophrenic patient care settings: impact of an atypical antipsychotic under long-acting injection formulation," *Encephale*, vol. 31, no. 2, pp. 235–246, 2005.

[29] H. Ascher-Svanum, B. Zhu, D. E. Faries et al., "The cost of relapse and the predictors of relapse in the treatment of schizophrenia," *BMC Psychiatry*, vol. 10, article no. 2, 2010.

[30] C. Mihalopoulos, M. Harris, L. Henry, S. Harrigan, and P. McGorry, "Is early intervention in psychosis cost-effective over the long term?" *Schizophrenia Bulletin*, vol. 35, no. 5, pp. 909–918, 2009.

[31] J. M. Kane, "Strategies for improving compliance in treatment of Schizophrenia by using a long-acting formulation of an antipsychotic: clinical studies," *Journal of Clinical Psychiatry*, vol. 64, no. 16, pp. 34–40, 2003.

[32] E. Parellada, R. Andrezina, V. Milanova et al., "Patients in the early phases of schizophrenia and schizoaffective disorders effectively treated with risperidone long-acting injectable," *Journal of Psychopharmacology*, vol. 19, no. 5, pp. 5–14, 2005.

[33] J. M. Kane, "Review of treatments that can ameliorate non-adherence in patients with schizophrenia," *Journal of Clinical Psychiatry*, vol. 67, no. 5, pp. 9–14, 2006.

[34] D. G. Robinson, M. G. Woerner, J. M. J. Alvir et al., "Predictors of treatment response from a first episode of schizophrenia or schizoaffective disorder," *American Journal of Psychiatry*, vol. 156, no. 4, pp. 544–549, 1999.

[35] K. L. Subotnik, K. H. Nuechterlein, J. Ventura et al., "Risperidone nonadherence and return of positive symptoms in the early course of schizophrenia," *American Journal of Psychiatry*, vol. 168, no. 3, pp. 286–292, 2011.

[36] J. A. Lieberman, "Pathophysiologic mechanisms in the pathogenesis and clinical course of schizophrenia," *Journal of Clinical Psychiatry*, vol. 60, no. 12, pp. 9–12, 1999.

[37] W. Gaebel and M. Riesbeck, "Revisiting the relapse predictive validity of prodromal symptoms in schizophrenia," *Schizophrenia Research*, vol. 95, no. 1–3, pp. 19–29, 2007.

[38] R. Bodén, L. Brandt, H. Kieler, M. Andersen, and J. Reutfors, "Early non-adherence to medication and other risk factors for rehospitalization in schizophrenia and schizoaffective disorder," *Schizophrenia Research*, vol. 133, no. 1–3, pp. 36–41, 2011.

[39] M. X. Patel and A. S. David, "Why aren't depot antipsychotics prescribed more often and what can be done about it?" *Advances in Psychiatric Treatment*, vol. 11, no. 3, pp. 203–213, 2005.

[40] J. Walburn, R. Gray, K. Gournay, S. Quraishi, and A. S. David, "Systematic review of patient and nurse attitudes to depot antipsychotic medication," *British Journal of Psychiatry*, vol. 179, pp. 300–307, 2001.

[41] J. Palazzolo, "Medical compliance and relapses in schizophrenia: from classical neuroleptics to APAP," *Annales Medico-Psychologiques*, vol. 167, no. 4, pp. 308–317, 2009.

[42] M. Jaeger and W. Rossler, "Attitudes towards long-acting depot antipsychotics: a survey of patients, relatives and psychiatrists," *Psychiatry Research*, vol. 175, no. 1-2, pp. 58–62, 2010.

[43] H. A. Nasrallah, "The case for long-acting antipsychotic agents in the post-CATIE era," *Acta Psychiatrica Scandinavica*, vol. 115, no. 4, pp. 260–267, 2007.

[44] J. Gilden, A. B.P. Staring, M. V. der Gaag, and C. L. Mulder, "Does Treatment Adherence Therapy reduce expense of healthcare use in patients with psychotic disorders? Cost-minimization analysis in a randomized controlled trial," *Schizophrenia Research*, vol. 133, no. 1–3, pp. 47–53, 2011.

[45] J. M. Kane and C. Garcia-Ribera, "Clinical guideline recommendations for antipsychotic long-acting injections," *British Journal of Psychiatry*, vol. 195, no. 52, pp. s63–s67, 2009.

[46] E. Stip, A. Abdel-Baki, D. Bloom, S. Grignon, and M.-A. Roy, "Long-acting injectable antipsychotics: an expert opinion from the Association des médecins psychiatres du Québec," *Canadian Journal of Psychiatry*, vol. 56, no. 6, pp. 367–376, 2011.

18

Weight Gain, Schizophrenia and Antipsychotics: New Findings from Animal Model and Pharmacogenomic Studies

Fabio Panariello,[1] Vincenzo De Luca,[1] and Andrea de Bartolomeis[2]

[1] *Department of Psychiatry, Centre for Addiction and Mental Health, University of Toronto, 250 College Street, Room 30, Toronto, ON, Canada M5T 1R8*
[2] *Dipartimento di Neuroscienze, Sezione di Psichiatria, Laboratorio di Psichiatria Molecolare, University of Napoli "Federico II", Via Pansini 5, 80131 Napoli, Italy*

Correspondence should be addressed to Fabio Panariello, fabiomdphd@gmail.com

Academic Editor: Nakao Iwata

Excess body weight is one of the most common physical health problems among patients with schizophrenia that increases the risk for many medical problems, including type 2 diabetes mellitus, coronary heart disease, osteoarthritis, and hypertension, and accounts in part for 20% shorter life expectancy than in general population. Among patients with severe mental illness, obesity can be attributed to an unhealthy lifestyle, personal genetic profile, as well as the effects of psychotropic medications, above all antipsychotic drugs. Novel "atypical" antipsychotic drugs represent a substantial improvement on older "typical" drugs. However, clinical experience has shown that some, but not all, of these drugs can induce substantial weight gain. Animal models of antipsychotic-related weight gain and animal transgenic models of knockout or overexpressed genes of antipsychotic receptors have been largely evaluated by scientific community for changes in obesity-related gene expression or phenotypes. Moreover, pharmacogenomic approaches have allowed to detect more than 300 possible candidate genes for antipsychotics-induced body weight gain. In this paper, we summarize current thinking on: (1) the role of polymorphisms in several candidate genes, (2) the possible roles of various neurotransmitters and neuropeptides in this adverse drug reaction, and (3) the state of development of animal models in this matter. We also outline major areas for future research.

1. Introduction

Schizophrenia is a chronic disabling mental illness that affects millions of people worldwide [1]. People with schizophrenia suffer increased rates of multiple medical problems [2–5]. Among these issues, weight gain is a common problem, and some epidemiologic data suggest that patients with mental illnesses are at greater risk of developing obesity estimated to be about 2 times more common in patients with schizophrenia (especially women) than the general population [6]. This is due to their life style inherent neglect of personal care (smoking behavior, high-fat diet), barriers to treatment of physical illness, side effects profile of antipsychotic medications, and genetic influences. Thus, it represents a notable example of genetic/environment interaction, but the extent of the involvement of each factor is unclear. Antipsychotic medications have been associated with considerable weight gain, but the mechanisms by which they increase weight and produce metabolic disturbances are not known [7–10]. Normal subjects have a BMI between 18.5 and 24.9 kg/m^2. Subjects with a BMI from 25 to 29.9 kg/m^2 are classified as overweight and from 30 to 39.9 kg/m^2 as obese. Patients with a BMI above 40 kg/m^2 are classified as extremely obese [11]. The importance of this side effect clearly arises from the following considerations: (1) a significant increase in weight gain may affect the compliance to pharmacotherapy, because it may add to the schizophrenia stigma the stigma of obesity and be indirectly responsible for psychosis relapses; (2) weight gain may increase the risk for diabetes type II; (3) weight gain can be associated with the metabolic syndrome, a very severe condition that has serious implications for overall health and survival due to an increased risk for cardiovascular and malignant disorders. Although clozapine and olanzapine are the second generation antipsychotics (SGAs) most frequently associated with weight gain, all of the antipsychotic agents seem to share this effect as a group to varying degrees that may be because each drug exerts different degree of action on the serotonergic, dopaminergic, cholinergic, histaminergic, and other neurotransmitter systems [12]. Several lines of evidence suggest that aripiprazole and ziprasidone are associated with the lowest weight gain risk [7]. SGAs have been considered for a very long time to be related to tremendous weight gain compared with first-generation antipsychotics (FGAs). Nevertheless, some studies have shown similar weight gain between these 2 groups of treatment. Among first-generation neuroleptics, low-potency fenotiazines may have grater liability for weight gain than butyrrophenones. Molindone and pimozide have been associated with loss of weight in short-term studies, even if the available data are in some way contrasting [8]. The significance of weight gain as relevant side effect of antipsychotics treatment, that can cause the lack of adherence in drug assumption, has been recently discussed by the authors of the Catie study. The rate of discontinuation due to weight gain or metabolic changes was more than twice as great for olanzapine as for the other study medications (9% versus 1% to 4%) [13]. Olanzapine caused significantly more weight gain than any of the other medicines, even after adjustment for duration of treatment [13]. Despite the growing literature on the clinical impact of weight gain and diabetes in schizophrenia during antipsychotics therapy, and the increasing number of pharmacogenetics studies targeting SNPs (single-nucleotide polymorphisms) [14–17] of candidate genes, few reports are focused, at preclinical level, on the potential molecular mechanisms that may be responsible or substantially contribute or can be correlated robustly to this crucial health issue in schizophrenia treatment. It should be recognized that a major problem in preclinical studies is the difficulty in inducing weight gain reliably in animal paradigm of chronic antipsychotics administration [18]. The major problems in that regard are that female, but not male, rodents appear to be sensitive to the weight-promoting effects of antipsychotics. In fact, after chronic antipsychotic treatments, female mice and rats [19–25] increase their weight. On the contrary in male rats, any weight changes are not observed [24, 26, 27]. Besides, weight gain in female rats seems to result from hyperphagia, while males do not change their food intake [19, 27]. It is a hypothesis that these differences in weight and food intake in female rats from males were due to different expressed hormones [28, 29]. These observations do not match the clinical situation in humans in which there are no differences in antipsychotics-induced weight gain and food intake in both males and females [8, 29]. It is even more surprising that compared to the major side effects of first-generation antipsychotics, that is, extrapiramidal movements and specially parkinsonism, no specific neurotransmitter, receptor, or transduction system has been significantly tracked down as the major responsible factor of antipsychotics-induced increase in weight, even after more than twenty years since the introduction in therapy of the first atypical antipsychotic drug, clozapine. The relationship between the occupancy of some receptors, claimed to be relevant for this side effect, and the real-world clinical evidence is still lacking of a clear demonstration and need to be explored more on both a preclinical and clinical level. However, continuing in the similitude, it needs to be acknowledged that also with the typicals, preferentially dopamine D2 blocking agents, there is an important movement disorder that has not been fully explained yet in molecular terms: tardive dyskinesia. Understanding the mechanism(s) related to the weight gain may require recognizing the following issues.

(1) It is important to underline that the molecular mechanism(s) responsible for weight gain could be unrelated to the molecular mechanisms of the antipsychotic action, but that cannot be completely ruled out that the two mechanisms may partially overlap. The recent discovery of significant interaction between orexin [30], a key molecule in food intake control, and dopamine indicate that the above-mentioned overlap is possible.

(2) Any step of the signal transduction pathway that is initiated by antipsychotic-receptor interaction is, at least potentially, a candidate target of the molecular mechanism responsible for the weight gain.

(3) Transcription factors are the amplifiers and regulators of the signal triggered by receptor activation, and it should be of great interest to explore those transcription factors that are related in the CNS with weight gain mechanism control [31].

(4) The receptor-binding profile of typical and atypical antipsychotics may predict, theoretically, the liability for weight gain; however, the real-world outcome may not confirm in straightforward manner the prediction. On the other side, receptors may be involved in the mechanism of weight gain even if they are not included in the receptor-binding profile of an antipsychotic compound. For instance, olanzapine may indirectly affect certain functions mediated by beta-adrenergic receptors even if has not a significant affinity for any of the beta-receptor subtypes [32].

(5) The dissection between central and peripheral mechanisms responsible of antipsychotics weight gain should also be considered.

(6) It should be acknowledged that the link between weight gain, metabolic syndrome, diabetes type II, and dyslipidemia is a complex matter, and it is conceivable that probably multiple mechanisms should be taken into account and that the weight gain-inducing mechanism may follow [33]. Also, it should be clearly noted that many statements regarding the mechanism of weight gain induced by atypical antipsychotics are surprisingly lacking robust and consistent experimental replication and should be cautiously translated to clinical practice.

2. Atypical Antipsychotics Receptor Profile and Weight Gain

Even if any step of the signal transduction pathway activated (or inhibited) by antipsychotics can be regarded as potential target responsible for the weight gain liability of these compounds, the interaction with membrane receptors is, probably, the first, functional relevant, step in their cellular and molecular mechanism that gives the right of clinical properties and profile of side effects. It should be acknowledged that trying to match receptor profile and compare the receptor-binding properties of each compound with weight gain liability is not a straightforward task. Several, probably too many, receptors have been considered putative candidates for the weight gain-inducing effect of atypical antipsychotics: among the others 5HT2cR, 5HT3R α2R, H1R, and β3R. It should not be forgotten that the involvement of membrane receptor in weight gain antipsychotics liability must include also those receptors that may modulate energy expenditure, and this makes the effort to track down the potential mechanisms even more difficult. Finally, it is a more realistic approach to consider that the weight gain side effects may be the result of the combined action of a certain antipsychotic compound on multiple receptors [34]. Despite these difficulties, the antipsychotics receptor profile may represent the most direct mechanistic connection between antipsychotic molecular effects and antipsychotics-induced weight gain. Typical antipsychotics are universally characterized by their antagonistic effect and high affinity for dopamine receptors, particularly D2 receptors [35]. Dopamine antagonism is believed to be the mechanism of these agents' ability to reduce positive symptoms of schizophrenia as well as their tendency to produce EPS [36]. Atypical antipsychotics, in contrast, are antagonists for both serotonin (5-hydroxytryptamine, 5-HT) and dopamine receptors. In general, atypical agents have an enhanced 5-HT2A/D2 affinity ratio and that helps explain why typical and atypical agents may have different clinical effects [37, 38]. The atypical antipsychotics generally have additional affinities for a variety of neurotransmitter receptor subtypes [39]. This complex pharmacology leads to interactions of varying intensity with numerous serotonergic, dopaminergic, histaminergic, adrenergic, and muscarinic acetylcholine receptors. In addition to having distinct binding profiles, some atypical antipsychotics have a unique effect on neurotransmitter receptor activity [40, 41]. While most parts of antipsychotics are dopamine antagonists that block dopaminergic systems throughout the brain, some newer agents, such as aripiprazole [42] and bifeprunox [43], act as partial dopamine agonists. Certain atypical antipsychotics also act as partial agonists at other sites in addition to dopamine receptor sites. Aripiprazole, ziprasidone, and bifeprunox, for example, each display partial agonism at 5-HT1A [44–46] receptors, and clozapine acts as a partial agonist at M1, M2, and M4 muscarinic receptors and an antagonist of M3 and M5 [47]. Similarly, different findings suggest that N-desmethylclozapine, the major active metabolite of clozapine, acts as a partial agonist at M5, a full agonist at M1, and an antagonist at M3 receptors [47].

3. Serotonin Signaling

The serotonin system has been regarded for long time as a chief player among neurotransmitters involved in food intake regulation, so it is not surprising that it has been also under scrutiny in the search for molecular mechanism responsible of antipsychotics weight gain considering also that second-generation antipsychotics differ substantially in serotonin receptor occupancy compared to first generation ones. 5-HT is a potent satiety signal; administration of 5-HT to rodents decreases food intake [48]. Agonists at the 5-HT1A and 5-HT2C receptors have opposing effects on food intake: 5-HT1A agonists increase food intake [49] and 5-HT2C agonists decrease it as well [50]. 5-HT2C antagonists have been shown to increase food intake [51] and also attenuate the decrease in food intake which is produced by 5-HT2C agonists [52–54] or sibutramine, a 5-HT and noradrenaline reuptake inhibitor [55]. Knockout of the 5-HT2C receptor in mice can result in obesity and increased feeding [56]. Thus, the 5HT2C, 5HT3, and 5HT1A are the receptors with the most elevated probability to be involved in the induction of weight gain based on their physiological characteristics. The most studied receptor is 5-HT2C. What is surprising, however, is that the correlation between some of these receptors and weight gain is all but straightforward when different new generations of antipsychotics are compared to each other. Ziprasidone for example is an antagonist at the 5HT2C receptor, but there are no demonstrated clinical evidence for its weight-gain liability. Different findings suggest that serotonin also regulate NPY, one of the most abundant neuropeptides in the brain with high levels in several brain areas [57]. The 5-HT1B/2C agonist mCPP produced decreases in food intake, maybe through the reduction in NPY levels in the paraventricular nucleus (PVN) of the hypothalamus [58]. This is an important area of the brain which is involved in food intake and body-weight regulation, and it is rich in 5-HT2C [59, 60]. Furthermore, there is evidence suggesting an interaction between 5-HT2C and leptin, a circulating hormone that is released by adipocytes in response to increased fat deposition to regulate body weight and that acts through receptors mapping in hypothalamus [61]. 5-HT2C antagonists attenuate the reduction in food intake produced by leptin [61]. There are a body of evidences that 5-HT2C receptor and NPY are also involved in antipsychotics-induced weight gain. Chronic administration of clozapine produced an increase in NPY-immunoreactive cell density in the rat arcuate nucleus [62] that could, at least in part, be due to antagonism of the 5-HT2C receptor resulting in disinhibition of the NPY neurons.

That the 5-HT2C receptor is directly involved in antipsychotics-induced weight gain is also demonstrated by pharmacogenetic observation such as the findings of Yuan et al. [63] that have identified several haplotypes of the promoter region of the 5-HT2C receptor gene which are associated with obesity and diabetes. Reynolds et al., in two different study [64, 65], have found that one 5-HT2C promoter polymorphism, −759*C/T*, is involved in developing weight gain during antipsychotics medication. In the first study, analyzed subjects (Chinese patients at first treatment) carrying the −759*T* allele had substantially lower weight gain following 10 weeks of treatment. In the second study, they have found that this association remains after 9 months of treatment in a group of first episode Caucasian patients. In the same study, the protective −759*T* allele was associated with higher concentrations of leptin.

4. Dopamine Signaling

Based on the pharmacodynamic profile of antipsychotics, dopamine has been considered the crucial target responsible for the efficacy of this class of compounds, and this may be true at least partially also for the new generation of antipsychotics since no compound devoid of D2R antagonism has been proved to be clinically effective in the treatment of schizophrenia [66]. Several lines of evidence also indicate that dopamine is involved in feeding behavior. (1) dorsal striatum and ventral striatum, both heavily innervated by dopamine, are related to the regulation of the caloric and rewarding effect of food, respectively [67]; (2) dopamine release is increased in certain areas of the brain, such as the accumbens, by palatable and sweet foods [68]; (3) dopamine may be critical in reward or in predicting the reward linked to food with high palatability [69]; (4) a reduced dopamine D2R availability measured with positron emission tomography and 11C Raclopride correlates with obesity in humans [67]. Moreover, the absence of dopamine production in the knockout mouse, which does not express tyrosine hydroxylase, does not inhibit motor capabilities to eat but causes an inability to initiate feeding; this ability can be restored by gene delivery of tyrosine hydroxylase into the striatum [70]. Dopamine release seems to have a site-specific action in food-intake regulation, such as in the nucleus accumbens, and it is associated with the reinforcement effect in feeding [71]. In the hypothalamus, dopamine release is associated with the duration of meal consumption, which is a factor in determining the feeding pattern. Hence, dopamine is required to initiate each meal and is thus associated with meal number and duration. Increased dopamine in the VMN, the area of neuroendocrine and autonomic regulation of metabolism, accompanies food intake. Medial hypothalamic lesions produce both hyperphagia and morbid obesity, suggesting that VMN dopamine is involved in regulating both food intake and the bodyweight setpoint [72–74].

The important contribution of dopamine to the regulation of food intake and feeding pattern has been shown in the medial hypothalamus by the study of both pre- and postsynaptic dopaminergic systems, as measured by in vivo microdialysis in experimental paradigms involving Zucker obese rat and its lean counterpart. Dopamine release is rapidly but transiently increased in the VMN during spontaneous eating in lean and obese rats, and this increase is more pronounced in obese rats, which consume larger meals [75]. When rats are deprived of food for 24 h, food intake brings about an immediate decrease of dopamine release to 65% of pre-eating levels in both lean and obese rats. These two findings show that release of dopamine is associated with both short-term (individual meals) and long-term (hunger) regulation of food intake. These data also suggest that during obesity, the presynaptic dopaminergic system adequately responds to the change of feeding status [73–75]. Dopamine acts on its receptors postsynaptically to modulate the activity of target neurons by stimulation or inhibition of adenylyl cyclase activity by D1 and D5 or D2 to D4 subtypes of receptors, respectively. The finding that hypothalamic neurons express both subtypes of dopaminergic receptors provides evidence that dopamine may activate or inhibit its target neurons based on the (1) function of the subtype and (2) level of the dopaminergic receptor expressed for a given metabolic condition under normal or pathologic conditions. D1 receptor, which normally is not abundantly expressed in the hypothalamus, was found highly expressed in the VMN of obese rats whereas D2 receptor was detected in the lean rat but at an undetectable level in the VMN of the obese Zucker rat [76]. The different levels of dopaminergic receptor expression in the two phenotypes may be related to the relatively low concentration of ligand (dopamine) in obese as opposed to lean rats, or it may directly depend on altered leptin signaling in postsynaptic neurons [76]. It is pointed out by different preclinical and clinical evidence that even with different degree, all clinically available antipsychotics have a certain degree of D2R occupancy. Beyond the clinical efficacy and extrapiramidal movements liability, the dopamine system has been investigated to much less extent for its implication in food regulation intake and weight gain during antipsychotic treatment. However, it should not be surprising that drugs that are with different degrees all antagonists of dopamine receptors may disrupt the normal physiology of dopamine-related feeding behavior, even if the precise mechanism by which dopamine could be primary affected is still elusive. On the other side, if dopamine is really involved in antipsychotics-induced weight gain, this possibility should be critically taken into account considered that dopamine depletion, at least in animals, is responsible of reducing food intake and that among antipsychotics with liability for weight gain, there are compounds with low affinity for dopamine D2 receptor. With regard to dopamine receptor involvement in antipsychotics-induced weight gain, it should be important to explore what extent the different dopamine receptors may contribute to feeding behavior and how antipsychotics with different D1-like and D2-like profile may differentially impact the body weight during the treatment. The putative role of dopamine system in the mechanism responsible for the weight gain is particularly puzzling, and the introduction in the pharmacotherapy of schizophrenia of antipsychotics with reported dopamine partial agonism does not help to clarify the issue. In 2005, it has been demonstrated that the administration of olanzapine (1–10 mg/kg p.o.) or aripiprazole (2.0–8.0 mg/kg p.o.) resulted in rapid and robust weight gain in rat taking the drugs compared to control animals whereas the liability for inducing prolactin elevation was substantially different, with olanzapine inducing a significantly increase in prolactin compared to control animals and aripirazole-treated animals [77]. The complexity of a "realistic" animal model of antipsychotics-induced weight gain is underscored by a series of experiments in which olanzapine and aripiprazole are compared. In a first experiment, the authors validated a pharmacologic isomorphism of olanzapine induced weight gain, by oral administration per 14 days, of olanzapine 5.0 mg/kg, twice per day, per os, in female Wistar rats [77]. As previously demonstrated with 8 mg/kg per 14 days olanzapine-induced a significant weight gain compared to control rats (vehicle treated) [78]. The weight gain was positively correlated with food intake, mirroring the increase in appetite in humans [79]; however, considering that weight gain can be detected starting from day 3 whereas food intake increase is detectable only from day 6, other factors should be taken into account in order to fully explain the mechanism of weight gain. In the second experiment, the different liability for inducing weight again and metabolic changes by antipsychotics with different receptor profile was challenged. The effect on weight gain of olanzapine compared to aripiprazole, a dopamine-partial agonist, was also studied in two different strains of rats: Wistar and Sprague Dawley. The utilization of two strains was introduced to gain information and evaluate the potential contribution of genetic background on antipsychotics-induced weight gain. Finally, in order to investigate the effect of housing conditions on food intake and weight gain, the authors compared the treatment with the two antipsychotics in rat singly and group housed [77]. Taking together all these findings suggest that DRD2 is a possible candidate gene for antipsychotics-induced weight gain. In 209 nondiabetic hypertensive and 174 gender-matched normotensive Chinese subjects, the DRD2 TaqI polymorphism was associated with obesity and hypertension [80].

Another gene belonging to dopamine pattern studied as a candidate gene for association study to obesity is the dopamine transporter gene. In a study, it was founded that the 10/10 genotype of the dopamine transporter gene has a 5.16 times higher likelihood of obesity in African-American smokers compared to the 9/9 or 9/10 genotype, while there was no association in non-Hispanic Whites [81].

5. Adrenergic Signaling

The role of the adrenergic system in the putative mechanism of antipsychotics-induced weight gain is elusive, even if a growing number of evidence indicate that both alpha and beta-adrenergic receptors are key molecules in the regulation of metabolic expenditure. Based on findings in animal models of obesity, the sympathoadrenal system has commonly been assumed to have a determining role in obesity development through its influence on regulation of energy expenditure. An earlier hypothesis was that sympathetic under activity, by reducing thermogenesis, might lead to weight gain in obesity, with some experimental observations supporting this view. One example was provided by surgical lesioning of the ventromedial hypothalamus in rodents, in which obesity was due to increased appetite and also to lowered sympathetic activity and obesity [82]. In regard of weight gain and body-weight homeostasis, it is proposed that excess in food intake is sensed by the brain which responds by a reduction of caloric assumption and by an increase in energy expenditure. This latter is mediated by sympathetic nervous system through the stimulation of adrenergic receptors on thermogenically active target tissues [83]. Taken one by one, single attempts including ablation of sympathetic nerves, the generation of genetically altered mice that are unable to synthesize catecholamines, and gene knockouts of individual β ARs have not resulted in obesity [84, 85]. It is possible that functional redundancy between the three known β ARs can justify the lack of complications caused by loss of all adrenergic signaling. To prove this hypothesis, Bachman et al. have created mice that are knockout for all three known β ARs (β-less) [86, 87]. This triple knockout mice that have lacked the $\beta1/\beta2/\beta3$-adrenoceptors developed a progressive obesity at adulthood. An involvement of the adrenergic system in antipsychotics-induced weight gain is suggested by pharmacogenetic investigations that have shown an association between the $\beta2$ adrenergic receptor gene polymorphisms and obesity. Although not undisputed [88, 89], two meta-analyses of a number of human studies have found the Trp64Arg polymorphism in the beta3-adrenergic receptor gene to be associated with obesity [90–92]. Several recent studies confirmed this association [93–96]. A pilot study of 73 subjects with schizophrenia [97] also found a trend (P = .10) between clozapine-related weight gain and the Trp64Arg beta3-adrenergic receptor gene, with the presence of the less frequent arginine allele predicting weight gain. The affinity of antipsychotic agents to the alpha1 adrenergic receptor also suggests that this gene may be a candidate for pharmacogenetic investigation of antipsychotics-induced weight gain. In addition, alpha 1-noradrenergic binding was inversely proportional to body weight gain [98], and in animal model of diet-induced obesity it was founded that lower levels of alpha 1-noradrenergic receptor in the hypothalamic ventromedial nucleus were expressed only in those rats that became obese. In a study involving 60 treatment-refractory patients with schizophrenia, Basile et al. [97] found a trend (P = .22) towards reduced clozapine-induced weight gain in individuals homozygous for the cysteine variant of the Arg347Cys polymorphism of the alpha 1-adrenergic receptor gene. With respect to drug-induced weight gain, no pre-clinical data are available on the effect of antipsychotics on central beta receptors. The two compounds with the highest liability for weight gain, clozapine and olanzapine, have no significant affinity for any of the beta receptors; however, it has been demonstrated that olanzapine-induced activation of prefrontal cortical neurons, analyzed by c-fos induction, is prevented by administration of the beta-receptor antagonist propanolol [99]. It has been hypothesized that olanzapine acting on presynaptic alpha 1 receptors may increase the release of norepinephrine in the prefrontal cortex and in turn activate adrenergic beta receptors [99]. It will be interesting to show a similar c-fos induction and propanolol prevention in neurons of CNS regions related to food intake or energy expenditure.

6. Hystamine Signaling

Hystamine is probably the neurotransmitter for which there are more available data on an involvement in food intake regulation. Histaminergic neurons are exclusively found in the tuberomammillary nucleus in the posterior hypothalamus but act through postsynaptic H1-receptors on almost all areas of the brain involved in energy homeostasis. Moreover, several reports have suggested that histamine (HA) is involved in the regulation of arousal state, locomotor activity, cardiovascular control, water intake, food intake, and memory formation on antihistaminic receptorial activity of antipsychotics. The propensity of antipsychotic agents to induce weight gain is addressed by different experimental on affinity for H1-receptor system. Many authors have founded that affinity for H1 receptors closely correlates with antipsychotics-induced weight gain [100]. Consistent with these data, other authors have demonstrated that histamine H1-receptor antagonism promotes feeding in rodents and that H1 knockout mice are prone to weight gain [101, 102]. Moreover, in this animal model is abolished clozapine augmentation of AMP kinase that is potentially stimulated in the hypothalamus by orexigenic antipsychotics and is involved in regulating food intake [103]. Also, leptin-induced food intake appears suppresses in H1 knockout mice. This data suggest that that hypothalamic histamine is a modulator of leptin activity [104, 105]. Furthermore, histamine release in CNS seems to be involved in lipolysis [106] and glycolysis [107] during energy-deficient states in animal studies. There are several novel H1-receptor polymorphisms that are been identified, including Leu449Ser [108], −17 C/T, −974 C/T, −1023 A/G, −1536-G/C [109], and Glu349Asp [110], but there is only one pharmacogenomic study focused on antipsychotics-induced weight gain that shows no association in 88 schizophrenic patients between the Glu349Asp variant of the HR-1 gene and weight gain after 4 months of treatment with clozapine [110], but the use of treatment-refractory schizophrenic as samples probably may have diminished the power of association study. Despite the relevance of these neurobiological factors, it is notable that different authors have pointed out that the drugs with high H1 receptor antagonism can lead to weight gain also for their sedative effects with consequent reduced mobility.

7. Cholinergic Signaling

Some evidence have suggested that the blockade of mACh exerted by different antipsychotics may lead to weight gain trough anticholinergic-induced dry mouth that has as a consequence an increase in the ingestion of high-calorie beverages. One study showed a significant reduction in muscarinic M2 receptor density in the dorsal vagal complex DVC and a significant increase in weight gain in rats after treatment with olanzapine but not with haloperidol [111].

The DVC comprises the dorsal motor nucleus of the vagus (DMV), nucleus of the tractus solitarius (NTS), and the area postrema (AP). The NTS is the primary site for innervation by vagal afferents from the gut, whilst the DMV is the site for primary efferents to the gut [112]. The DVC is also a target for the inhibitory effect of leptin on food intake [113]. There is evidence that the DVC is also involved in detecting and responding to hunger and satiety signals. This is an indirect involvement of cholinergic transmission in weight gain induced by antipsychotics mechanism. Nevertheless, neither remarkable weight gain nor diabetes mellitus has reported the use of typical anticholinergic drugs, such as scopolamine. This finding reinforce the data of Matsui-Sakata et al. [114] that in a meta-analysis pointed out that the affinities to mACh receptors of the antipsychotics were very low and correlates with H1 receptor occupancy. As a consequence, mACh receptor occupancy is likely to be a confounding factor in analysis of the cause of antipsychpotics-induced weight gain.

8. Cannabinoid Signaling

The endocannabinoid system consists of cannabinoid receptors, endocannabinoids, and a set of endocannabinoid synthesising and degrading enzymes. Early roles for the endocannabinoid system were ascribed based on the location of the endocannabinoid receptors. In the early 1990s, two cannabinoid receptors, belonging to the family of G-protein coupled receptors, had been cloned cannabinoid receptor type 1 (CB1) and cannabinoid receptor type 2 (CB2), and the two major endogenous cannabinoids (the so-called endocannabinoids) were identified as arachidonoyl ethanolamine (anandamide, AEA) and 2-arachidonoyl glycerol (2-AG). Therefore, the abundance of CB1 receptors in the brain suggested a role as an important modulator of neuronal functions, and the fact that CB2 receptors are mainly expressed in the immune system suggested an immune modulatory role. In addition to other functions, endocannabinoids have been shown to induce a dose-dependent orexigenic effect and thus mimic the hyperphagic effect produced by THC [115]. More importantly, it has been demonstrated not only that changes in endocannabinoids production occur with respect to the feeding state of the animal, for example, increasing between meals, reaching a critical level in order to trigger the motivation to feed, and then falling rapidly following access to food, but that these changes are localised to specific areas of the brain directly involved in modulating feeding behaviour, such as the nucleus accumbens [115]. Some authors hypothesize that the endocannabinoid system may display an incentive action to increase the incentive value of the food regardless of the quality of the macronutrients [116, 117]. Others speculate about the orosensory rewarding properties of endocannabinoids [118]. In other words, endocannabinoids may stimulate a preference for highly palatable food. Interestingly, CB1 receptors are colocalised with dopamine D1 and D2 receptors in the rat limbic forebrain and crosstalk between the endocannabinoid and the dopaminergic system in the control of reward for tasty food has recently been documented using dopamine D1 receptor antagonists which reduce the orexigenic stimulus induced by THC [119]. Several findings in rodents point to a pivotal role of the hypothalamus as the integrating centre for the anabolic signals induced by endocannabinoids [120]. In that regard, recent evidence suggests that endocannabinoids act within various hypothalamic nuclei to influence other neurons that produce peptides that influence food intake. In lateral hypothalamus, one finds the following.

(1) It has been demonstrated that AEA increases and AM251 (a CB1 antagonist) decreases depolarization-induced neuropeptide Y (NPY) release in hypothalamic rat explants, suggesting that NPY may contribute to the orexigenic action of endocannabinoids—possibly via modulation of an intermediate factor involved in NPY release [121].

(2) CB1 receptor stimulation strongly augments the orexin-A-stimulated intracellular pathway, and this effect can be blocked by the CB1 receptor antagonist rimonabant, suggesting a positive orexigenic role for CB1 in this neural population [122].

(3) In models of obesity such as *ob/ob* and *db/db* mice, characterised by an impairment of leptinergic signalling, it has been shown an increase of (pathological) levels of endocannabinoids at the hypothalamus. A single intravenous (i.v.) injection of leptin in these animals was able to reduce the overproduction of endocannabinoids [123].

(4) Recently, it has been also characterised the interactions among endocannabinoids, leptin, and melanocortin-concentrating hormone (MCH) within the limbic system: MCH neurons are inhibited by GABAergic inputs from the limbic system and endocannabinoids act to reduce GABA release, and thus may stimulate the excitability of MCH neurons, leading to an increase in food intake [123, 124].

(5) Endocannabinoids also interact with a-melanocyte-stimulating hormone (MSH) and cocaine- and amphetamine-related transcript(CART). This is a neuropeptide highly expressed in the hypothalamus and nucleus accumbens. Hypothalamic CART has been associated with food intake and body weight control [125].

The hypothalamic paraventricular nucleus (PVN) may represent another site within the brain where endocannabinoids interact with orexigenic and anorexigenic neurons. Here, it has been clearly demonstrated that endocannabinoids released from parvocellular neurons act at presynaptic CB1 receptors to decrease glutamatergic transmission onto CRH-releasing neurons, resulting in an inhibition of CRH release. Recent findings suggest that the orexigenic crosstalk between endocannabinoids and ghrelin signalling may represent a novel target for the pharmacological treatment of obesity [126]. In order to investigate the role of cannabinoid system in antipsychotics-induced weight gain, Weston-Green et al. have investigated whether different antipsychotic drugs (olanzapine, haloperidol, aripiprazole, or vehicle) alter cannabinoid receptor-binding density in the DVC in female Sprague-Dawley rats treated in both acute (1 week) and chronic (12 weeks) paradigms [127]. Using quantitative autoradiographic methods, they have found that acute olanzapine induced a significant 39% decrease in cannabinoid receptor binding compared to controls, whilst short-term aripiprazole and haloperidol had no significant effect. In addition, chronic olanzapine treatment induced a significant 46% decrease in cannabinoid receptor binding compared to controls, and aripiprazole slightly decreased cannabinoid receptor binding (12%), whilst haloperidol had no effect [127]. These results coincide with the clinical setting in which patients treated with olanzapine exhibit higher weight gain than aripiprazole [128] and haloperidol [129]. However, due to the low abundance of CB2 receptors in the DVC, it is probable that the findings observed in this study was mostly to the CB1 receptor. This study supports a role for brainstem cannabinoid receptors in the mechanisms of antipsychotic-induced weight gain. In contrast with Weston-green et al., Theisen et al. [130], in a recent work, using radioligand-binding assays to compare the binding affinities of clozapine, olanzapine, and haloperidol for candidate receptors potentially involved in AP-induced weight gain, have not found significant binding rate to cannabinoid receptor 1.

9. Insulin, Leptine, and Other Neuropeptide Signaling

In 1979, it was demonstrated in nonhuman primates that insulin infused into the CNS caused a significant decline in food intake and body weight. Woods et al. [131] proposed that insulin served as an "adiposity signal" that links the behavior of feeding with size of adipose stores [131]. In the mid-1990s, it was identified leptin as another candidate hormone working in adiposity signal [132] and has been well characterized as a regulator of energy homeostasis. The presence of insulin in the CNS was reported in 1979 [133]. Although negligible quantities of insulin can be synthesized locally, many studies established that the predominant amount of insulin in the CNS can be accounted for by receptor-mediated transport into the CNS by blood [134]. Receptors for both insulin and leptin are widely expressed throughout the CNS, but the major target of these two hormons is the medial hypothalamus [134]. Although the leptin receptor is present as different splice-variant isoforms in the CNS, the form OBRb has the major role in its metabolic action [135]. The obese *db/db* mouse and Zucker *fa/fa* rat represent naturally occurring "knockouts" of the leptin receptor that have helped to validate the importance of CNS leptin action in energy homeostasis. Leptin and insulin have multiple effects on energy homeostasis through activation of key hypothalamic nuclei and peptides to regulate energy balance such as neuropeptide-Y (NPY), POMC and its product α-melanocyte-stimulating hormone (α-MSH), and the melanocortin antagonist, AgRP [136, 137]. POMC and AgRP are selectively expressed in neurons of the ARC nucleus colocalized with receptors for insulin and leptin, and different data suggested that leptin and insulin act on ARC to increase melanocortin and decrease AgRP to regulate food intake and energy balance [138]. Recent evidence suggest that there are other key players in modulation of food intake influenced by insulin and leptin in a direct or indirect way. Among these, are notable

Orexin A and melanin concentrating hormone (MCH), both with orexigenic function. Additionally, Orexin A may be an important factor in the effects of drugs of abuse and for the rewarding effects of food [137]. The orexins (hypocretins) are a family of hypothalamic neuropeptides that are selectively expressed in neurons of the classical "feeding area" of the lateral hypothalamus and perifornical area (LH/PFA) [139, 140]. The orexins (orexin A and orexin B) arise from the precursor peptide prepro-orexin by proteolytic processing.

Orexins bind and activate two closely related G-protein-coupled receptors, orexin 1 receptor (OX1R) and orexin 2 receptor (OX2R) [139]. Despite the small number of orexin cells, orexin axons are distributed throughout the brain [141, 142]. The orexins are potent regulators of feeding and other metabolic processes and of arousal [143, 144]; in addition, intracerebral orexin administration increases food intake [145]. In a study of Fadel et al. (2002) [146], the authors have demonstrated in animal experimental paradigm that *fos* expression was induced in orexin neurons by APDs that cause significant weight gain but not by those APDs with low weight-gain liability. However, amphetamine also activated orexin neurons, but clozapine markedly increased *fos* expression in orexin neurons that innervate the PFC whereas amphetamine had a weak effect. This findings suggest that it is likely that changes in the activity of afferents or hormonal signals to these orexin neurons determine the differential response. The identity of these afferents is unknown, but may include the PFC and nucleus accumbens, regions that receive dopaminergic projections from the A10 cell group and project to the LH/PFA [147, 148]. Moreover, the receptors that are targeted by APDs that induce weight gain may be present on orexin neurons or on afferents to the orexin neurons, such as neurons of the PFC and play an important role. Alternatively, peripherally derived signals may be critical. Several data suggested the presence of specific CNS circuitry which is either directly or indirectly connected with hypothalamic circuitry to modulate feeding behavior. Components of this circuitry could contribute also to complex behaviors like food seeking and food intake and include portions of the cerebral cortex, hippocampus, amygdala, and the striatonigral pathway, which is implicated in transposing motivational aspects of stimuli into motor responses, as well as hedonic evaluation of the stimulus and associative learning. The major neurotransmitter pathways associated with motivation and hedonics are mesolimbic dopamine (DA) and certain CNS opioid pathways. In terms of neural connectivity, the hypothalamus is linked to the motivational circuitry of the CNS, and numerous mono- and multisynaptic pathways between different components of the limbic circuitry and the hypothalamus have been identified [149]. Food intake can be driven by energy demands, that is, "homeostatic" feeding and by the palatability or pleasure associated with eating a preferred food, "non-homeostatic" feeding [150]. The behavior associated with non-homeostatic feeding is in part regulated by the mesolimbic dopamine system. Berridge et al. have identified nucleus accumbens (NAc) dopamine projections, that receive projection of DA neurons from VTA as central to "wanting" and has been implicated in the motivating, rewarding, reinforcing, and incentive salience properties of natural stimuli such as food and water as well as drugs of abuse [151]. The neural mechanisms of food reward are believed to be similar, if not identical, to drug rewards.

At least, Ghrelin is a newly discovered appetite-stimulating peptide that has a role in the regulation of feeding behaviour. It is primarily secreted by the stomach and duodenum, and it has been implicated in both mealtime hunger and the long-term regulation of body weight. Ghrelin is currently recognized as the main endogenous ligand for growth hormone secretagogue receptors. The levels of circulating ghrelin are increased under conditions of starvation and in anorexia nervosa, but decreased under conditions of feeding and in obesity. Ghrelin and leptin may have opposite actions in the regulation of body weight. The link between atypical antipsychotic treatment and elevated serum ghrelin levels is not clear so far, but a dysregulation of the central feedback mechanism can be hypothesized. Murashita et al. in an interesting work have suggested that olanzapine may directly act on the secretion of ghrelin and induce appetite, resulting in weight gain [152].

10. Animal Model of Weight Gain after Antipsychotics Administration

A critical approach to the search for a molecular mechanism of antipsychotics weight gain should start recognizing that the results from animal models have been not consistent and that the paradigms may not fulfill the hypothesis: quite a paradox for compounds whose action on CNS can be modeled with relatively sufficient approximation. On the other side, a reliable animal model of antipsychotics-induced weight gain should be particularly helpful considering that this side effect cannot be completely predicted on the basis of the receptor-binding profile of an antipsychotic agent. The importance of animal models is underlined also by a recent consensus development on antipsychotics drugs, obesity, and diabetes, and it is recommended in order to determine whether the above disorders are due to a central peripheral mechanisms. Several caveats needs to be taken into account analyzing animal models: (1) the route of administration, (2) the day-time of administration, (3) the duration of the treatment, (4) the dose-equivalent to human dose, and (5) species difference, in some of these methodological issues may be relevant for the modeling of increased food intake whereas others for the reproduction of the metabolic dysregulation that me be responsible of weight gain in patients taking atypical antipsychotics.

The route of administration is usually i.p. or i.m. injection, and only few studies have used oral administration and the cleavage method. Chronic injection and cavage may represent a stressful condition that can interfere with food-intake regulation and should be carefully controlled. The day time of drug administration may be relevant considering that rodents have an inverse day-night rhythm compared to human, and this method of treatment may have consequences on food intake. The antipsychotic dose administered is chosen mainly based on the dopamine D2 occupancy and on the behavioral effects of the compound. The effect of certain antipsychotics on metabolism and weight gain in different species may be different from the dose responsible for the CNS effects. The duration of the treatment may be a crucial issue too; the mean duration of chronic animal studies is about three–four weeks, the time frame in which is believed the antipsychotic action begins to appear. However, the metabolic effects in human appear clearly after 10 weeks of treatment and are usually reported within this frame time. Finally, few studies have been conducted in a "head-to-head" antipsychotics-administration paradigm that includes more than two antipsychotics. The results of animal studies conducted have been in some cases surprising. Both olanzapine (2.5–5 mg/kg/day) and haloperidol (0.08–0.31 mg/kg/day) administered by cavage for three weeks to male and female Wistar rats induced a significant weight gain in female rats only, failing to reproduce the clinical situation where olanzapine has been shown to increase weight gain significantly more than haloperidol in both genders. Moreover, the low but not the high dose of olanzapine caused a significant increase in food intake in female rats [153]. If antipsychotics influence food intake and this effect may in turn be responsible for the weight gain, how the meals pattern is changed? In other words, what is modified the feeding rate or the meal size or both? The meals pattern of free feeding in rats has been studied by Lee and Clifton who have investigated meal behavior in Lister hooded rats after the i.p administration of haloperidol (0.05–0.2 mg/kg), clozapine (1–10 mg/kg), olanzapine (0.3–3.0 mg/kg), and analysis of feeding rate and meal size in the interval of time between 2 h and 48 h after the drug injection [154]. Haloperidol and clozapine, but not olanzapine, produced a transitory increase in food intake in the 2 h following drug administration. A rapid compensatory response to the initial period of hyperphagia was indicated by the unchanged total amount of food intake after six hours. Haloperidol produced a substantial enhancement of meal sizes at intermediate doses whereas higher doses were related to a decrease in meal size Clozapine and olanzapine showed no tendency to enhance meal sizes, and the highest doses of olanzapine and haloperidol decreased meal sizes. This study indicates that feeding rates and meal sizes at least in this experimental paradigm are under control of different mechanisms [154]. Are animal models useful in dissecting the effect of low and high antipsychotics dose? Although risperidone has been associated with less weight gain than clozapine, risperidone treatment leads to a greater increase in the body mass of patients than conventional treatment with an antipsychotic such as haloperidol.

A study from Ota et al. (2002) revealed an intriguing biphasic response to low and high doses of risperidone with respect of weight gain [155]. In this study, rats were injected twice a day with risperidone 0.005 mg/kg, 0.05 mg/kg, and 0.5 mg/kg for 21 days, the body weight was measured, and the expression of leptin and uncoupling protein 1 (UCP-1) were quantitated with Real-Time PCR. Leptin is mainly expressed in the white adipose tissue (WAT); UCP-1 is a protein promoting energy expenditure in the Brown Adipose Tissue (BAT). Risperidone 0.005 mg/kg increased food intake and the rate of body weight gain, as well as *leptin* gene expression in WAT. Risperidone 0.5 mg/kg caused a reduction in body weight and an increase in UCP-1 expression. It appears clear that a critical issue in developing a realistic animal model of weight-gain induction after chronic treatment with antipsychotics should rely on a "quasi-naturalistic" modality of drug administration. As already mentioned, the injection of the drug allows a precise delivery of the daily dosage; however, it may be stressful for the animal and have a negative impact on the behavioral outcome; on the other side, administering the drug with the food is also biased by the need to house the animal in a single cage that may mimic an isolation paradigm. A new method of oral antipsychotics administration in individual rats has recently been proposed [156]. The animals (male Sprague Dowley rats) were trained to drink 2 ml of 5% sucrose solution from a disposable syringe on a daily basis for 1 week or until each animal had taken the 2 ml of fluid from the syringe on three consecutive days. After three week of training, all the animals were adapted to drink the solution. At this point, the treatment was initiated according to the experimental protocol: the animal were divided in four groups, haloperidol (2 mg/kg), clozapine (20 kg/mg), diazepam (0.5 mg/kg), or vehicle solution (control treatment) were administered; all the drugs were dissolved in a 5% sucrose solution and were administered for 4 or 7 weeks. The results of the behavioral testing (vacuous chewing movuments, grooming disengage test, chocolate disengage test, and motivational test) was consistent with each drug treatment. After four weeks, only the animals treated with diazepam group showed a significant weight gain compared to controls and to all other treatments; however, after seven weeks, all the animals treated with an active compound showed a similar increase in body weight significantly different from the control group. The animals that were treated for four weeks and then withdrawn from the treatment were not significantly different in body weight from the rats of the control group. This study indicates that this novel method of drug administration may be considered reliable and specifically suitable for studying antipsychotics-induced weight gain, avoiding the potential bias due to the cavage or drug injection [156].

11. Weight Gain and Insulin Function in Animal Model

In addition to weight gain, patients treated with atypical compounds display various metabolic disturbances including increased serum triglycerides and total cholesterol as well as decreased high-density lipoprotein cholesterol [157]. Several other studies have reported anomalous responses to the oral glucose tolerance test and elevated fasting insulin levels after treatment consistent with insulin resistance [158]. Initially, these alterations in glucose regulation and other metabolic parameters were seen as secondary to the weight gain linked to atypical antipsychotic use. However, rapid induction of hyperglycemia, sometimes accompanied by ketoacidosis, has been reported in patients on clozapine and olanzapine without weight gain challenged this notion [159]. This line of evidence suggests a direct, drug-related effect that is independent of changes resulting from weight gain. Despite the burgeoning clinical literature on the possibility that atypical antipsychotics may induce diabetes, few studies have tackled in an animal model, in vivo, the relationship between second-generation APS, weight gain, and pancreatic function. The effect on weight gain, abdominal fat, insulin sensitivity, pre- and post- administration of olanzapine (dose target.15 mg/day) o or risperidone (dose target 5 mg/day) has been investigated in mongrel dog compared to a "neutral" treatment (gel capsules) [160]. Abdominal MRI, euglicemic hyperisnsulinemic clamp (measuring haepatic and insulin sensitivity) and a stepwise beta-cell stimulation (monitoring pancreatic beta-cell response) were performed. This study not only reveals differential effects of two atypical antipsychotics on adiposity and hepatic insulin resistance but also shows for the first time a substantial effect of one antipsychotic to impair pancreatic β-cell function. Animals treated with olanzapine exhibited greater (+5.9%) weight gain than which (+3.9%) were observed with RIS. The authors also found that observed body-weight changes are not explained solely by alterations in food intake, but it reflects treatment effects on both caloric intake and energy expenditure. MRI analyses revealed that dogs treated with olanzapine developed substantial adiposity that greatly exceeded observed changes in control animals. At variance, ripseridone caused more modest increases. In regard of glucose metabolism, in this study, the authors have pointed out that dogs treated with olanzapine exhibited severe hepatic insulin resistance (reduced above 75%). This differs with the more modest declines with risperidone or placebo. While olanzapine-induced hepatic insulin resistance may reflect a primary hepatic defect, other sites of action are also plausible. This study revealed a dramatic impairment in β-cell compensation during olanzapine treatment. Both drugs induced similar whole-body insulin resistance, yet only riperidone responded with compensatory upregulation of β-cell sensitivity. Since insulin secretion can be neurally regulated, one possibility is that negative effects of olanzapine on β-cell compensation may be mediated by its known central actions as a dopamine antagonist. Moreover, it is unknown if a similar dopamine-mediated neuropancreatic axis exists for pancreatic endocrine secretion. Since studies have suggested that weight gain and therapeutic response resulting from clozapine treatment may be correlated [161], Zhao et al. in their interesting work have examined behavioral and biochemical effects of clozapine [162].

They have measured startle response and prepulse inhibition of the startle reflex in untreated mice and 68-day clozapine-treated mice. They have found that clozapine treatment significantly reduced the startle response but did not potentiate prepulse inhibition. In the same work, they have also treated mice with clozapine (2 mg/kg/day) for 3 days, 25 days, and 68 days. These treatments developed a sustained insulin insensitivity, which resulted in impaired plasma glucose clearance as measured by intraperitoneal glucose-tolerance test without significant weight gain. Indeed, impaired plasma glucose clearance was observed at day 3 and persisted for the entire 68-day period of clozapine treatment. This suggests that clozapine was effective not only in behavioral changes as measured by the startle response magnitude but also in systemic metabolic alterations. If the mechanistic relationship between weight gain and diabetes induced by antipsychotics has been investigated only in few animal studies, the mechanism by which second generation-antipsychotics may disrupt the normal metabolic function and cause glucose disturbance has been investigated in *in vitro* experiments mainly addressing the effects of antipsychotics on glucose transport and glucose sensing [163, 164]. Trying to make sense of the preclinical and *in vitro* data on the relationship between putative mechanisms responsible of weight gain and diabetes in schizophrenics patients treated with second-generation antipsychotics, one should take into account the important observation that diabetes may be a disorder that is related with pathophysiology of schizophrenia and as underlined recently by Citrome. He has assessed that the presence of a diagnosis of schizophrenia in itself is a risk factor, prompting the Canadian Diabetes Association to recommend routine screening for diabetes for all who have that disorder. Lifetime risk of developing diabetes may in fact be quite high for certain groups, as estimated by the Centers for Disease Control and Prevention, where the estimated lifetime risk of developing diabetes for individuals born in 2000 appears to be 32.8% for males and 38.5% for females, with the highest estimated lifetime risk for diabetes being among Hispanics (males 45.4%, females 52.5%) [165]. Moreover, in its recent meta-analysis, the same author did not not demonstrate a significantly increased risk of diabetes during treatment with second-generation antipsychotics compared with first-generation drugs [165]. This finding suggests that probably basic studies have overscored the importance of the disorders in glucose metabolism induced by second-generation antipsychotics and probably underlie that insulin resistance and schizophrenia have a common substrate.

12. Conclusions

Weight gain due to antipsychotic medication is associated with significant physical and psychological morbidity. Individuals with schizophrenia treated with antipsychotics have concerns about weight gain and weight management, like the general population, and express a desire to be more active. Driven by the public health impact of obesity, substantial progress has recently been made in the basic understanding of the regulation of appetite and body weight, including the identification of genetic polymorphisms and other markers of obesity risk. Newer studies are focusing on elucidating the fundamental mechanisms of weight gain through pharmacogenomic approaches and evaluating changes in energy homeostasis, metabolism, and energy intake and expenditure during antipsychotic treatment. As psychiatric practice moves into an era of personalized medicine, the ability to identify risk markers, besides those related to demographic characteristics or the drug itself, will not only help clinicians to screen out patients at high risk for weight gain and metabolic changes, but potentially allow earlier access to higher-risk medications for patients who do not possess vulnerability markers. Medications such as olanzapine and clozapine carry significant metabolic burdens, but are effective treatments for some patients who do not respond to other antipsychotics. The elucidation of mechanisms by which antipsychotic medications impact metabolic parameters remains important for quantification of patient risk, to inform the frequency and targets of metabolic monitoring during antipsychotic therapy, and to permit the development of novel agents without these limitations.

References

[1] K. T. Mueser and S. R. McGurk, "Schizophrenia," *The Lancet*, vol. 363, no. 9426, pp. 2063–2072, 2004.

[2] J. B. Dynes, "Mental health–cause of death in schizophrenia," *Virginia Medical Monthly*, vol. 96, no. 6, p. 3340, 1969.

[3] B. Felker, J. J. Yazel, and D. Short, "Mortality and medical comorbidity among psychiatric patients: a review," *Psychiatric Services*, vol. 47, no. 12, pp. 1356–1363, 1996.

[4] S. Mukherjee, P. Decina, V. Bocola, F. Saraceni, and P. Scapicchio, "Diabetes mellitus in schizophrenic patients," *Comprehensive Psychiatry*, vol. 37, no. 1, pp. 68–73, 1996.

[5] S. Brown, "Excess mortality of schizophrenia. A meta-analysis," *British Journal of Psychiatry*, vol. 171, pp. 502–508, 1997.

[6] S. Saddichha, N. Manjunatha, S. Ameen, and S. Akhtar, "Effect of olanzapine, risperidone, and haloperidol treatment on weight and body mass index in first-episode schizophrenia patients in India: a randomized, double-blind, controlled, prospective study," *Journal of Clinical Psychiatry*, vol. 68, no. 11, pp. 1793–1798, 2007.

[7] S. Leucht, C. Corves, D. Arbter, R. R. Engel, C. Li, and J. M. Davis, "Second-generation versus first-generation antipsychotic drugs for schizophrenia: a meta-analysis," *The Lancet*, vol. 373, no. 9657, pp. 31–41, 2009.

[8] D. B. Allison, J. L. Mentore, M. Heo et al., "Antipsychotic-induced weight gain: a comprehensive research synthesis," *American Journal of Psychiatry*, vol. 156, no. 11, pp. 1686–1696, 1999.

[9] J. Bobes, J. Rejas, M. Garcia-Garcia et al., "Weight gain in patients with schizophrenia treated with risperidone, olanzapine, quetiapine or haloperidol: results of the EIRE study," *Schizophrenia Research*, vol. 62, no. 1-2, pp. 77–88, 2003.

[10] H. Nasrallah, "A review of the effect of atypical antipsychotics on weight," *Psychoneuroendocrinology*, vol. 28, no. 1, pp. 83–96, 2003.

[11] "Expert panel on the identification, evaluation, and treatment of overweight and obesity in adults," 1998.

[12] R. S. McIntyre, S. M. McCann, and S. H. Kennedy, "Antipsychotic metabolic effects: weight gain, diabetes mellitus, and lipid abnormalities," *Canadian Journal of Psychiatry*, vol. 46, no. 3, pp. 273–281, 2001.

[13] T. C. Manschreck and R. A. Boshes, "The CATIE schizophrenia trial: results, impact, controversy," *Harvard Review of Psychiatry*, vol. 15, no. 5, pp. 245–258, 2007.

[14] M. J. Arranz and J. De Leon, "Pharmacogenetics and pharmacogenomics of schizophrenia: a review of last decade of research," *Molecular Psychiatry*, vol. 12, no. 8, pp. 707–747, 2007.

[15] A. K. Malhotra, T. Lencz, C. U. Correll, and J. M. Kane, "Genomics and the future of pharmacotherapy in psychiatry," *International Review of Psychiatry*, vol. 19, no. 5, pp. 523–530, 2007.

[16] V. De Luca, D. J. Müller, R. Hwang et al., "HTR2C haplotypes and antipsychotics-induced weight gain: X-linked multimarker analysis," *Human Psychopharmacology*, vol. 22, no. 7, pp. 463–467, 2007.

[17] V. De Luca, D. J. Mueller, A. De Bartolomeis, and J. L. Kennedy, "Association of the HTR2C gene and antipsychotic induced weight gain: a meta-analysis," *International Journal of Neuropsychopharmacology*, vol. 10, no. 5, pp. 697–704, 2007.

[18] A. J. Goudie, G. D. Cooper, and J. C. G. Halford, "Antipsychotic-induced weight gain," *Diabetes, Obesity and Metabolism*, vol. 7, no. 5, pp. 478–487, 2005.

[19] A. A. Arjona, S. X. Zhang, B. Adamson, and R. J. Wurtman, "An animal model of antipsychotic-induced weight gain," *Behavioural Brain Research*, vol. 152, no. 1, pp. 121–127, 2004.

[20] T. Baptista, E. Araujo de Baptista, N. M. K. NG. Ying Kin et al., "Comparative effects of the antipsychotics sulpiride or risperidone in rats. I: bodyweight, food intake, body composition, hormones and glucose tolerance," *Brain Research*, vol. 957, no. 1, pp. 144–151, 2002.

[21] M. J. Fell, J. C. Neill, and K. M. Marshall, "Effects of the classical antipsychotic haloperidol and atypical antipsychotic risperidone on weight gain, the oestrous cycle and uterine weight in female rats," *European Neuropsychopharmacology*, vol. 14, no. 5, pp. 385–392, 2004.

[22] A. J. Goudie, J. A. Smith, and J. C. G. Halford, "Characterization of olanzapine-induced weight gain in rats," *Journal of Psychopharmacology*, vol. 16, no. 4, pp. 291–296, 2002.

[23] G. Kaur and S. K. Kulkarni, "Studies on modulation of feeding behavior by atypical antipsychotics in female mice," *Progress in Neuro-Psychopharmacology and Biological Psychiatry*, vol. 26, no. 2, pp. 277–285, 2002.

[24] B. Pouzet, T. Mow, M. Kreilgaard, and S. Velschow, "Chronic treatment with antipsychotics in rats as a model for antipsychotic-induced weight gain in human," *Pharmacology Biochemistry and Behavior*, vol. 75, no. 1, pp. 133–140, 2003.

[25] G. D. Cooper, L. C. Pickavance, J. P. H. Wilding, J. C. G. Halford, and A. J. Goudie, "A parametric analysis of olanzapine-induced weight gain in female rats," *Psychopharmacology*, vol. 181, no. 1, pp. 80–89, 2005.

[26] T. Baptista, A. Mata, L. Teneud, M. De Quijada, H.-W. Han, and L. Hernandez, "Effects of long-term administration of clozapine on body weight and food intake in rats," *Pharmacology Biochemistry and Behavior*, vol. 45, no. 1, pp. 51–54, 1993.

[27] J. Minet-Ringuet, P. C. Even, B. Guesdon, D. Tomé, and R. De Beaurepaire, "Effects of chronic neuroleptic treatments on nutrient selection, body weight, and body composition in the male rat under dietary self-selection," *Behavioural Brain Research*, vol. 163, no. 2, pp. 204–211, 2005.

[28] T. Baptista, Q. Contreras, L. Teneud et al., "Mechanism of the neuroleptic-induced obesity in female rats," *Progress in Neuro-Psychopharmacology and Biological Psychiatry*, vol. 22, no. 1, pp. 187–198, 1998.

[29] T. Baptista, D. Reyes, and L. Hernández, "Antipsychotic drugs and reproductive hormones relationship to body weight regulation," *Pharmacology Biochemistry and Behavior*, vol. 62, no. 3, pp. 409–417, 1999.

[30] A. Stefanidis, A. N.A. Verty, A. M. Allen, N. C. Owens, M. A. Cowley, and B. J. Oldfield, "The role of thermogenesis in

antipsychotic drug-induced weight gain," *Obesity*, vol. 17, no. 1, pp. 16–24, 2009.
[31] V. Srivastava, S. N. Deshpande, V. L. Nimgaonkar, B. Lerer, and B. K. Thelma, "Genetic correlates of olanzapine-induced weight gain in schizophrenia subjects from north India: role of metabolic pathway genes," *Pharmacogenomics*, vol. 9, no. 8, pp. 1055–1068, 2008.
[32] H. Ujike, A. Nomura, Y. Morita et al., "Multiple genetic factors in olanzapine-induced weight gain in schizophrenia patients: a cohort study," *Journal of Clinical Psychiatry*, vol. 69, no. 9, pp. 1416–1422, 2008.
[33] J. W. Newcomer, "Metabolic syndrome and mental illness," *American Journal of Managed Care*, vol. 13, no. 11, pp. S170–S177, 2007.
[34] H. A. Nasrallah, "Atypical antipsychotic-induced metabolic side effects: insights from receptor-binding profiles," *Molecular Psychiatry*, vol. 13, no. 1, pp. 27–35, 2008.
[35] P. G. Strange, "Antipsychotic drugs: importance of dopamine receptors for mechanisms of therapeutic actions and side effects," *Pharmacological Reviews*, vol. 53, no. 1, pp. 119–133, 2001.
[36] R. Kaiser, P.-B. Tremblay, F. Klufmöller, I. Roots, and J. Brockmöller, "Relationship between adverse effects of antipsychotic treatment and dopamine D2 receptor polymorphisms in patients with schizophrenia," *Molecular Psychiatry*, vol. 7, no. 7, pp. 695–705, 2002.
[37] N. C. Di Pietro and J. K. Seamans, "Dopamine and serotonin interactions in the prefrontal cortex: insights on antipsychotic drugs and their mechanism of action," *Pharmacopsychiatry*, vol. 40, supplement 1, pp. S27–S33, 2007.
[38] T. Kuroki, N. Nagao, and T. Nakahara, "Neuropharmacology of second-generation antipsychotic drugs: a validity of the serotonin-dopamine hypothesis," *Progress in Brain Research*, vol. 172, pp. 199–212, 2008.
[39] J. Horacek, V. Bubenikova-Valesova, M. Kopecek et al., "Mechanism of action of atypical antipsychotic drugs and the neurobiology of schizophrenia," *CNS Drugs*, vol. 20, no. 5, pp. 389–409, 2006.
[40] G. P. Reynolds, "Receptor mechanisms in the treatment of schizophrenia," *Journal of Psychopharmacology*, vol. 18, no. 3, pp. 340–345, 2004.
[41] S. Miyamoto, G. E. Duncan, C. E. Marx, and J. A. Lieberman, "Treatments for schizophrenia: a critical review of pharmacology and mechanisms of action of antipsychotic drugs," *Molecular Psychiatry*, vol. 10, no. 1, pp. 79–104, 2005.
[42] P. G. Strange, "Antipsychotic drug action: antagonism, inverse agonism or partial agonism," *Trends in Pharmacological Sciences*, vol. 29, no. 6, pp. 314–321, 2008.
[43] A. Newman-Tancredi, D. Cussac, and R. Depoortère, "Neuropharmacological profile of bifeprunox: merits and limitations in comparison with other third-generation antipsychotics," *Current Opinion in Investigational Drugs*, vol. 8, no. 7, pp. 539–554, 2007.
[44] A. D. Stark, S. Jordan, K. A. Allers et al., "Interaction of the novel antipsychotic aripiprazole with 5-HT1A and 5-HT2A receptors: functional receptor-binding and in vivo electrophysiological studies," *Psychopharmacology*, vol. 190, no. 3, pp. 373–382, 2007.
[45] V. Audinot, A. Newman-Tancredi, D. Cussac, and M. J. Millan, "Inverse agonist properties of antipsychotic agents at cloned, human (h) serotonin (5-HT)1B and h5-HT1D receptors," *Neuropsychopharmacology*, vol. 25, no. 3, pp. 410–422, 2001.
[46] A. Dekeyne, J.-M. Rivet, A. Gobert, and M. J. Millan, "Generalization of serotonin (5-HT)1A agonists and the antipsychotics, clozapine, ziprasidone and S16924, but not haloperidol, to the discriminative stimuli elicited by PD128,907 and 7-OH-DPAT," *Neuropharmacology*, vol. 40, no. 7, pp. 899–910, 2001.
[47] A. J. Prus, A. L. Pehrson, S. D. Philibin, J. T. Wood, S. A. Vunck, and J. H. Porter, "The role of M1 muscarinic cholinergic receptors in the discriminative stimulus properties of N-desmethylclozapine and the atypical antipsychotic drug clozapine in rats," *Psychopharmacology*, vol. 203, no. 2, pp. 295–301, 2009.
[48] J. E. Blundell and M. B. Leshem, "The effect of 5 hydroxytryptophan on food intake and on the anorexic action of amphetamine and fenfluramine," *Journal of Pharmacy and Pharmacology*, vol. 27, no. 1, pp. 31–37, 1975.
[49] C. T. Dourish, P. H. Hutson, and G. Curzon, "Characteristics of feeding induced by the serotonin agonist 8-hydroxy-2-(di-n-propylamino) tetralin (8-OH-DPAT)," *Brain Research Bulletin*, vol. 15, no. 4, pp. 377–384, 1985.
[50] S. P. Vickers, K. R. Benwell, R. H. Porter, M. J. Bickerdike, G. A. Kennett, and C. T. Dourish, "Comparative effects of continuous infusion of mCPP, Ro 60-0175 and d-fenfluramine on food intake, water intake, body weight and locomotor activity in rats," *British Journal of Pharmacology*, vol. 130, no. 6, pp. 1305–1314, 2000.
[51] D. W. Bonhaus, K. K. Weinhardt, M. Taylor et al., "RS-102221: a novel high affinity and selective, 5-HT(2C) receptor antagonist," *Neuropharmacology*, vol. 36, no. 4-5, pp. 621–629, 1997.
[52] H. C. Jackson, M. C. Bearham, L. J. Hutchins, S. E. Mazurkiewicz, A. M. Needham, and D. J. Heal, "Investigation of the mechanisms underlying the hypophagic effects of the 5-HT and noradrenaline reuptake inhibitor, sibutramine, in the rat," *British Journal of Pharmacology*, vol. 121, no. 8, pp. 1613–1618, 1997.
[53] P. G. Clifton, M. D. Lee, and C. T. Dourish, "Similarities in the action of Ro 60-0175, a 5-HT(2c) receptor agonist, and d-fenfluramine on feeding patterns in the rat," *Psychopharmacology*, vol. 152, no. 3, pp. 256–267, 2000.
[54] A. Hayashi, M. Suzuki, M. Sasamata, and K. Miyata, "Agonist diversity in 5-HT2C receptor-mediated weight control in rats," *Psychopharmacology*, vol. 178, no. 2-3, pp. 241–249, 2005.
[55] A. Hayashi, R. Sonoda, Y. Kimura et al., "Antiobesity effect of YM348, a novel 5-HT2C receptor agonist, in Zucker rats," *Brain Research*, vol. 1011, no. 2, pp. 221–227, 2004.
[56] L. H. Tecott, L. M. Sun, S. F. Akana et al., "Eating disorder and epilepsy in mice lacking 5-HT(2C) serotonin receptors," *Nature*, vol. 374, no. 6522, pp. 542–546, 1995.
[57] J. P. Redrobe, Y. Dumont, A. Fournier, G. B. Baker, and R. Quirion, "Role of serotonin (5-HT) in the antidepressant-like properties of neuropeptide Y (NPY) in the mouse forced swim test," *Peptides*, vol. 26, no. 8, pp. 1394–1400, 2005.
[58] S. Dryden, Q. Wang, H. M. Frankish, and G. Williams, "Differential effects of the 5-HT(1B/2C) receptor agonist mCPP and the 5-HT(1A) agonist flesinoxan on hypothalamic neuropeptide Y in the rat: evidence that NPY may mediate serotonin's effects on food intake," *Peptides*, vol. 17, no. 6, pp. 943–949, 1996.
[59] D. Abramowski, M. Rigo, D. Duc, D. Hoyer, and M. Staufenbiel, "Localization of the 5-hydroxytryptamine(2C) receptor protein in human and rat brain using specific

antisera," *Neuropharmacology*, vol. 34, no. 12, pp. 1635–1645, 1995.
[60] D. A. Clemett, T. Punhani, M. S. Duxon, T. P. Blackburn, and K. C. F. Fone, "Immunohistochemical localisation of the 5-HT(2C) receptor protein in the rat CNS," *Neuropharmacology*, vol. 39, no. 1, pp. 123–132, 2000.
[61] A. Hay-Schmidt, L. Helboe, and P. J. Larsen, "Leptin receptor immunoreactivity is present in ascending serotonergic and catecholaminergic neurons of the rat," *Neuroendocrinology*, vol. 73, no. 4, pp. 215–226, 2001.
[62] S. L. Kirk, M. Cahir, and G. P. Reynolds, "Clozapine, but not haloperidol, increases neuropeptide Y neuronal expression in the rat hypothalamus," *Journal of Psychopharmacology*, vol. 20, no. 4, pp. 577–579, 2006.
[63] X. Yuan, K. Yamada, S. Ishiyama-Shigemoto, W. Koyama, and K. Nonaka, "Identification of polymorphic loci in the promoter region of the serotonin 5-HT(2c) receptor gene and their association with obesity and Type II diabetes," *Diabetologia*, vol. 43, no. 3, pp. 373–376, 2000.
[64] L. A. Templeman, G. P. Reynolds, B. Arranz, and L. San, "Polymorphisms of the 5-HT2C receptor and leptin genes are associated with antipsychotic drug-induced weight gain in Caucasian subjects with a first-episode psychosis," *Pharmacogenetics and Genomics*, vol. 15, no. 4, pp. 195–200, 2005.
[65] G. P. Reynolds, Z.-J. Zhang, and X.-B. Zhang, "Association of antipsychotic drug-induced weight gain with a 5-HT2C receptor gene polymorphism," *The Lancet*, vol. 359, no. 9323, pp. 2086–2087, 2002.
[66] S. Kapur and G. Remington, "Dopamine D2 receptors and their role in atypical antipsychotic action: still necessary and may even be sufficient," *Biological Psychiatry*, vol. 50, no. 11, pp. 873–883, 2001.
[67] G.-J. Wang, N. D. Volkow, J. Logan et al., "Brain dopamine and obesity," *The Lancet*, vol. 357, no. 9253, pp. 354–357, 2001.
[68] P. Martel and M. Fantino, "Mesolimbic dopaminergic system activity as a function of food reward: a microdialysis study," *Pharmacology Biochemistry and Behavior*, vol. 53, no. 1, pp. 221–226, 1996.
[69] P. S. Grigson and R. C. Twining, "Cocaine-induced suppression of saccharin intake: a model of drug-induced devaluation of natural rewards," *Behavioral Neuroscience*, vol. 116, no. 2, pp. 321–333, 2002.
[70] M. S. Szczypka, M. A. Rainey, D. S. Kim et al., "Feeding behavior in dopamine-deficient mice," *Proceedings of the National Academy of Sciences of the United States of America*, vol. 96, no. 21, pp. 12138–12143, 1999.
[71] E. Anderzhanova, M. Covasa, and A. Hajnal, "Altered basal and stimulated accumbens dopamine release in obese OLETF rats as a function of age and diabetic status," *American Journal of Physiology—Regulatory Integrative and Comparative Physiology*, vol. 293, no. 2, pp. R603–R611, 2007.
[72] M. M. Meguid, S. O. Fetissov, M. Varma et al., "Hypothalamic dopamine and serotonin in the regulation of food intake," *Nutrition*, vol. 16, no. 10, pp. 843–857, 2000.
[73] M. M. Meguid, S. O. Fetissov, V. Blaha, and Z.-J. Yang, "Dopamine and serotonin VMN release is related to feeding status in obese and lean Zucker rats," *NeuroReport*, vol. 11, no. 10, pp. 2069–2072, 2000.
[74] S. O. Fetissov, M. M. Meguid, G. Miyata, G. F. Torelli, and M. Shafiroff, "VMN dopaminergic graft and feeding pattern in obese Zucker rats," *International Journal of Obesity*, vol. 24, no. 3, pp. 376–381, 2000.
[75] S. O. Fetissov, M. M. Meguid, M. Shafiroff, G. Miyata, and G. F. Torelli, "Dopamine in the VMN of the hypothalamus is important for diurnaldistribution of eating in obese male Zucker rats," *Nutrition*, vol. 16, no. 1, pp. 65–66, 2000, Erratum in: Nutrition 2000 May;16(5):343.
[76] S. O. Fetissov, M. M. Meguid, T. Sato, and L.-H. Zhang, "Expression of dopaminergic receptors in the hypothalamus of lean and obese Zucker rats and food intake," *American Journal of Physiology—Regulatory Integrative and Comparative Physiology*, vol. 283, no. 4, pp. R905–R910, 2002.
[77] M. Kalinichev, C. Rourke, A. J. Daniels et al., "Characterisation of olanzapine-induced weight gain and effect of aripiprazole vs olanzapine on body weight and prolactin secretion in female rats," *Psychopharmacology*, vol. 182, no. 2, pp. 220–231, 2005.
[78] A. J. Goudie, J. A. Smith, and J. C. G. Halford, "Characterization of olanzapine-induced weight gain in rats," *Journal of Psychopharmacology*, vol. 16, no. 4, pp. 291–296, 2002.
[79] D. Gothelf, B. Falk, P. Singer et al., "Weight gain associated with increased food intake and low habitual activity levels in male adolescent schizophrenic inpatients treated with olanzapine," *American Journal of Psychiatry*, vol. 159, no. 6, pp. 1055–1057, 2002.
[80] G. N. Thomas, J. A. J. H. Critchley, B. Tomlinson, C. S. Cockram, and J. C. N. Chan, "Relationships between the TaqI polymorphism of the dopamine D2 receptor and blood pressure in hyperglycaemic and normoglycaemic Chinese subjects," *Clinical Endocrinology*, vol. 55, no. 5, pp. 605–611, 2001.
[81] L. H. Epstein, J. L. Jaroni, R. A. Paluch et al., "Dopamine transporter genotype as a risk factor for obesity in African-American smokers," *Obesity Research*, vol. 10, no. 12, pp. 1232–1240, 2002.
[82] G. A. Bray, "Autonomic and endocrine factors in the regulation of energy balance," *Federation Proceedings*, vol. 45, no. 5, pp. 1404–1410, 1986.
[83] J. J. Lima, H. Feng, L. Duckworth et al., "Association analyses of adrenergic receptor polymorphisms with obesity and metabolic alterations," *Metabolism*, vol. 56, no. 6, pp. 757–765, 2007.
[84] K. Yasuda, T. Matsunaga, T. Adachi, N. Aoki, G. Tsujimoto, and K. Tsuda, "Adrenergic receptor polymorphisms and autonomic nervous system function in human obesity," *Trends in Endocrinology and Metabolism*, vol. 17, no. 7, pp. 269–275, 2006.
[85] H. R. Peterson, M. Rothschild, C. R. Weinberg, R. D. Fell, K. R. McLeish, and M. A. Pfeifer, "Body fat and the activity of the autonomic nervous sytem," *New England Journal of Medicine*, vol. 318, no. 17, pp. 1077–1083, 1988.
[86] E. S. Bachman, H. Dhillon, C.-Y. Zhang et al., "βAR signaling required for diet-induced thermogenesis and obesity resistance," *Science*, vol. 297, no. 5582, pp. 843–845, 2002.
[87] E. S. Bachman, T. G. Hampton, H. Dhillon et al., "The metabolic and cardiovascular effects of hyperthyroidism are largely independent of β-adrenergic stimulation," *Endocrinology*, vol. 145, no. 6, pp. 2767–2774, 2004.
[88] D. B. Allison and M. Heo, "Meta-analysis of linkage data under worst-case conditions: a demonstration using the human OB region," *Genetics*, vol. 148, no. 2, pp. 859–865, 1998.
[89] D. B. Allison, M. Heo, M. S. Faith, and A. Pietrobelli, "Meta-analysis of the association of the Trp64Arg polymorphism in the $\beta 3$ adrenergic receptor with body mass index,"

International Journal of Obesity, vol. 22, no. 6, pp. 559–566, 1998.
[90] T. Fujisawa, H. Ikegami, Y. Kawaguchi, and T. Ogihara, "Meta-analysis of the association of Trp64 arg polymorphism of β3- adrenergic receptor gene with body mass index," *Journal of Clinical Endocrinology and Metabolism*, vol. 83, no. 7, pp. 2441–2444, 1998.
[91] J. Hoffstedt, O. Poirier, A. Thörne et al., "Polymorphism of the human beta3-adrenoceptor gene forms a well-conserved haplotype that is associated with moderate obesity and altered receptor function," *Diabetes*, vol. 48, no. 1, pp. 203–205, 1999.
[92] P. Arner and J. Hoffstedt, "Adrenoceptor genes in human obesity," *Journal of Internal Medicine*, vol. 245, no. 6, pp. 667–672, 1999.
[93] N. P. Endo, H. Yanagi, C. Hirano, H. Hamaguchi, S. Tsuchiya, and S. Tomura, "Association of Trp64Arg polymorphism of the beta3-adrenergic receptor gene and no association of Gln223Arg polymorphism of the leptin receptor gene in Japanese schoolchildren with obesity," *International Journal of Obesity and Related Metabolic Disorders*, vol. 24, no. 4, pp. 443–449, 2000.
[94] N. P. Thomas, B. Tomlinson, J. C. Chan, R. P. Young, and J. A. Critchley, "The Trp64Arg polymorphism of the beta3-adrenergic receptor gene and obesity in Chinese subjects with components of the metabolic syndrome," *International Journal of Obesity and Related Metabolic Disorders*, vol. 24, no. 5, pp. 545–551, 2000.
[95] T. Oizumi, M. Daimon, T. Saitoh et al., "Genotype Arg/Arg, but not Trp/Arg, of the Trp64Arg polymorphism of the beta(3)-adrenergic receptor is associated with type 2 diabetes and obesity in a large Japanese sample," *Diabetes Care*, vol. 24, no. 9, pp. 1579–1583, 2001.
[96] P. Strazzullo, R. Iacone, A. Siani et al., "Relationship of the Trp64Arg polymorphism of the beta3-adrenoceptor gene to central adiposity and high blood pressure: interaction with age. Cross-sectional and longitudinal findings of the Olivetti prospective heart study," *Journal of Hypertension*, vol. 19, no. 3, pp. 399–406, 2001.
[97] V. S. Basile, M. Masellis, R. S. McIntyre, H. Y. Meltzer, J. A. Lieberman, and J. L. Kennedy, "Genetic dissection of atypical antipsychotic-induced weight gain: novel preliminary data on the pharmacogenetic puzzle," *Journal of Clinical Psychiatry*, vol. 62, supplement 23, pp. 45–66, 2001.
[98] C. A. Wilmot, A. C. Sullivan, and B. E. Levin, "Effects of diet and obesity on brain α1- and α2-noradrenergic receptors in the rat," *Brain Research*, vol. 453, no. 1-2, pp. 157–166, 1988.
[99] K. Ohashi, T. Hamamura, Y. Lee, Y. Fujiwara, H. Suzuki, and S. Kuroda, "Clozapine- and olanzapine-induced Fos expression in the rat medial prefrontal cortex is mediated by β-adrenoceptors," *Neuropsychopharmacology*, vol. 23, no. 2, pp. 162–169, 2000.
[100] A. Matsui-Sakata, H. Ohtani, and Y. Sawada, "Receptor occupancy-based analysis of the contributions of various receptors to antipsychotics-induced weight gain and diabetes mellitus," *Drug Metabolism and Pharmacokinetics*, vol. 20, no. 5, pp. 368–378, 2005.
[101] T. Masaki, H. Yoshimatsu, S. Chiba, T. Watanabe, and T. Sakata, "Targeted disruption of histamine H1-receptor attenuates regulatory effects of leptin on feeding, adiposity, and UCP family in mice," *Diabetes*, vol. 50, no. 2, pp. 385–391, 2001.
[102] T. Masaki, S. Chiba, T. Yasuda et al., "Involvement of hypothalamic histamine H1 receptor in the regulation of feeding rhythm and obesity," *Diabetes*, vol. 53, no. 9, pp. 2250–2260, 2004.
[103] P. Seeman, J. Schwarz, J.-F. Chen et al., "Psychosis pathways converge via D2High dopamine receptors," *Synapse*, vol. 60, no. 4, pp. 319–346, 2006.
[104] E. A. Jørgensen, T. W. Vogelsang, U. Knigge, T. Watanabe, J. Warberg, and A. Kjaer, "Increased susceptibility to diet-induced obesity in histamine-deficient mice," *Neuroendocrinology*, vol. 83, no. 5-6, pp. 289–294, 2006.
[105] T. Ishizuka, S. Nomura, H. Hosoda, K. Kangawa, T. Watanabe, and A. Yamatodani, "A role of the histaminergic system for the control of feeding by orexigenic peptides," *Physiology and Behavior*, vol. 89, no. 3, pp. 295–300, 2006.
[106] J. Bugajski and Z. Janusz, "Lipolytic responses induced by intracerebroventricular administration of histamine in the rat," *Agents and Actions*, vol. 11, no. 1-2, pp. 147–150, 1981.
[107] T. Sakata, Y. Tamari, M. Kang, and H. Yoshimatsu, "2-Deoxy-D-glucose suppresses food intake through activation of hypothalamic histamine in rats," *American Journal of Physiology—Regulatory Integrative and Comparative Physiology*, vol. 267, part 2, pp. R616–R618, 1994.
[108] M. J. Arranz, J. Munro, J. Birkett et al., "Pharmacogenetic prediction of clozapine response," *The Lancet*, vol. 355, no. 9215, pp. 1615–1616, 2000.
[109] D. Mancama, M. J. Arranz, J. Munro et al., "Investigation of promoter variants of the histamine 1 and 2 receptors in schizophrenia and clozapine response," *Neuroscience Letters*, vol. 333, no. 3, pp. 207–211, 2002.
[110] C.-J. Hong, C.-H. Lin, Y. W.-Y. Yu, S.-C. Chang, S.-Y. Wang, and S.-J. Tsai, "Genetic variant of the histamine-1 receptor (glu349asp) and body weight change during clozapine treatment," *Psychiatric Genetics*, vol. 12, no. 3, pp. 169–171, 2002.
[111] C. Deng, G. L. Weston-Green, M. Han, and X. F. Huang, "Olanzapine treatment decreases the density of muscarinic M2 receptors in the dorsal vagal complex of rats," *Progress in Neuro-Psychopharmacology and Biological Psychiatry*, vol. 31, no. 4, pp. 915–920, 2007.
[112] G. J. Schwartz, "The role of gastrointestinal vagal afferents in the control of food intake: current prospects," *Nutrition*, vol. 16, no. 10, pp. 866–873, 2000.
[113] H. J. Grill, M. W. Schwartz, J. M. Kaplan, J. S. Foxhall, J. Breininger, and D. G. Baskin, "Evidence that the caudal brainstem is a target for the inhibitory effect of leptin on food intake," *Endocrinology*, vol. 143, no. 1, pp. 239–246, 2002.
[114] A. Matsui-Sakata, H. Ohtani, and Y. Sawada, "Receptor occupancy-based analysis of the contributions of variousreceptors to antipsychotics-induced weight gain and diabetes mellitus," *Drug Metabolism and Pharmacokinetics*, vol. 20, no. 5, pp. 368–378, 2005.
[115] D. Jesudason and G. Wittert, "Endocannabinoid system in food intake and metabolic regulation," *Current Opinion in Lipidology*, vol. 19, no. 4, pp. 344–348, 2008.
[116] S. P. Vickers and G. A. Kennett, "Cannabinoids and the regulation of ingestive behaviour," *Current Drug Targets*, vol. 6, no. 2, pp. 215–223, 2005.
[117] T. J. De Vries and A. N. M. Schoffelmeer, "Cannabinoid CB1 receptors control conditioned drug seeking," *Trends in Pharmacological Sciences*, vol. 26, no. 8, pp. 420–426, 2005.
[118] Y. Avraham, A. B. Menachem, A. Okun et al., "Effects of the endocannabinoid noladin ether on body weight, food consumption, locomotor activity, and cognitive index in mice," *Brain Research Bulletin*, vol. 65, no. 2, pp. 117–123, 2005.

[119] J. A. López-Moreno, G. González-Cuevas, G. Moreno, and M. Navarro, "The pharmacology of the endocannabinoid system: functional and structural interactions with other neurotransmitter systems and their repercussions in behavioral addiction," *Addiction Biology*, vol. 13, no. 2, pp. 160–187, 2008.

[120] M. Bjursell, A.-K. Gerdin, C. J. Lelliott et al., "Acutely reduced locomotor activity is a major contributor to Western diet-induced obesity in mice," *American Journal of Physiology—Endocrinology and Metabolism*, vol. 294, no. 2, pp. E251–E260, 2008.

[121] K. M. Gamber, H. Macarthur, and T. C. Westfall, "Cannabinoids augment the release of neuropeptide Y in the rat hypothalamus," *Neuropharmacology*, vol. 49, no. 5, pp. 646–652, 2005.

[122] I. Crespo, R. Gómez de Heras, F. Rodríguez de Fonseca, and M. Navarro, "Pretreatment with subeffective doses of Rimonabant attenuates orexigenic actions of orexin A-hypocretin 1," *Neuropharmacology*, vol. 54, no. 1, pp. 219–225, 2008.

[123] V. Di Marzo, S. K. Goparaju, L. Wang et al., "Leptin-regulated endocannabinoids are involved in maintaining food intake," *Nature*, vol. 410, no. 6830, pp. 822–825, 2001.

[124] S. Arora and A. , "Role of neuropeptides in appetite regulation and obesity—a review," *Neuropeptides*, vol. 40, no. 6, pp. 375–401, 2006.

[125] D. Osei-Hyiaman, M. Depetrillo, J. Harvey-White et al., "Cocaine- and amphetamine-related transcript is involved in the orexigenic effect of endogenous anandamide," *Neuroendocrinology*, vol. 81, no. 4, pp. 273–282, 2005.

[126] M. P. Viveros, F. R. de Fonseca, F. J. Bermudez-Silva, and J. M. McPartland, "Critical role of the endocannabinoid system in the regulation of food intake and energy metabolism, with phylogenetic, developmental, and pathophysiological implications," *Endocrine, Metabolic and Immune Disorders—Drug Targets*, vol. 8, no. 3, pp. 220–230, 2008.

[127] K. Weston-Green, X.-F. Huang, M. Han, and C. Deng, "The effects of antipsychotics on the density of cannabinoid receptors in the dorsal vagal complex of rats: implications for olanzapine-induced weight gain," *International Journal of Neuropsychopharmacology*, vol. 11, no. 6, pp. 827–835, 2008.

[128] D. Naber and M. Lambert, "Aripiprazole: a new atypical antipsychotic with a different pharmacological mechanism.," *Progress in Neuro-Psychopharmacology and Biological Psychiatry*, vol. 28, no. 8, pp. 1213–1219, 2004.

[129] R. B. Zipursky, H. Gu, A. I. Green et al., "Course and predictors of weight gain in people with first-episode psychosis treated with olanzapine or haloperidol," *British Journal of Psychiatry*, vol. 187, pp. 535–543, 2005.

[130] F. M. Theisen, M. Haberhausen, M. A. Firnges et al., "No evidence for binding of clozapine, olanzapine and/or haloperidol to selected receptors involved in body weight regulation," *Pharmacogenomics Journal*, vol. 7, no. 4, pp. 275–281, 2007.

[131] S. C. Woods, M. Chavez, C. R. Park et al., "The evaluation of insulin as a metabolic signal influencing behavior via the brain," *Neuroscience and Biobehavioral Reviews*, vol. 20, no. 1, pp. 139–144, 1996.

[132] R. Cancello, A. Tounian, C. Poitou, and K. Clément, "Adiposity signals, genetic and body weight regulation in humans," *Diabetes and Metabolism*, vol. 30, no. 3 I, pp. 215–227, 2004.

[133] M. Van Houten and B. I. Posner, "Insulin binds to brain blood vessels in vivo," *Nature*, vol. 282, no. 5739, pp. 623–625, 1979.

[134] D. P. Figlewicz Lattemann and S. C. Benoit, "Insulin, leptin, and food reward: update 2008," *American Journal of Physiology—Regulatory Integrative and Comparative Physiology*, vol. 296, no. 1, pp. R9–R19, 2009.

[135] J. H. Peters, S. M. Simasko, and R. C. Ritter, "Modulation of vagal afferent excitation and reduction of food intake by leptin and cholecystokinin," *Physiology and Behavior*, vol. 89, no. 4, pp. 477–485, 2006.

[136] S. Arora and A. , "Role of neuropeptides in appetite regulation and obesity—a review," *Neuropeptides*, vol. 40, no. 6, pp. 375–401, 2006.

[137] E. Valassi, M. Scacchi, and F. Cavagnini, "Neuroendocrine control of food intakec," *Nutrition, Metabolism & Cardiovascular Diseases*, vol. 18, no. 2, pp. 158–168, 2008.

[138] R. S. Ahima, Y. Qi, and N. S. Singhal, "Chapter 9: adipokines that link obesity and diabetes to the hypothalamus," *Progress in Brain Research*, vol. 153, pp. 155–174, 2006.

[139] T. Sakurai, A. Amemiya, M. Ishii et al., "Orexins and orexin receptors: a family of hypothalamic neuropeptides and G protein-coupled receptors that regulate feeding behavior," *Cell*, vol. 92, no. 4, pp. 573–585, 1998.

[140] L. De Lecea, T. S. Kilduff, C. Peyron et al., "The hypocretins: hypothalamus-specific peptides with neuroexcitatory activity," *Proceedings of the National Academy of Sciences of the United States of America*, vol. 95, no. 1, pp. 322–327, 1998.

[141] C. Peyron, D. K. Tighe, A. N. Van Den Pol et al., "Neurons containing hypocretin (orexin) project to multiple neuronal systems," *Journal of Neuroscience*, vol. 18, no. 23, pp. 9996–10015, 1998.

[142] Y. Date, Y. Ueta, H. Yamashita et al., "Orexins, orexigenic hypothalamic peptides, interact with autonomic, neuroendocrine and neuroregulatory systems," *Proceedings of the National Academy of Sciences of the United States of America*, vol. 96, no. 2, pp. 748–753, 1999.

[143] J. T. Willie, R. M. Chemelli, C. M. Sinton, and M. Yanagisawa, "To eat or to sleep? Orexin in the regulation of feeding and wakefulness," *Annual Review of Neuroscience*, vol. 24, pp. 429–458, 2001.

[144] J. G. Sutcliffe and L. De Lecea, "The hypocretins: excitatory neuromodulatory peptides for multiple homeostatic systems, including sleep and feeding," *Journal of Neuroscience Research*, vol. 62, no. 2, pp. 161–168, 2000.

[145] C. M. B. Edwards, S. Abusnana, D. Sunter, K. G. Murphy, M. A. Ghatei, and S. R. Bloom, "The effect of the orexins on food intake: comparison with neuropeptide Y, melanin-concentrating hormone and galanin," *Journal of Endocrinology*, vol. 160, no. 3, pp. R7–R12, 1999.

[146] J. Fadel, M. Bubser, and A. Y. Deutch, "Differential activation of orexin neurons by antipsychotic drugs associated with weight gain," *Journal of Neuroscience*, vol. 22, no. 15, pp. 6742–6746, 2002.

[147] S. R. Sesack and B. S. Bunney, "Pharmacological characterization of the receptor mediating electrophysiological responses to dopamine in the rat medial prefrontal cortex: a microiontophoretic study," *Journal of Pharmacology and Experimental Therapeutics*, vol. 248, no. 3, pp. 1323–1333, 1989.

[148] L. Heimer, D. S. Zahm, L. Churchill, P. W. Kalivas, and C. Wohltmann, "Specificity in the projection patterns of accumbal core and shell in the rat," *Neuroscience*, vol. 41, no. 1, pp. 89–125, 1991.

[149] P. C. Holland and G. D. Petrovich, "A neural systems analysis of the potentiation of feeding by conditioned stimuli," *Physiology & Behavior*, vol. 86, no. 5, pp. 747–761, 2005.

[150] M. F. Barbano, M. Le Saux, and M. Cador, "Involvement of dopamine and opioids in the motivation to eat: influence of palatability, homeostatic state, and behavioral paradigms," *Psychopharmacology*, vol. 203, no. 3, pp. 475–487, 2009.

[151] K. C. Berridge and E. S. Valenstein, "What psychological process mediates feeding evoked by electrical stimulation of the lateral hypothalamus?" *Behavioral Neuroscience*, vol. 105, no. 1, pp. 3–14, 1991.

[152] M. Murashita, I. Kusumi, T. Inoue et al., "Olanzapine increases plasma ghrelin level in patients with schizophrenia," *Psychoneuroendocrinology*, vol. 30, no. 1, pp. 106–110, 2005.

[153] B. Pouzet, T. Mow, M. Kreilgaard, and S. Velschow, "Chronic treatment with antipsychotics in rats as a model for antipsychotic-induced weight gain in human," *Pharmacology Biochemistry and Behavior*, vol. 75, no. 1, pp. 133–140, 2003.

[154] M. D. Lee and P. G. Clifton, "Meal patterns of free feeding rats treated with clozapine, olanzapine, or haloperidol," *Pharmacology Biochemistry and Behavior*, vol. 71, no. 1-2, pp. 147–154, 2002.

[155] M. Ota, K. Mori, A. Nakashima et al., "Peripheral injection of risperidone, an atypical antipsychotic, alters the bodyweight gain of rats," *Clinical and Experimental Pharmacology and Physiology*, vol. 29, no. 11, pp. 980–989, 2002.

[156] S. B. Schleimer, G. A. R. Johnston, and J. M. Henderson, "Novel oral drug administration in an animal model of neuroleptic therapy," *Journal of Neuroscience Methods*, vol. 146, no. 2, pp. 159–164, 2005.

[157] J. W. Newcomer, "Metabolic considerations in the use of antipsychotic medications: a review of recent evidence," *Journal of Clinical Psychiatry*, vol. 68, no. 1, pp. 20–27, 2007.

[158] A. N. Elias and H. Hofflich, "Abnormalities in Glucose Metabolism in Patients with Schizophrenia Treated with Atypical Antipsychotic Medications," *American Journal of Medicine*, vol. 121, no. 2, pp. 98–104, 2008.

[159] D. C. Henderson, E. Cagliero, P. M. Copeland et al., "Elevated hemoglobin A1c as a possible indicator of diabetes mellitus and diabetic ketoacidosis in schizophrenia patients receiving atypical antipsychotics," *Journal of Clinical Psychiatry*, vol. 68, no. 4, pp. 533–541, 2007.

[160] M. Ader, S. P. Kim, K. J. Catalano et al., "Metabolic dysregulation with atypical antipsychotics occurs in the absence of underlying disease: a placebo-controlled study of olanzapine and risperidone in dogs," *Diabetes*, vol. 54, no. 3, pp. 862–871, 2005.

[161] H. Y. Meltzer, E. Perry, and K. Jayathilake, "Clozapine-induced weight gain predicts improvement in psychopathology," *Schizophrenia Research*, vol. 59, no. 1, pp. 19–27, 2003.

[162] Z. Zhao, H. Ksiezak-Reding, S. Riggio, V. Haroutunian, and G. M. Pasinetti, "Insulin receptor deficits in schizophrenia and in cellular and animal models of insulin receptor dysfunction," *Schizophrenia Research*, vol. 84, no. 1, pp. 1–14, 2006.

[163] D. S. Dwyer, H. B. Pinkofsky, Y. Liu, and R. J. Bradley, "Attachment of PC12 cells to adhesion substratum induces the accumulation of glucose transporters (GLUTs) and stimulates glucose metabolism," *Neurochemical Research*, vol. 23, no. 8, pp. 1107–1116, 1998.

[164] X.-H. Lu and D. S. Dwyer, "Second-generation antipsychotic drugs, olanzapine, quetiapine, and clozapine enhance neurite outgrowth in PC12 cells via PI3K/AKT, ERK, and pertussis toxin-sensitive pathways," *Journal of Molecular Neuroscience*, vol. 27, no. 1, pp. 43–64, 2005.

[165] L. L. Citrome, R. I.G. Holt, W. M. Zachry et al., "Risk of treatment-emergent diabetes mellitus in patients receiving antipsychotics," *Annals of Pharmacotherapy*, vol. 41, no. 10, pp. 1593–1603, 2007.

19

Sex Differences in Facial, Prosodic, and Social Context Emotional Recognition in Early-Onset Schizophrenia

Julieta Ramos-Loyo,[1] Leonor Mora-Reynoso,[1]
Luis Miguel Sánchez-Loyo,[2] and Virginia Medina-Hernández[3]

[1] *Instituto de Neurociencias, CUCBA, Universidad de Guadalajara, 44130 Guadalajara, JAL, Mexico*
[2] *Departamento de Neurociencias, CUCS, Universidad de Guadalajara, 44130 Guadalajara, JAL, Mexico*
[3] *Centro Comunitario de Salud Mental No. 1, Guadalajara, 45150 Zapopan, JAL, Mexico*

Correspondence should be addressed to Julieta Ramos-Loyo, jramos@cencar.udg.mx

Academic Editor: Susana Ochoa

The purpose of the present study was to determine sex differences in facial, prosodic, and social context emotional recognition in schizophrenia (SCH). Thirty-eight patients (SCH, 20 females) and 38 healthy controls (CON, 20 females) participated in the study. Clinical scales (BPRS and PANSS) and an Affective States Scale were applied, as well as tasks to evaluate facial, prosodic, and within a social context emotional recognition. SCH showed lower accuracy and longer response times than CON, but no significant sex differences were observed in either facial or prosody recognition. In social context emotions, however, females showed higher empathy than males with respect to happiness in both groups. SCH reported being more identified with sad films than CON and females more with fear than males. The results of this study confirm the deficits of emotional recognition in male and female patients with schizophrenia compared to healthy subjects. Sex differences were detected in relation to social context emotions and facial and prosodic recognition depending on age.

1. Introduction

Sex differences in schizophrenia regarding to clinical, neuroanatomical, cognitive, emotional and social domains have been reported (i.e.,[1–6]). With respect to psychopathological characteristics, male patients suffer more acute symptoms than females, with higher prevalence of paranoid symptoms, aggression, and antisocial behavior [7]. The latter, on the other hand, show more affective disorders, such as anxiety and depression [8], as well as sudden changes in appetite, weight, and sexual activity [9]. Schizophrenic females also show a less deteriorative course during the illness [10], a better premorbid adjustment in the social, sexual, and marital domains, and improved outcomes with a higher index of spontaneous remissions and better treatment response than males, probably due to the protector effects of sexual hormones [11–13]. Other authors have pointed out that females are more capable of living independently, while male patients are more used to living in sheltered houses [13]. Furthermore, males present a higher number of hospitalizations and greater deterioration; thus, their outcomes and social reintegration tend to be unfavourable [7].

Some studies have reported sex differences in cognitive functions in schizophrenia [3, 14–16]. Results of these studies suggest that females perform better than males in executive functions, visual working memory, verbal memory, and learning. In this regard, schizophrenic females may be less vulnerable to cognitive deficits than their males counterparts although the former still show lower performance than healthy controls on different tasks [6, 17–20]. However, studies regarding sex differences in affect recognition in cases of schizophrenia are scarce. One showed that schizophrenic females outperform males when asked to label negative facial emotions, a skill that may contribute to improving their abilities in social life [21]. Weiss et al. [22] found that males with schizophrenia tend to interpret neutral faces as anger, while females interpret them as sadness. In addition, females outperform schizophrenic males in emotional prosodic and semantic processing [23]. In another study, an effect of sex was found in both facial and prosodic emotional recognition performance, where schizophrenic females were observed to be more accurate than men though they still presented difficulties in these processes when compared to control subjects [24].

Regarding sex differences in affect recognition abilities in healthy subjects, several studies have revealed that females generally outperform males, especially for negative facial emotional expressions [25–31]. Sex differences in emotional prosody have also been reported, showing that females can integrate both semantic content and emotional intonation information more quickly than males [32].

Results from various studies that included males exclusively or males and females together have demonstrated that schizophrenics show impairments in recognizing, expressing and regulating emotions [33–39]. Impairments in facial emotional recognition in schizophrenic patients are present from early stages of the illness and are greater for negative emotional stimuli, especially for fear and disgust [34, 40–42]. Difficulties in prosodic recognition have also been described in schizophrenia mainly for sadness and fear [23, 34, 36, 38, 43]. However, few studies have explored emotional recognition deficits in schizophrenic patients within social contexts. Studying impairments in emotional recognition in all modalities is relevant since this element contributes to abnormal social functioning, mainly in patients with a predominancy of negative symptoms [44, 45].

The question here is whether schizophrenic patients present similar sex differences for emotional recognition to those found in healthy subjects, based on an assessment of three modalities: facial, prosodic, and within a social context. Studying these three different modalities in the same subjects will make it possible to ascertain whether recognition disorders are similar in visual and prosodic recognition, as a general effect on emotion, and if they are present in a more ecological and complex modality, that is, a social context in which people express similar or different emotions in a dynamic behavioural pattern. It is possible than it in social contexts, the disorders observed in specific visual or auditory modalities could be compensated to recognize an expressed emotion, based on the conjunction of different sensory information. Furthermore, this approach will be able to evaluate other socioemotional aspects, such as the empathy level experienced by an observer while watching a film. Given the foregoing, one would expect that schizophrenic patients would show a poorer performance than healthy controls in emotional recognition tasks and, moreover, that females would show a greater preservation of emotional recognition than men.

Based on the findings reviewed above, the aim of the present study was to determine the existence of sex differences in facial, prosodic, and social context emotional recognition in patients with schizophrenia when compared to healthy controls.

2. Methods

2.1. Participants. Schizophrenic patients were recruited from the Guadalajara Mental Health Center of the Mexican Social Security Institute (IMSS). Thirty-eight paranoid schizophrenic patients (SCH 20 females and 18 males) with recent onset illness (from 6 months to 4 years) and 38 healthy control subjects (CON, 20 females and 18 males) matched with the patients for age (18–45 years) and years of formal education (minimum 9 years) met the inclusion criteria. Patients who had been submitted to electroconvulsive therapy within the previous 6 months, or had presented severe psychiatric comorbidity, were not included in the sample. All subjects were right-handed, according to Annette's test [46] but showed no neurological or chronic-degenerative disorders, addictions, carcinoma, diabetes, or infections.

In addition, the female menstrual cycle was considered when programming the evaluations, such that they were distributed similarly across the different menstrual phases. This was done in order to avoid hormonal effects on emotional recognition, since some authors [47] have found that females perform more accurately in recognizing emotional expressions of fear during the preovulatory phase compared to the menstrual phase. Also, better recognition of emotions was found in the follicular phase, in association with stronger amygdala and orbitofrontal activation in females [48, 49].

Patients were clinically assessed in two moments by an experienced psychiatrist, taking into account their clinical medical history and the international DSM-IV criteria [50]. Symptoms were rated by means of the Brief Psychiatric Rating Scale (BPRS, [51]) and the Positive and Negative Symptom Scale (PANSS, [52]).

The study was approved by the Ethic Committees of the IMSS and the Neuroscience Institute of the University of Guadalajara and was conducted according to Code of Ethics of the World Medical Association (Declaration of Helsinki). All subjects gave their informed consent before participating in the study.

2.2. Procedure. Patients arrived at the hospital in acute stage. In that moment, the first psychopathological assessment was conducted. The second psychopathological assesment was carried out during a remission stage under neuroleptic treatment. In this second session, the Affective States Scale was applied. This scale was also applied to control subjects. Subsequently, facial, prosodic, and social context emotional tasks were counterbalanced administered to the participants.

2.2.1. Clinical Assessment. The first psychopathological assessment was conducted when patients arrived to the psychiatric hospital in acute condition without medication for their first admission due to diagnoses of schizophrenia. Thereafter, patients remained at the hospital for at least 15 days. The second assesment was conducted after approximately 15 days of hospitalization (females $X = 14.25 \pm 4.12$, males $X = 15.33 \pm 5.58$), once positive symptom were remitted under pharmacological treatment with typical (haloperidol: 15 mg/day) or atypical (olanzapine: 10 mg/day) neuroleptics.

With the two completed assessments, it was possible to test whether there were clinical sex differences in both the acute phase and/or after a similar neuroleptic treatment with an equal dosage for all patients. A structured clinical interview was also applied to all subjects, as well as the laterality test [46] to confirm right handedness. These procedures were performed by one of the researchers, who is an experienced psychiatrist (VMH). Only the BPRS and PANSS were applied in both sessions.

2.2.2. Affective States Scale. The Affective States Scale was applied to controls and patients, in order to determine their basal emotional state, as this could influence their performance on the emotional recognition tasks. At the beginning of the evaluation session, participants were asked to judge their personal emotional state on a continuous linear scale ranking from 0 to 10 cm in two subscales: (1) pleasant: animated, inspired, enchanted, comfortable, happy, pleased, cheerful, and calm and; (2) unpleasant: uncomfortable, angry, sad, afflicted, frightened, tense, annoyed, and worried [53].

2.2.3. Facial Emotional Recognition Task. This test has been used previously in other studies, both in schizophrenic patients and epileptic patients [36, 54]. Facial emotional expressions of 8 models (4 males and 4 females) from Ekman and Friesen [55] were presented on a computer screen (15 in). Each model portrayed six basic emotions (happiness, sadness, anger, fear, surprise, and disgust) and one emotionally neutral expression. Participants were seated at a distance of 60 cm from the computer screen. They were instructed to press a key and, at the same time, to label the emotion that each stimulus represented, performing it as precisely and quickly as possible. Presentation of each one of the 56 stimuli lasted until the subject responded with a maximum of 2000 ms. A list with the possible emotional expressions represented in the photographs was shown to them previously, and it was confirmed that they had understood the instructions completely. Also rehearsal essays were performed before the task. Response times were recorded on a computer at the moment the subjects pressed the key. The answers were written down by hand by the experimenter.

A facial identity recognition task was presented. The goal of this task was to control for possible difficulties in face configuration processing in schizophrenics that may affect emotional recognition. Participants were asked to press a key when a previously indicated person appeared (28%) on the computer screen, with no regard for the emotional expression. Presentation of each of the 56 stimuli lasted until the subject responded with a maximum of 2000 ms. number of correct responses and response times were recorded in the computer.

2.2.4. Prosodic Emotional Recognition Task. This test consisted of 32 sentences in Spanish presented on a computer. The semantic content of the sentences was emotionally neutral but were spoken with different affective prosody—happy, sad, angry, and fear—by two professional radio announcers, one male and one female (e.g., "The table is square"; "The moon is a satellite"). The stimuli with different emotional intonation were presented randomly. Participants were asked to label the emotional tone expressed in the sentences, given a list with the four possible emotions. Answers were recorded by the experimenter to determine the number of correct responses. This task has been used in other experiments, and tested previously in a normal sample [36, 54].

2.2.5. Social Context Emotional Recognition Task. Four films with an approximate duration of 2 min were presented. All in Spanish, without music; they included several characters, and the dialogues represented situations for each one of the four aforementioned emotions (happiness, sadness, anger and fear). The films had been used in a previous study [36] and were presented randomly on a computer screen (15 in). Each participant was seated at a distance of 60 cm while watching the stimuli. At the end of each film, participants were asked to respond to a questionnaire to determine their ability to describe the scene, identify the emotions expressed by the principal and secondary characters, and indicate their perception of the intensity with which the characters experienced that emotion. In addition, participants were asked to indicate their emotional reaction when watching each film and the intensity they experienced (empathy). To evaluate the emotional intensity of the characters and that experienced by participants, an emotional scale, similar to the Emotional States Scale mentioned above, was applied to the participants. It consisted of a continuous line 10 cm long, on which they had to make a mark; the lowest intensity corresponded to the extreme left (0 cm) and the greatest intensity to the extreme right (10 cm).

2.2.6. Statistical Analysis. In order to measure sex differences in clinical symptomatology, one-way Analysis of Variance (ANOVA) test was applied for BPRS and PANSS. Two-way ANOVAs for independent groups were used in order to compare the data obtained from SCH and CON groups (Factor A) as a function of sex (Factor B) for: (a) sociodemographic data (b) Affective States Scale scores: for pleasant and unpleasant (c) identity and (d) social context emotional recognition: attribution of intensity to emotional expression of the principal character and empathy level experienced by the participant. A three-way ANOVA—A: groups; B: sexes; C: emotions—for mixed designs was applied to analyze the facial emotional recognition task: number of correct responses and response times and prosodic recognition task: number of correct responses. In order to assess the effect of age on facial and prosodic recognition, an Analysis of Covariance (ANCOVA) was applied, since females were older than males. Significant levels were adjusted using the Greenhouse-Geisser epsilon correction for factors, and corrected P values are reported. The percentage of congruent responses with that represented in the scene, identification with the principal character, and association of the scenes with their personal life were evaluated by means of a chi square test.

Table 1: Sociodemographic characteristics from healthy controls (CON) and schizophrenic patients (SCH).

	CON				SCH			
	Females (n = 20)		Males (n = 18)		Females (n = 20)		Males (n = 18)	
	$\overline{X}$	SD	$\overline{X}$	SD	$\overline{X}$	SD	$\overline{X}$	SD
Age (years)	34.20	±9.46	26.06	±7.16	36.15	±7.01	27.06	±7.22
Formal education (years)	13.87	±2.62	13.88	±2.83	13.87	±2.87	12.36	±2.58
	% Subjects							
Single	30%		55%		35%		61%	
Married or stable partner	60%		33%		40%		33%	
Widow	0%		0%		5%		0%	
Divorced/separated	10%		11%		20%		6%	
Occupation	% Subjects							
Student	25%		33%		0%		22%	
Employee	5%		50%		45%		50%	
Professional	10%		17%		15%		6%	
House worker	55%		0%		30%		0%	
None	0%		0%		5%		22%	
Others (commerce)	5%		0%		5%		0%	

Table 2: Clinical characteristics of the schizophrenic patients; BPRS and PANSS were applied twice, first in the acute phase (1) and later in the remission phase (2).

	Females (n = 20)		Males (n = 18)	
	$\overline{X}$	DS	$\overline{X}$	DS
Number of Hospitalizations	1.65	±1.18	1.44	±.61
Duration of illness (months)	22.50	±16.87	24.44	±13.57
Days of Hospitalization at the time of evaluation	14.25	±4.12	15.33	±5.58
BPRS (1)	44.89	±16.46	45.94	±7.32
PANSS positive (1)	24.00	±7.10	25.66	±5.96
PANSS negative (1)	21.52	±7.16	23.33	±7.06
PANSS general (1)	36.16	±9.48	37.16	±6.4
PANSS global (1)	81.75	±19.40	86.16	±10.6
BPRS (2)	24.52	±7.61	25.29	±8.04
PANSS positive (2)	8.36	±4.25	9.56	±2.92
PANSS negative (2)*	11.47	±5.18	14.93	±3.67
PANSS general (2)	20.42	±8.96	22.00	±2.36
PANSS global (2)	44.73	±9.56	47.35	±7.94

* $P < .03$.

3. Results

3.1. Sociodemographic Data. Age was significantly different between sexes ($F(1,72) = 23.10$, $P < .001$). Schizophrenic females (SCHf) were about 8 years older than males (SCHm) and, as a result, the matched control females (CONf) compared to males (CONm). No differences were found in years of formal education (Table 1).

3.2. Clinical Characteristics. With regard to the initial psychopathological assessment, no differences either in BPRS or PANSS were found in the patient group. In the second assessment, SCHm showed higher scores than SCHf only on the Negative Symptoms Subscale ($F(1,34) = 2.23$, $P < .03$). (see Table 2).

There were no differences between SCHf and SCHm in the number of previous hospitalizations, duration of illness, number of days between the initial and second evaluations, or in the type of medication. Two SCHf and two SCHm were medicated with 15 mg/day of haloperidol (250 chlorpromazine equivalent) while 18 SCHf and 16 SCHm were taking 10 mg/day of olanzapine (200 chlorpromazine equivalent).

3.3. Affective States Scale. There were no significant differences between SCH and CON, or between males and females, on the pleasant affective states subscale ($F(1,72) = 0.06$, $P < .79$); however, the SCH group reported higher unpleasant affectivity than CON ($F(1,72) = 16.53$, $P < .001$), both in the case of males and females at the beginning of the assessment session. No sex differences were observed. (Figure 1).

3.4. Emotional Recognition

3.4.1. Facial Recognition. There were no significant differences on the identity control task between CON and SCH, or between sexes in terms of the number of correct responses and response times.

Figure 2 shows that SCH achieved a lower number of correct responses for all emotions with the exception of happiness ($F(1,72) = 13.74$, $P < .001$) compared to CON as a main factor. With regard to sex, the statistical analysis did not reach significant values. Females in both groups CON and SCH, showed a tendency to have a higher number of correct responses in sadness recognition than males. The factor of emotions showed significant differences ($F(6,432) = 36.92$, $P < .001$) in the number of correct responses. As expected, happiness had the highest values and fear the lowest (Figure 2).

With respect to response times, SCH were slower to recognize all the emotions than CON ($F(1,72) = 7.36$, $P < .008$). There was no significant effect of sex. Response times were also significant between emotions ($F(6,432) = 24.27$, $P < .001$), with happiness showing the fastest response times (Figure 2). There were no significant interactions for either the number of correct responses or response times.

When age was considered as a covariate, the number of correct responses was still significant for emotions ($F(6,432) = 3.1$, $P < .01$) and for groups ($F(1,72) = 12.81$, $P < .001$). Although gender did not reach the level of significant differences, when age is considered as a covariate, it showed a trend ($F(1,72) = 3.58$, $P < .06$). There were no significant interactions between factors.

3.4.2. Prosodic Recognition. There were significant differences between emotions on the prosodic recognition task ($F(3,1892) = 31.21$, $P < .001$). SCH showed a significantly lower number of correct responses in prosodic emotional recognition than CON ($F(1,72) = 16.53$, $P < .001$) as a main factor. In addition, an interaction of emotion by group was found ($F(3,1892) = 4.24$, $P < .01$). No sex differences were observed. As can be seen in Figure 3, the easiest emotion to recognize was happiness, whereas the most difficult one was fear. SCH showed a lower number of correct responses than CON with respect to all emotions. In addition, results demonstrate that only for SCH was recognizing sadness as difficult as identifying fear.

The ANCOVA with age, included as a covariate, revealed a significant effect ($F(1,71) = 9.05$, $P < .004$). The significant differences between emotions in prosodic recognition disappeared ($F(1,71) = 2.21$, $P < .10$). The main effect for group remained, with SCH showing a significantly lower number of correct responses in prosodic emotional recognition than CON ($F(1,72) = 15.79$, $P < .001$). Although no sex differences were observed, an interaction of group by gender was found ($F(1,71) = 4.06$, $P < .04$). A Pearson correlation analysis between the global number of correct responses and age revealed a significant negative correlation only for SCHm ($r = -0.52$, $P < .005$).

3.4.3. Social Context Emotional Recognition. All the participants in CON and SCH groups were able to recognize all the emotions expressed by the characters in the 4 films.

With respect to the intensity of the emotions expressed by the principal character, there were no differences between CON and SCH or between the sexes, but a significant interaction of group by sex ($F(1,72) = 4.18$, $P < .04$) revealed that SCHm attributed less intensity to the expression of happiness by the principal character than CONm. Both CON and SCH females attributed a higher intensity to the expression of happiness by the secondary character ($F(1,72) = 9.35$, $P < .003$) and reported greater empathy with the characters in the films when they expressed happiness, compared to males in both groups ($F(1,72) = 11.94$, $P < .001$) (see Figure 4).

A higher percentage of females compared to males in both groups reported identifying with the principal character in the case of fear ($P < .001$); and a higher percentage of SCH females and males identified more closely with sadness ($P < .05$, $P < .001$, resp.), compared to CON. Similar results were found in fear and sadness in terms of the percentage of subjects when they relate the films scenes to their personal lives ($P < .001$ in all cases) (Figure 5).

4. Discussion

The purpose of the present study was to determine sex differences in schizophrenic patients with regards to emotional recognition, considering three modalities: facial, prosodic and in a socioemotional context, as well as to confirm impairments in those modalities in early onset schizophrenic patients.

4.1. Sociodemographic and Clinical Characteristics. As has been reported by Kraepelin in 1919, and other authors have replicated [2, 3, 56], both illness onset and first hospital admission occurred later in schizophrenic females than in males by approximately 8 years. More males than females were single or had no stable partner; half of the patients, both females and males had jobs; some males were students, while some females were homemakers. In general, patients showed adequate social functioning, perhaps due to the recent onset of the illness.

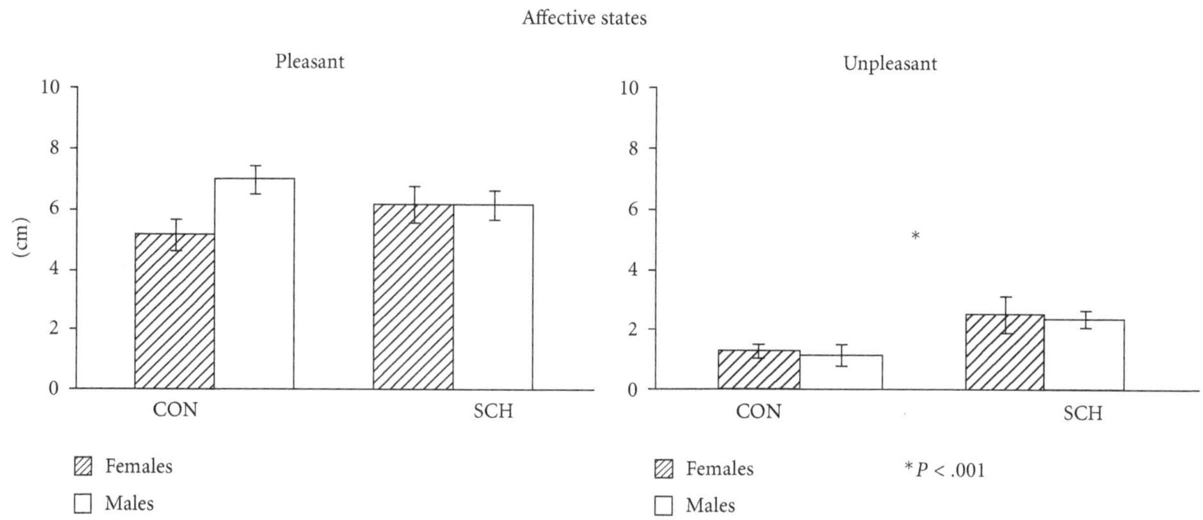

FIGURE 1: Means and standard errors on the pleasant and unpleasant Affective States Scale in controls (CON) and schizophrenic patients (SCH). SCH group reported higher unpleasant affectivity than CON.

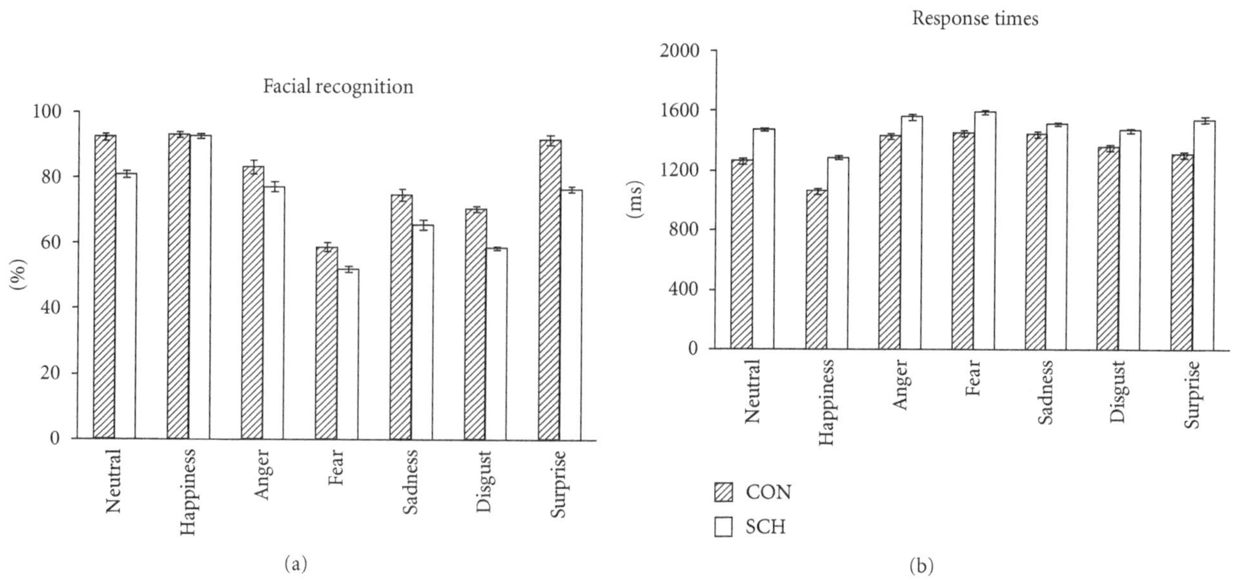

FIGURE 2: Means and standard errors of the percentage of correct responses and response times in the facial emotional recognition tasks for the control (CON) and schizophrenic groups (SCH).

Regarding psychiatric symptoms, no differences were observed between the sexes when the patients arrived at the hospital in the acute phase of the illness. Although other studies have affirmed that males present more acute symptomatology, and a higher prevalence of paranoid symptoms, aggression and antisocial behaviour [7] compared to females, we did not find similar results.

However, in the second psychopathological assessment, during the remission stage, males showed higher scores of negative symptoms than females. The better outcomes for the latter have been associated with better responses to treatment, a higher number of spontaneous remissions and the later onset of the illness, compared to males [7, 13, 15]. Rao and Kölsch [57] have attributed the higher severity in negative symptoms in males to lower concentrations of estradiol.

Turning to emotional states, we observed no differences by sex in the Affective States Scale scores. While both groups showed higher scores on the pleasant scale in comparison to the unpleasant scale, schizophrenics reported a higher level of unpleasant states. This finding is significant, since a negative emotional state could work as a marker for

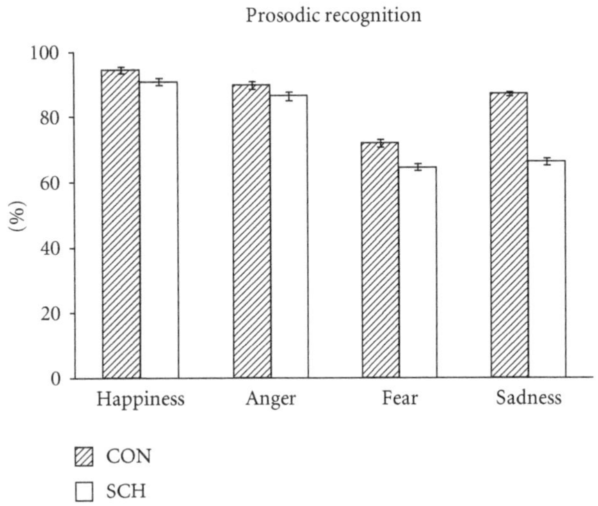

FIGURE 3: Means and standard errors for the percentage of correct responses in the prosodic emotional recognition task for males and females from the control (CON) and schizophrenic groups (SCH).

overlooked negative emotions on neutral faces. For instance, studies in depressive patients have described that they tend to attribute sadness to faces showing neutral expressions [58].

In conclusion, sex differences in schizophrenic patients were observed only in negative symptoms in the remission stage after medication, with a higher level in males than females.

4.2. Facial Emotional Recognition. Schizophrenic patients showed lower accuracy than controls in the recognition of all emotions, with the exception of expressions of happiness. The main effect for group remained when age was introduced as a covariate, indicating an independence of emotional recognition abilities in relation to age. In addition, the schizophrenic patients presented longer response times. These findings agree with those reported by several other studies in which deficits in facial emotional recognition in schizophrenic were found [38, 39]. It has been documented that people with schizophrenia commit more errors in recognizing fear, disgust and sadness, though they have no problem in recognizing happiness, an emotion that is more easily recognized than others [26, 59]. The fact that there were no difficulties in identity recognition suggests that this is not a problem in facial configuration processing.

Another issue has to do with response time. It is commonly accepted that schizophrenic patients generally show a slower processing on most type of tasks, including facial emotional recognition. In previous studies, we have found slower reaction times in male schizophrenics than healthy controls in odd-ball tasks using letters and emotional faces as stimuli [60], as well as on identity and emotional tasks [61]. In addition, longer reaction times (RT) were correlated with higher level of symptomatology and lower number of correct responses on both tasks [60].

On the question of differences between the sexes in emotional recognition, the variation found did not reach significant values. However, when age was introduced as a covariate, a trend was observed in the sense of a better performance in females than males. Other studies have reported better facial emotional recognition in females than males (i.e., [26, 62, 63]). In particular, it has been reported that healthy females outperform males in recognizing sad faces, while males perform better when it comes to identifying fear [31].

4.3. Emotional Prosody. In this research, schizophrenics showed lower accuracy in prosodic emotional recognition than controls as a whole. These results are congruent with those of other studies [34] that also found significant deficits in sadness and fear prosodic recognition in schizophrenics.

In a previous study, we have also found difficulties in prosodic recognition of happiness and sadness in chronic resistant schizophrenics without treatment [36]. However, a significant improvement was observed in the patients after they took olanzapine, as was a reduction in depression, though only for happiness prosodic expressions [36]. The effect of medication is relevant, since almost all the schizophrenics in the present study had taken olanzapine for at least 15 days when they were evaluated; therefore, accuracy in identifying happiness may have improved.

Regarding sex differences in prosodic recognition, no differences were found as long as age was not considered as a covariate; however, when it was, a significant group by gender interaction was found. In addition, a negative correlation between accuracy and age was observed only for schizophrenic males. These results suggest that prosodic recognition depends on age, mainly in schizophrenic males, as their performance worsens as age increases.

The prosodic stimuli used in this work had the particularity that the sentences were semantically neutral, such that the participants only had to pay attention to the emotional prosody. It is relevant because Schirmer et al. [32, 64] proposed that sex differences in emotional prosody depend on whether the subjects are asked to pay attention only to prosody and not to semantic information in the sentence. When the subjects pay attention to semantic content and emotional intonation simultaneously, females can integrate the two types of information more quickly than males, but when they only have to attend to emotional prosody, there are not sex differences. In daily life, speech contains both types of information that must be processed simultaneously, so it would be useful to evaluate emotional prosody processing when semantic information is also present, or even when there is incongruence between them.

Disorders in prosodic emotional recognition are related to difficulties in maintaining social interaction, which leads to social withdrawal even in healthy young adults [65]. In this sense, these disorders would result in lower social adaptive behavior in schizophrenic males than females as age increases.

4.4. Emotional Recognition in a Social Context. Understanding information on socioemotional contexts requires several abilities, including, as a first step, recognizing facial and body

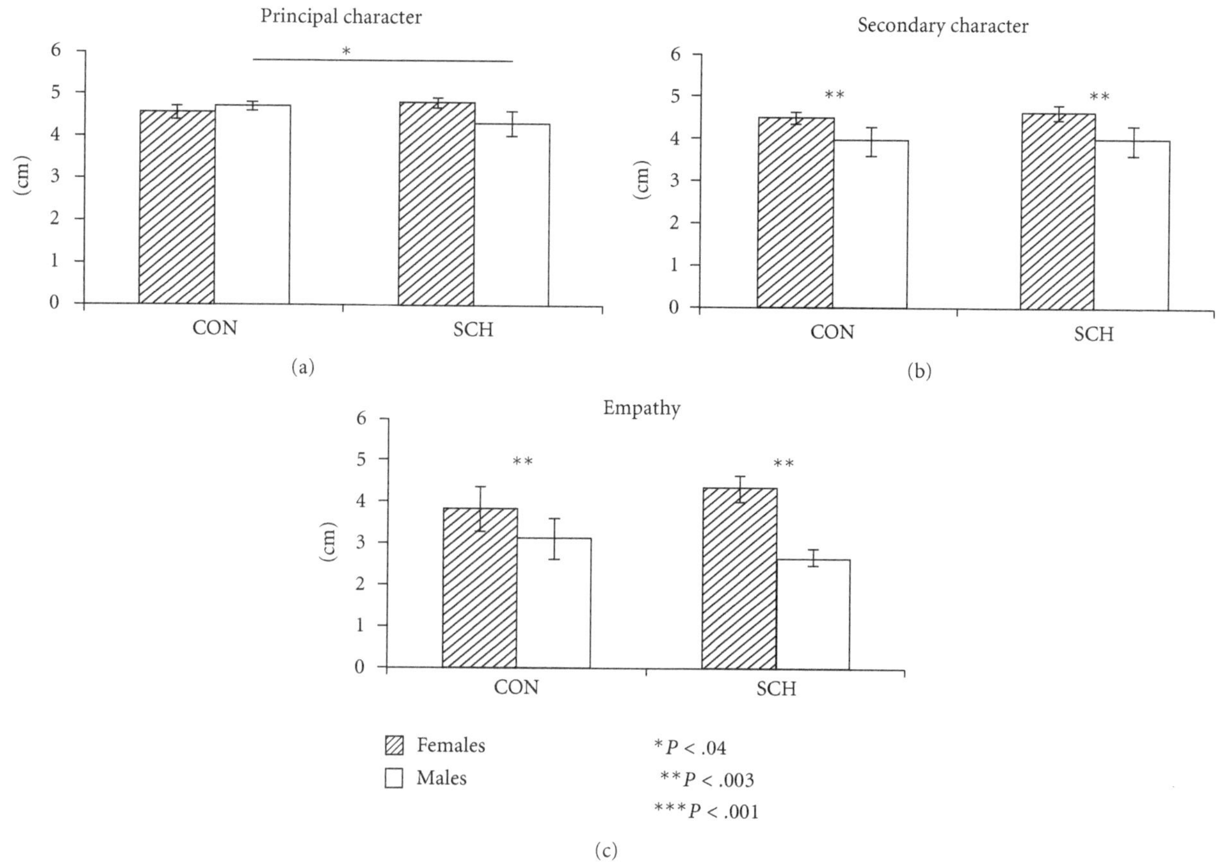

FIGURE 4: Means and standard errors for intensity level attributed to happiness expression from the principal and second characters and the empathy level experienced during the happiness film for females and males of the control (CON) and schizophrenic groups (SCH).

expressions and emotional prosody, and second, integrating those different types of emotional information. In addition, it requires interpreting all the emotional information within a context that includes, on the one hand, physical and spatial features, but more importantly, the ability to infer mental states and intentions from other individuals, in order to predict their behaviour and interpret the significance of personal relationships, as well as the effect of one's own behavioral responses on others. The final step refers to the empathetic abilities needed to understand the feelings of others (for reviews [66, 67]).

With regard to the recognition of the emotion represented in the films, all participants were capable of reporting their content congruently. These may be due to the fact that there are several simultaneous sensory inputs that allow the patients to compensate possible difficulties in any particular input channel. However, schizophrenic males attributed less intensity to the expression of happiness by the principal character than control males. In addition, both CON and SCH females attributed higher intensity to the expression of happiness by the secondary character. A higher percentage of females compared to males in both groups reported identifying with the principal character in the case of fear, while schizophrenic females and males identified more strongly with sadness than did controls. Similar results were found in the percentage of subjects when they were asked to relate the films scenes with their personal lives. Furthermore, both control and schizophrenic females reported a greater intensity of empathetic feelings during the happiness film. These results are consistent with those of a previous study carried out by Grossman and Wood [68] in which females reported experiencing emotions with greater intensity than males in findings that correlated with higher electromyograph activity.

Both female and male patients showed higher identification with the principal character in sadness films and reported that this scene related more closely to their personal lives than did controls. This may be related to the more unpleasant emotional state reported by the patients on the Affective Scale.

In a previous study conducted with similar facial, prosodic, and social context stimuli, we found that schizophrenic people showed difficulties in making social judgments as to what was happening in the scene, and in attributing intentions to the characters portrayed [36].

The role of emotions in formation and maintenance of interpersonal relationships is crucial. Not surprisingly, then, disturbances in an individual's emotions have important social consequences [69]. Understanding facial expressions in others makes it possible to form a representation of

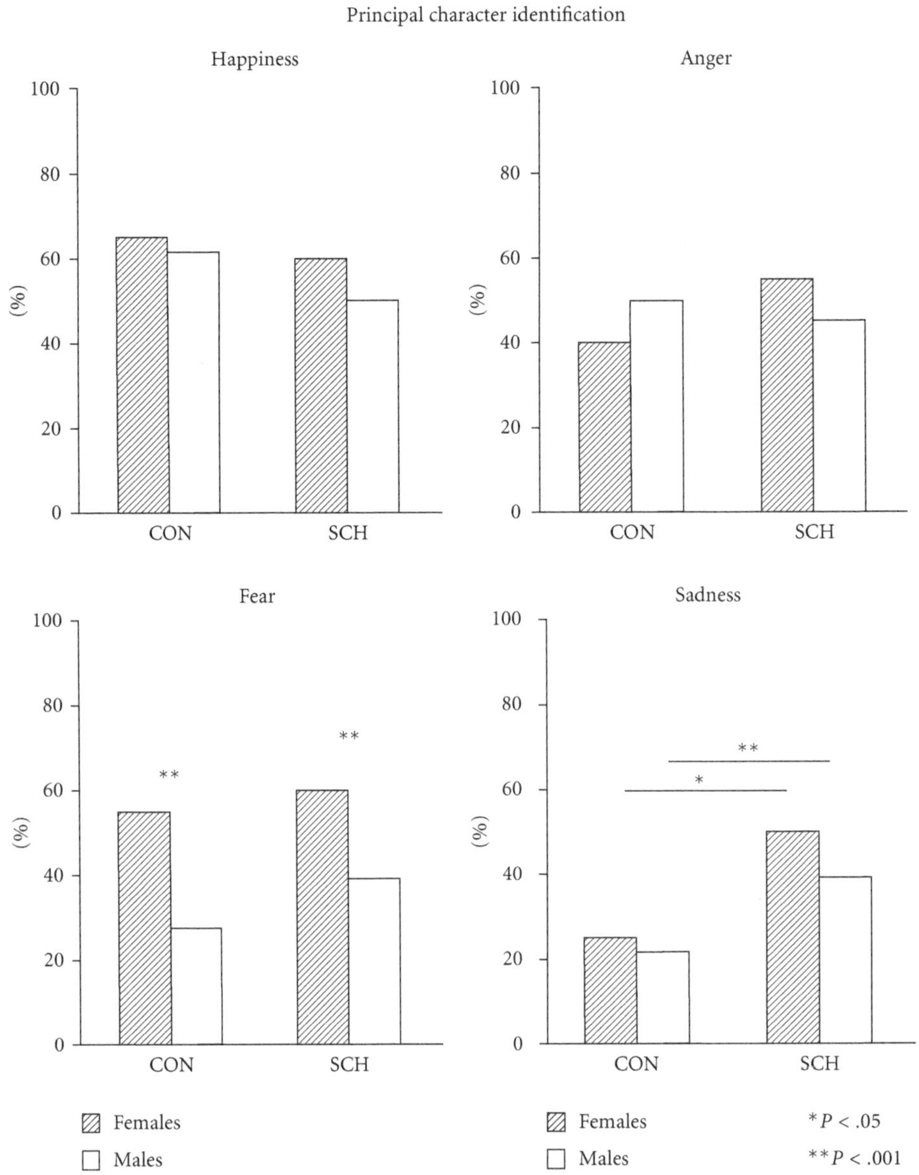

FIGURE 5: Percentage of controls (CON) and schizophrenic patients (SCH) that reported being identified with the principal character.

their intentions and emotional states and then respond accordingly in an adaptive way. Although there exists an important relationship between emotional recognition and adequate social development [69], it is also suggested that other cognitive abilities, such as executive functions, are fundamental to interpreting emotions in a scene where the role of lateral prefrontal cortex is predominant [70, 71].

It is important to conduct studies with complex emotions such as proud, shame, guilt, frustration, and so forth, because, in daily life, patients are continuously exposed to not only basic emotions, but also complex ones. It is possible that when exposed to such complex emotional expressions schizophrenics would show greater impairment and more pronounced differences between sexes.

This study took into account the fact that there are many variables that can influence emotional recognition performance; however, controlling for all such variables made it difficult to recruit a larger sample. For this reason, there is some question as to what degree these findings could be generalized to a larger population.

In summary, in the results of the present study, both females and males schizophrenic patients showed poorer performance than controls in terms of visual and prosodic modalities with respect to almost all emotions, except for happiness. However, when placed in the social context portrayed in the films, patients with schizophrenia were able to recognize all the emotions, suggesting that simultaneous sensory inputs may allow them to compensate for the difficulties that can appear when information is processed by independent input channels. Schizophrenic patients reported that they identified more with sad films than did controls, a finding that may be related to a more unpleasant emotional state. Schizophrenic females and males presented similar impairments with regards to facial and prosodic emotional recognition compared to CON, though upon considering age as a covariate, schizophrenic males showed poorer performance as age increased. However, in the social context of emotions, females showed higher empathy in relation to happiness than males in both groups and attributed a greater intensity of happiness to the secondary characters. As well, control and schizophrenic females identified more with fear than males.

Knowledge of emotional impairments in schizophrenia may be useful in designing therapeutic strategies, by taking into account the emotions that present greater difficulties in a particular sensory modality. It would be important to attend not only to emotional recognition of faces and prosody impairments, but to the way the patients interpret those emotions in order to improve formation and maintenance of interpersonal relationships. Together with other findings, the data from this study suggest that both in clinical management and research most take into account sexual differences in schizophrenic patients.

Acknowledgments

This work was supported by a Grant from CONACyT (40883). Authors want to thank Paul Kersey for the English correction.

References

[1] M. C. Angermeyer, L. Kuhn, and J. M. Goldstein, "Gender and the course of schizophrenia: differences in treated outcomes," *Schizophrenia Bulletin*, vol. 16, no. 2, pp. 293–307, 1990.

[2] A. Leung and P. Chue, "Sex differences in schizophrenia, a review of the literature," *Acta Psychiatrica Scandinavica*, vol. 101, no. 401, supplement, pp. 3–38, 2000.

[3] H. Häfner, "Gender differences in schizophrenia," *Psychoneuroendocrinology*, vol. 28, no. 2, pp. 17–54, 2003.

[4] J. Edwards, P. E. Pattison, H. J. Jackson, and R. J. Wales, "Facial affect and affective prosody recognition in first-episode schizophrenia," *Schizophrenia Research*, vol. 48, no. 2-3, pp. 235–253, 2001.

[5] R. E. Gur, B. I. Turetsky, P. E. Cowell et al., "Temporolimbic volume reductions in schizophrenia," *Archives of General Psychiatry*, vol. 57, no. 8, pp. 769–775, 2000.

[6] M. Torniainen, J. Suvisaari, T. Partonen et al., "Sex differences in cognition among persons with schizophrenia and healthy first-degree relatives," *Psychiatry Research*, vol. 188, no. 1, pp. 7–12, 2011.

[7] Z. Z. Cernovsky, J. A. Landmark, and R. L. O'Reilly, "Symptom patterns in schizophrenia for men and women," *Psychological Reports*, vol. 80, no. 3, pp. 1267–1271, 1997.

[8] J. M. Goldstein, "Sex, hormones and affective arousal circuitry dysfunction in schizophrenia," *Hormones and Behavior*, vol. 50, no. 4, pp. 612–622, 2006.

[9] T. H. McGlashan and K. K. Bardenstein, "Gender differences in affective, schizoaffective, and schizophrenic disorders," *Schizophrenia Bulletin*, vol. 16, no. 2, pp. 319–329, 1990.

[10] K. K. Bardenstein and T. H. McGlashan, "Gender differences in affective, schizoaffective, and schizophrenic disorders. A review," *Schizophrenia Research*, vol. 3, no. 3, pp. 159–172, 1990.

[11] H. Y. Meltzer, J. Rabinowitz, M. A. Lee et al., "Age at onset and gender of schizophrenic patients in relation to neuroleptic resistance," *American Journal of Psychiatry*, vol. 154, no. 4, pp. 475–482, 1997.

[12] R. Halari, V. Kumari, R. Mehrotra, M. Wheeler, M. Hines, and T. Sharma, "The relationship of sex hormones and cortisol with cognitive Functioning in schizophrenia," *Journal of Psychopharmacology*, vol. 18, no. 3, pp. 366–374, 2004.

[13] L. A. Lindamer, A. Bailey, W. Hawthorne et al., "Gender differences in characteristics and service use of public mental health patients with schizophrenia," *Psychiatric Services*, vol. 54, no. 10, pp. 1407–1409, 2003.

[14] L. J. Seidman, J. M. Goldstein, J. M. Goodman et al., "Sex differences in olfactory identification and Wisconsin card sorting performance in schizophrenia: relationship to attention and verbal ability," *Biological Psychiatry*, vol. 42, no. 2, pp. 104–115, 1997.

[15] J. M. Goldstein and B. G. Link, "Gender and the expression of schizophrenia," *Journal of Psychiatric Research*, vol. 22, no. 2, pp. 141–155, 1988.

[16] J. H. Gruzelier, "Syndromes of schizophrenia and schizotypy, hemispheric imbalance and sex differences: implications for developmental psychopathology," *International Journal of Psychophysiology*, vol. 18, no. 3, pp. 167–178, 1994.

[17] K. L. Narr, P. M. Thompson, T. Sharma, J. Moussai, A. F. Cannestra, and A. W. Toga, "Three-dimensional mapping of temporal-limbic regions and the lateral ventricles in schizophrenia: gender effects," *Society of Biological Psychiatry*, vol. 50, pp. 87–97, 2001.

[18] P. R. Szeszko, R. D. Strous, R. S. Goldman et al., "Neuropsychological correlates of hippocampal volumes in patients experiencing a first episode of schizophrenia," *American Journal of Psychiatry*, vol. 159, no. 2, pp. 217–226, 2002.

[19] J. M. Goldstein, L. J. Seidman, J. M. Goodman et al., "Are there sex differences in neuropsychological functions among patients with schizophrenia?" *American Journal of Psychiatry*, vol. 155, no. 10, pp. 1358–1364, 1998.

[20] M. Albus, W. Hubmann, F. Mohr et al., "Are there gender differences in neuropsychological performance in patients with first-episode schizophrenia?" *Schizophrenia Research*, vol. 28, no. 1, pp. 39–50, 1997.

[21] M. R. M. Scholten, A. Aleman, B. Montagne, and R. S. Kahn, "Schizophrenia and processing of facial emotions: sex matters," *Schizophrenia Research*, vol. 78, no. 1, pp. 61–67, 2005.

[22] E. M. Weiss, C. G. Kohler, C. M. Brensinger et al., "Gender differences in facial emotion recognition in persons with chronic schizophrenia," *European Psychiatry*, vol. 22, no. 2, pp. 116–122, 2007.

[23] M. R. M. Scholten, A. Aleman, and R. S. Kahn, "The processing of emotional prosody and semantics in schizophrenia: relationship to gender and IQ," *Psychological Medicine*, vol. 38, no. 6, pp. 887–898, 2008.

[24] K. Kucharska-Pietura, A. S. David, M. Masiak, and M. L. Phillips, "Perception of facial and vocal affect by people with schizophrenia in early and late stages of illness," *British Journal of Psychiatry*, vol. 187, pp. 523–528, 2005.

[25] R. Campbell, K. Elgar, J. Kuntsi et al., "The classification of 'fear' from faces is associated with face recognition skill in women," *Neuropsychologia*, vol. 40, no. 6, pp. 575–584, 2002.

[26] G. Kirouac and F. Y. Doré, "Accuracy and latency of judgment of facial expressions of emotions," *Perceptual and Motor Skills*, vol. 57, no. 3, pp. 683–686, 1983.

[27] J. A. Hall, "Gender effects in decoding nonverbal cues," *Psychological Bulletin*, vol. 85, no. 4, pp. 845–857, 1978.

[28] E. Hampson, S. M. van Anders, and L. I. Mullin, "A female advantage in the recognition of emotional facial expressions: test of an evolutionary hypothesis," *Evolution and Human Behavior*, vol. 27, no. 6, pp. 401–416, 2006.

[29] Q. Rahman, G. D. Wilson, and S. Abrahams, "Sex, sexual orientation, and identification of positive and negative facial affect," *Brain and Cognition*, vol. 54, no. 3, pp. 179–185, 2004.

[30] J. F. Thayer and B. H. Johnsen, "Sex differences in judgement of facial affect: a multivariate analysis of recognition errors," *Scandinavian Journal of Psychology*, vol. 41, no. 3, pp. 243–246, 2000.

[31] M. K. Mandal and S. Palchoudhury, "Perceptual skill in decoding facial affect," *Perceptual and Motor Skills*, vol. 60, no. 1, pp. 96–98, 1985.

[32] A. Schirmer, S. A. Kotz, and A. D. Friederici, "Sex differentiates the role of emotional prosody during word processing," *Cognitive Brain Research*, vol. 14, no. 2, pp. 228–233, 2002.

[33] F. Schneider, R. C. Gur, R. E. Gur, and D. L. Shtasel, "Emotional processing in schizophrenia: neurobehavioral probes in relation to psychopathology," *Schizophrenia Research*, vol. 17, no. 1, pp. 67–75, 1995.

[34] J. Edwards, P. E. Pattison, H. J. Jackson, and R. J. Wales, "Facial affect and affective prosody recognition in first-episode schizophrenia," *Schizophrenia Research*, vol. 48, no. 2-3, pp. 235–253, 2001.

[35] P. J. Johnston, M. Katsikitis, and V. J. Carr, "A generalised deficit can account for problems in facial emotion recognition in schizophrenia," *Biological Psychology*, vol. 58, no. 3, pp. 203–227, 2001.

[36] G. Y. Ibarraran-Pernas, L. E. Cerdan, M. A. Guevara, and J. Ramos Loyo, "Olanzapine effects on emotional recognition in treatment refractory schizophrenics," *Actas Espanolas de Psiquiatria*, vol. 31, no. 5, pp. 256–262, 2003.

[37] A. M. Kring, S. L. Kerr, and K. S. Earnst, "Schizophrenic patients show facial reactions to emotional facial expressions," *Psychophysiology*, vol. 36, no. 2, pp. 186–192, 1999.

[38] J. Edwards, H. J. Jackson, and P. E. Pattison, "Emotion recognition via facial expression and affective prosody in schizophrenia: a methodological review," *Clinical Psychology Review*, vol. 22, no. 6, pp. 789–832, 2002.

[39] C. G. Kohler, J. B. Walker, E. A. Martin, K. M. Healey, and P. J. Moberg, "Facial emotion perception in schizophrenia: a meta-analytic review," *Schizophrenia Bulletin*, vol. 36, no. 5, pp. 1009–1019, 2010.

[40] C. G. Kohler and E. A. Martin, "Emotional processing in schizophrenia," *Cognitive Neuropsychiatry*, vol. 11, no. 3, pp. 250–271, 2006.

[41] B. Bediou, P. Krolak-Salmon, M. Saoud et al., "Facial expression and sex recognition in schizophrenia and depression," *Canadian Journal of Psychiatry*, vol. 50, no. 9, pp. 525–533, 2005.

[42] R. E. Gur, C. G. Kohler, J. D. Ragland et al., "Flat affect in schizophrenia: relation to emotion processing and neurocognitive measures," *Schizophrenia Bulletin*, vol. 32, no. 2, pp. 279–287, 2006.

[43] D. R. Bach, K. Buxtorf, D. Grandjean, and W. K. Strik, "The influence of emotion clarity on emotional prosody identification in paranoid schizophrenia," *Psychological Medicine*, vol. 39, no. 6, pp. 927–938, 2009.

[44] A. S. Bellack, R. L. Morrison, J. T. Wixted, and K. T. Mueser, "An analysis of social competence in schizophrenia," *British Journal of Psychiatry*, vol. 156, pp. 809–818, 1990.

[45] J. H. Poole, F. C. Tobias, and S. Vinogradov, "The functional relevance of affect recognition errors in schizophrenia," *Journal of the International Neuropsychological Society*, vol. 6, no. 6, pp. 649–658, 2000.

[46] M. Annette, *Left, Right, Hand and Brain: The Right Shift Theory*, Hillsdale, Editors, New York, NY, USA, 1985.

[47] R. Pearson and M. B. Lewis, "Fear recognition across the menstrual cycle," *Hormones and Behavior*, vol. 47, no. 3, pp. 267–271, 2005.

[48] B. Derntl, C. Windischberger, S. Robinson et al., "Facial emotion recognition and amygdala activation are associated with menstrual cycle phase," *Psychoneuroendocrinology*, vol. 33, no. 8, pp. 1031–1040, 2008.

[49] X. Protopopescu, H. Pan, M. Altemus et al., "Orbitofrontal cortex activity related to emotional processing changes across the menstrual cycle," *Proceedings of the National Academy of Sciences of the United States of America*, vol. 102, no. 44, pp. 16060–16065, 2005.

[50] APA, American Psychiatric Association, *Manual Diagnóstico y Estadístico de los Trastornos Mentales. DSM-IV*, Masson, Barcelona, Spain, 1994.

[51] J. E. Overall and D. R. Gorham, "The brief psychiatric rating scale," *Psychological Reports*, vol. 10, pp. 799–812, 1962.

[52] S. R. Kay, A. Fiszbein, and L. A. Opler, "The positive and negative syndrome scale (PANSS) for schizophrenia," *Schizophrenia Bulletin*, vol. 13, no. 2, pp. 261–276, 1987.

[53] J. Ramos, M. A. Guevara, A. Martínez et al., "Evaluation of the affective states evoked by music," *Revista Mexicana de Psicologia*, vol. 13, no. 2, pp. 131–145, 1996.

[54] A. Sanz-Martín, M. A. Guevara, M. Corsi-Cabrera, R. Ondarza-Rovira, and J. Ramos-Loyo, "Differential effect of left and right temporal lobectomy on emotional recognition and experience in patients with epilepsy," *Revista de Neurologia*, vol. 42, no. 7, pp. 391–398, 2006.

[55] P. Ekman and W. V. Friesen, *Pictures of Facial Affect*, Consulting Psychologists Press, Palo Alto, Calif, USA, 1986.

[56] R. R. J. Lewine, E. F. Walker, R. Shurett, J. Caudle, and C. Haden, "Sex differences in neuropsychological functioning among schizophrenic patients," *American Journal of Psychiatry*, vol. 153, no. 9, pp. 1178–1184, 1996.

[57] M. L. Rao and H. Kölsch, "Effects of estrogen on brain development and neuroprotection—Implications for negative symptoms in schizophrenia," *Psychoneuroendocrinology*, vol. 28, no. 2, pp. 83–96, 2003.

[58] P. Luck and C. F. Dowrick, "Don't look at me in that tone of voice: disturbances in the perception of emotion in facial expression and vocal intonation by depressed patients," *Primary Care Mental Health*, vol. 2, pp. 99–106, 2004.

[59] P. J. Johnston, H. Devir, and F. Karayanidis, "Facial emotion processing in schizophrenia: no evidence for a deficit specific to negative emotions in a differential deficit design," *Psychiatry Research*, vol. 143, no. 1, pp. 51–61, 2006.

[60] J. Ramos-Loyo, L. F. Cerdán, and M. A. Guevara, "Evaluation of olanzapine effects on attention and emotional recognition processes through event related potentials in treatment refractory schizophrenics," in *Focus on Nonverbal Communication Research*, R. L. Finley, Ed., pp. 215–236, Nova Science Publisher, New York, NY, USA, 2007.

[61] J. Ramos-Loyo, A. A. González-Garrido, L. M. Sánchez-Loyo, V. Medina, and C. Basar-Eroglu, "Event-related potentials

and event-related oscillations during identity and facial emotional processing in schizophrenia," *International Journal of Psychophysiology*, vol. 71, no. 1, pp. 84–90, 2009.

[62] L. F. Barrett, L. Robin, P. R. Pietromonaco, and K. M. Eyssell, "Are women the "More Emotional" sex? Evidence from emotional experiences in social context," *Cognition and Emotion*, vol. 12, no. 4, pp. 555–578, 1998.

[63] R. E. Gur, C. McGrath, R. M. Chan et al., "An fMRI study of facial emotion processing in patients with schizophrenia," *American Journal of Psychiatry*, vol. 159, no. 12, pp. 1992–1999, 2002.

[64] A. Schirmer, S. A. Kotz, and A. D. Friederici, "On the role of attention for the processing of emotions in speech: sex differences revisited," *Cognitive Brain Research*, vol. 24, no. 3, pp. 442–452, 2005.

[65] J. S. Carton, E. A. Kessler, and C. L. Pape, "Nonverbal decoding skills and relationship well-being in adults," *Journal of Nonverbal Behavior*, vol. 23, no. 1, pp. 91–100, 1999.

[66] M. J. Green, P. J. Uhlhaas, and M. Coltheart, "Context processing and social cognition in schizophrenia," *Current Psychiatry Reviews*, vol. 1, pp. 11–21, 2005.

[67] S. M. Couture, D. L. Penn, and D. L. Roberts, "The functional significance of social cognition in schizophrenia: a review," *Schizophrenia Bulletin*, vol. 32, pp. S44–S63, 2006.

[68] M. Grossman and W. Wood, "Sex differences in intensity of emotional experience: a social role interpretation," *Journal of Personality and Social Psychology*, vol. 65, no. 5, pp. 1010–1022, 1993.

[69] C. Hooker and S. Park, "Emotion processing and its relationship to social functioning in schizophrenia patients," *Psychiatry Research*, vol. 112, no. 1, pp. 41–50, 2002.

[70] V. P. Bozikas, M. H. Kosmidis, D. Anezoulaki, M. Giannakou, and A. Karavatos, "Relationship of affect recognition with psychopathology and cognitive performance in schizophrenia," *Journal of the International Neuropsychological Society*, vol. 10, no. 4, pp. 549–558, 2004.

[71] J. R. Gray, T. S. Braver, and M. E. Raichle, "Integration of emotion and cognition in the lateral prefrontal cortex," *Proceedings of the National Academy of Sciences of the United States of America*, vol. 99, no. 6, pp. 4115–4120, 2002.

Jumping to Conclusions Is Associated with Paranoia but Not General Suspiciousness: A Comparison of Two Versions of the Probabilistic Reasoning Paradigm

Steffen Moritz,[1] Niels Van Quaquebeke,[2] and Tania M. Lincoln[3]

[1] *Department of Psychiatry and Psychotherapy, University Medical Center Hamburg-Eppendorf, Martinistraße 52, 20246 Hamburg, Germany*
[2] *Department of Management and Economics, Kuehne Logistics University, Hamburg, Germany*
[3] *Department of Psychology, University of Hamburg, Hamburg, Germany*

Correspondence should be addressed to Steffen Moritz, moritz@uke.de

Academic Editor: Robin Emsley

Theoretical models ascribe jumping to conclusions (JTCs) a prominent role in the pathogenesis of paranoia. While many earlier studies corroborated this account, some newer investigations have found no or only small associations of the JTC bias with paranoid symptoms. The present study examined whether these inconsistencies in part reflect methodological differences across studies. The study was built upon the psychometric high-risk paradigm. A total of 1899 subjects from the general population took part in an online survey and were administered the Paranoia Checklist as well as one of two different variants of the probabilistic reasoning task: one variant with a traditional instruction (a) and one novel variant that combines probability estimates with decision judgments (b). Factor analysis of the Paranoia Checklist yielded an unspecific suspiciousness factor and a psychotic paranoia factor. The latter was significantly associated with scores indicating hasty decision making. Subjects scoring two standard deviations above the mean of the Paranoia Checklist showed an abnormal data-gathering style relative to subjects with normal scores. Findings suggest that the so-called decision threshold parameter is more sensitive than the conventional JTC index. For future research the specific contents of paranoid beliefs deserve more consideration in the investigation of decision making in schizophrenia as JTC seems to be associated with core psychosis-prone features of paranoia only.

1. Introduction

Research on neuropsychological dysfunctions in schizophrenia (e.g., memory and executive dysfunction) has been increasingly extended by studies on cognitive biases [1–3]. Cognitive biases represent preferences, subtle distortions, and styles of information processing rather than neural deficits or mere inaccuracy [1]. An emerging literature has elucidated that persons with delusions tend to jump to conclusions [3, 4], are over-confident in their incorrect decisions [5–9], and show attributional biases [10–12], for example, a preference for monocausal inferences [13], and a bias against disconfirmatory evidence [14–18]. Some of these biases have been found to correlate with positive symptoms (i.e., delusions and hallucinations), which according to many clinicians represent the core of the disorder. Cognitive training programs such as the Social Cognition and Interaction Training (SCIT) [19, 20], the Maudsley Review Training Program [21] or the Metacognitive Training for Psychosis (MCT) [22, 23] have begun to translate these insights into practice: patients learn to withhold strong judgment in the face of ambiguous evidence and to be more flexible in their decision making.

The present study is primarily concerned with JTC which is usually assessed with the so-called beads or probabilistic reasoning task [24]. This task requires the subject to deduce from which of two containers a string of beads has been drawn. Typically, containers contain beads in an opposing ratio (e.g., 90 : 10 versus 10 : 90). Decisions after only one or two beads are counted as evidence for JTC. Since its introduction, numerous variants have been developed using different numbers of containers, material (e.g., beads/containers, fish/lakes, adjectives/personality traits, sheep/herds), mode of administration (e.g., real beads/containers versus computerized tasks), ratios (e.g., 90 : 10, 85 : 15, 80 : 20) and types of response (simulated decisions, probability assessment or concurrent measurement of probabilities and decisions) or manipulated other facets of the task. Notwithstanding these alterations, the evidence for JTC has been quite robust across many studies: numerous investigations found an association of JTC with (paranoid) delusions or dimensions of delusions, such as delusion conviction [25–30]. While an older review of Fine et al. [4] concludes that "a tendency to gather less evidence in the beads task is reliably associated with the presence of delusional symptomatology" (p. 46), some (more recent) studies have not been able to detect substantial associations with paranoid or delusional symptomatology [31–34] and there is mixed evidence whether nonclinical subjects scoring high on paranoia display JTC [35, 36]. In one study, JTC was pronounced in currently deluded patients but still detectable in nondeluded ones [37]. In contrast, Lincoln and colleagues [29] found JTC in acute but not remitted patients, whereby the association between JTC and delusions vanished when negative symptoms were accounted for. Few studies have looked at the impact of different themes of delusions on jumping to conclusions. An earlier study from the group of Garety and Freeman reported a rather specific association between JTC and persecutory delusions [38], whereas a novel study of the same group [39] found that grandiose delusions were more associated with JTC than persecutory delusions (as assessed with a 85 : 15% variant).

Two large recent studies are particularly noteworthy in our view as they were unable to secure substantial differences on the prevalence of JTC in patients versus controls. One study [40, 41] on 85 patients with schizophrenia and 25 healthy controls revealed no greater JTC in patients than in controls. Moreover, the amount of JTC was not moderated by the severity of positive symptomatology. Likewise, in the to date largest study on cognitive biases in schizophrenia ($N = 289$ patients), patients showed more JTC relative to 55 controls only at statistical trend level [42]. Correlations with positive symptoms were significant but small.

The two aforementioned studies both used a more complex version of the probabilistic reasoning task so that methodological differences to the conventional task may at least partially account for the inconsistent findings. First, the task used fish/lakes instead of beads/jars [30] which, however, can be regarded as a minor modification as this setup is quite intuitive and has elucidated group differences in other studies [43]. Perhaps more important, the novel task requested subjects to perform two judgments: first they were asked to provide an estimate of the probability that a (sequence of) fish is from lake A or B and then whether they would decide for one of the lakes or not. The parallel assessment of probability and decision serves the purpose to assess the decision threshold of schizophrenia patients as it has been put forward that people with schizophrenia may reason like *bad statisticians* who do not rely on high levels of probability before a decision is accepted (e.g., 95% as usually in statistics), but are satisfied with lower levels [6, 44–46]. A lowered acceptance threshold automatically increases the number of erroneous hypotheses. In line with this contention, different studies have demonstrated that patients with schizophrenia had a much lower significance threshold (i.e., liberal acceptance account). For example, in a study modeled after the "Who wants to be a millionaire" quiz [47], patients had a minimal decision threshold of 54% versus 70% in controls (mean decision threshold: 86% versus 93%) which resulted in a higher error rate. A low decision threshold has been replicated using other tasks as well and has also been found to be rather specific to schizophrenia patients [48]. Interestingly, a low decision threshold has been shown to be more sensitive to group differences than the original JTC parameters, such as draws to decision [49]. While we deem the measurement of decision thresholds an important advancement in the research on reasoning in schizophrenia, asking subjects to estimate probabilities might have fostered additional checks of the available evidence and thereby delayed decisions. Moreover, unlike the traditional variant this task did not request high confidence in the decision in order to dissociate probability and decision making. It may be argued that overconfidence in a quick decision may be more pathological and potentially discriminating across groups than just any quick decision [50].

Another reason for the heterogeneity of findings may relate to the different methods used to measure paranoia. While some studies used expert ratings like the Positive and Negative Syndrome Scale (PANSS); [51], others have used self-rating scales like the Peters' Delusions Inventory (PDI); [52] or the Paranoia Checklist [53]. Perhaps more importantly, paranoia is a multidimensional phenomenon that can be characterized along different aspects like content (e.g., suspiciousness versus Schneiderian symptoms), conviction, distress, and impact on behavior [54]. It deserves consideration that the JTC bias might be associated with some but not all of these aspects.

The present study was the first to conduct a head-to-head comparison of a version modeled after the traditional variant of the beads task [24] and a new paradigm that assesses probability estimates and decision judgments within one task [43]. We were interested to see if the pattern of results and psychopathological correlates is comparable across tasks.

Based on the notion that paranoia is represented along a continuum in the general population and some evidence [25, 36, 55] for a "dose-response relationship" between level of psychosis liability and JTC [35], we adopted a so-called psychometric high risk approach: subjects selected from a large population sample scoring higher than two standard deviations (SDs) above the mean of the Paranoia Checklist (see Section 2) were compared to a sample with scores not higher than 0.5 standard deviations above the mean [25, 56, 57]. The second aim was to examine if JTC is related to specific aspects of paranoia. To meet this purpose, we conducted a factor analysis on the Paranoia Checklist and correlated core parameters of the probabilistic reasoning tasks with the factor scores.

2. Methods

2.1. Participants and Procedure. Participants were recruited via the WiSo-panel, an academic online service in Germany that allows researchers to advertise their studies to potential participants. Recent research has demonstrated that this and similar services (e.g., Mturk or Studyresponse in the USA) provide reliable means of collecting data [58–60]. A total of 7,947 subjects from the general population were invited for participation in the study which was conducted over the internet using the software package "Unipark" [61]. Of these, 1,899 (24%) completed all tasks relevant for the present study. Subjects' age, gender, and educational level were drawn from the WiSo-panel data base. Before the experiments started, subjects were asked to provide informed consent. Then, the survey proceeded with items on perceptions of ethical leadership in organizations, all of which are unrelated to the present study and will be presented elsewhere. After that, the 18-item Paranoia Checklist [53] was administered which assesses paranoid beliefs. Good psychometric properties of the German version have been demonstrated in previous studies [62, 63]. At the end of the survey, each subject was randomly presented with one out of two versions of the fish task. For both versions the order of events was fixed mirroring the primary ratio of the lakes (both 80 : 20% versus 20 : 80%; the fourth and the ninth fish were in the color of the nondominant lake (lake B)). Upon a decision for lake A or B (the subject could decide either for lake A or B or make no decision) the task and the entire study were terminated. In both variants each new fish was highlighted with an arrow and shown along with previously caught fish. Moreover, the ratio of fish was explicitly shown on each slide to minimize the influence of memory. The two versions were as follows.

(a) For the Traditional Variant, the Subject Was Shown the Following Instruction. "Below you see two lakes with red and green fish. Lake A: 80% red fish and 20% green. Lake B: 80% green fish and 20% red. A fisherman randomly chooses one of the two lakes and then fishes from this lake only. Based on the caught fish, you should decide whether the fisherman caught fish from lake A or B. Important: (1) The fisherman catches fish from one lake only. (2) He throws the fish back after each catch. The ratio of green and red fish stays the same. (3) You can catch as many fish as you need to be completely sure as to which lake the fisherman has chosen."

(b) In the Extended Condition, Subjects Were Provided the Following Instruction (High Confidence in the Decision Was Not Explicitly Requested). "Below you see two lakes with orange and gray fish. Lake A: 80% orange fish and 20% gray. Lake B: 80% gray fish and 20% orange. A fisherman randomly chooses one of the two lakes and then fishes from this lake only. After each new catch, please make the following judgments: (1) What is the probability that the fish are being caught from lake A or lake B (0–100%)? (2) Do you have enough information to decide on one particular lake? Important: The fisherman catches fish from one lake only. He throws the fish back after each catch. The ratio of orange and gray fish stays the same."

As outlined before, we adopted a psychometric high-risk approach [56], whereby the performance of participants scoring at least 2 standard deviations above the mean of the Paranoia Checklist is contrasted with participants with scores not higher than 0,5 SD above the mean of the sample.

3. Results

3.1. Background and Experimental Data. Demographic, psychopathological, and experimental characteristics of the sample are displayed in Table 1. Most participants were female, around 40 years old and had a high educational level. The Paranoia Checklist total score was comparable to prior studies [64, 65]. No differences emerged between subsamples (i.e., the subsamples undergoing the traditional versus the extended version) on background and psychopathological scores. However, there were significant differences between the traditional and the extended version of the fish task: the rate of JTC was higher in the extended variant relative to the traditional task. Accordingly, the number of draws-to-decision (DTD) was lower in the extended task. The minimal probability required for a decision in the extended task was 74%. This parameter could be computed for the extended variant only.

Table 2 contrasts performance on the probabilistic reasoning tasks for participants who scored at least two standard deviations above the mean of the Paranoia Checklist and those with scores below a cut-off point of half a standard deviation above the mean. All comparisons were significant indicating a higher JTC bias, a smaller number of DTD, and a lowered decision threshold in the high scorers. In the novel variant, participants with high paranoia scores provided lower probability ratings after fish #1.

3.2. Correlations. To explore whether core parameters of the probabilistic reasoning task are differentially correlated with paranoia, we submitted the Paranoia Checklist to a principal component analysis with varimax rotation. Both the scree-plot and the Kaiser-Guttmann criterion (extraction of factors with eigenvalues > 1) suggested a two-factor solution (see Table 3) which explained approximately two thirds of the variance (64%). The Bartlett's test of sphericity was significant, $\chi^2(153) = 25566{,}82$; $P < .001$. The Kaiser-Meyer-Olkin measure suggested a good fit (.95). Factor 1 (eigenvalue = 6.63) explained 37% of the variance and was named "unspecific suspiciousness" as it was primarily loaded by (low threshold) items covering "normal" suspicion such as "There might be negative comments being circulated about me." The second factor (eigenvalue = 4.90) explained 27% of the variance and was named "psychotic paranoia" as it was primarily loaded by (high-threshold) items covering clearly pathological forms of delusions such as "I can detect coded messages about me in the press/TV/radio." These items dealt with conspiracy and Schneiderian first-rank symptoms (i.e., permeability of ego boundaries). Factor scores of the Paranoia Checklist were saved to the matrix

TABLE 1: Demographic, psychopathological, and experimental characteristics of the two samples. Percentages, means, and standard deviations (in brackets).

	Traditional variant ($n = 961$)	Extended variant ($n = 938$)	Statistics
Demographics			
Gender (female/male)	61%/39%	60%/40%	$\chi^2(1) = 0.74$; $P > .7$
Age in years	43.15 (15.72)	43.00 (15.12)	$t(1897) = 0.24$; $P > .8$
Educational level (below 13th grade/13th grade/university degree)	35%/27%/38%	37%/26%/37%	$\chi^2(1) = 0.29$; $P > .8$
Paranoia Checklist			
Total score	26.44 (11.67)	26.88 (11.32)	$t(1897) = 0.82$; $P > .4$
Unspecific suspiciousness (regression score; see factor analysis)	−.02 (1.00)	.02 (.99)	$t(1897) = 0.81$; $P > .4$
Psychotic paranoia (regression score)	−.00 (1.01)	.01 (.99)	$t(1897) = 0.29$; $P > .7$
Probabilistic reasoning			
JTC (1st fish)	37%	66%	$\chi^2(1) = 163.98$; $P < .001$
JTC (1st or 2nd fish)	52%	74%	$\chi^2(1) = 99.63$; $P < .001$
Draws to decision	3.13 (2.56)	2.18 (2.29)	$t(1897) = 8.49$; $P < .001$
Decision threshold in %	—	73.93% (19.56)	—

Note. JTC: jumping to conclusions.

TABLE 2: Comparison between high (≥2 SD) and low scorers (≤0.5 SD) on the Paranoia Checklist with respect to performance on the probabilistic reasoning tasks. Percentages, means, and standard deviations (in brackets).

Traditional variant	High scorers ($n = 68$)	Low scorers ($n = 485$)	Statistics
Draws to decision	2.65 (2.68)	3.46 (2.62)	$t(551) = 2.37$; $P = .02$
JTC (1st fish)	60%	29%	$\chi^2(1) = 27.18$; $P < .001$
JTC (1st or 2nd fish)	63%	45%	$\chi^2(1) = 7.82$; $P = .005$
Initial probability (after the 1st fish)	—	—	—
Decision threshold in %	—	—	—
Extended variant	**High scorers ($n = 68$)**	**Low scorers ($n = 449$)**	**Statistics**
Draws to decision	1.76 (2.07)	2.31 (2.28)	$t(515) = 2.01$; $P = .047$
JTC (1st fish)	81%	61%	$\chi^2(1) = 10.27$; $P = .001$
JTC (1st or 2nd fish)	85%	71%	$\chi^2(1) = 6.40$; $P = .01$
Initial probability (after the 1st fish)	62.95 (24.00)	69.20 (18.63)	$t(497)^* = 2.39$; $P = .05$
Decision threshold in %	65.21 (24.80)	75.63 (18.42)	$t(486)^* = 3.94$; $P < .001$

Note. SD: standard deviation; JTC: jumping to conclusions; *some subjects did not provide probabilistic estimates.

and correlated with the JTC measures. Table 4 shows that none of the probability reasoning parameters correlated substantially with the first factor. In fact, the correlations for the traditional variant were small ($rs < .1$) but negative, that is, in the opposite direction than expected (i.e., higher questionnaire scores were related to lower JTC). Vice versa, the second factor was correlated with all JTC indexes in the predicted direction. The decision threshold was the only parameter that was also correlated with the Paranoia Checklist total score. All correlational differences for the two factor scores with the experimental parameters were (highly) significant (at least $P < .05$).

4. Discussion

The present work was motivated by recent studies [41, 42] suggesting that JTC in schizophrenia may not be as robust as long claimed. We set out to investigate whether this line of research reflects an instance of the so-called decline effect [66] or methodological differences across studies. As mentioned before, the psychopathological correlates of JTC are not fully uncovered. We were especially interested in the question of whether the traditional instruction of the probabilistic reasoning task [24] would be more potent than a new variant of the task which requires the joint assessment of probability judgments and decisions. Recently, this extended variant produced some conflicting findings which—among other yet unknown factors—may mirror two things: first, asking for subjective probability may caution subjects and thus delay decision making even in otherwise hasty individuals. Secondly, the extended variant does not request high confidence for judgments so that even more cautious individuals may well decide after only few items.

Results show that the prevalence of JTC was higher in the extended condition challenging the hypothesis that asking for probability levels cautions subjects and attenuates

Table 3: Factor solution for the 18 items of the Paranoia Checklist. The first factor is named "unspecific suspiciousness," the second factor "psychotic paranoia." Factor loadings above 0.6 are set in bold type.

Paranoia Checklist items	Components	
	Factor 1 unspecific suspiciousness	Factor 2 psychotic paranoia
There might be negative comments being circulated about me.	**.830**	.123
Bad things are being said about me behind my back.	**.813**	.228
People communicate about me in subtle ways.	**.748**	.345
People deliberately try to irritate me.	**.738**	.320
People might be hostile towards me.	**.729**	.306
I need to be on my guard against others.	**.721**	.138
Someone I know has bad intentions towards me.	**.663**	.430
People are trying to make me upset.	**.663**	.353
Strangers and friends look at me critically.	**.653**	.247
People would harm me if given an opportunity.	**.638**	.470
People are laughing at me.	**.610**	.354
I can detect coded messages about me in the press/TV/radio.	.131	**.865**
I am under threat from others.	.222	**.844**
There is a possibility of a conspiracy against me.	.367	**.790**
My actions and thoughts might be controlled by others.	.245	**.780**
Someone I don't know has bad intentions towards me.	.444	**.653**
I have a suspicion that someone has it in for me.	.578	.594
I might be being observed or followed.	.499	.560

Table 4: Correlation between different parameters on the probabilistic reasoning tasks with the two factors and the total score of the Paranoia Checklist across the two subsamples and the total pooled sample. Means and standard deviations (in brackets).

	Unspecific suspiciousness	Psychotic paranoia	Paranoia Checklist total score
Traditional variant			
JTC (1st fish)	−.077*	.221***	.062+
JTC (1st or 2nd fish)	−.099**	.154***	.006
Draws to decision	.098**	−.136***	.003
Decision threshold in %	—	—	—
Extended variant			
JTC (1st fish)	−.025	.142***	.059+
JTC (1st or 2nd fish)	−.035	.132***	.046
Draws to decision	.012	−.122***	−.059+
Decision threshold in %	−.014	−.186***	−.119***
Entire sample, both versions pooled			
JTC (1st fish)	−.044+	.177***	.064(**)
JTC (1st or 2nd fish)	−.063**	.142***	.028
Draws to decision	.054*	−.129***	−.029
Decision threshold in %	—	—	—

Note. JTC: jumping to conclusions.
+$P \leq .1$, *$P \leq .05$, **$P \leq .01$, ***$P \leq .001$.

the level of JTC. Overall, the correlational pattern of experimental variables with paranoid delusions or the difference between high and normal scorers was comparable across tasks. Interestingly, even the traditional version produced a higher prevalence of JTC than is usually expected, which might be due to the administration mode over the internet.

Factor analysis of the Paranoia Scale yielded two factors that resemble the two subscales of the Green et al. Paranoid Thought Scales (GPTS) [67]: a core paranoid dimension and a dimension measuring suspiciousness/social reference. The most important result in our view was that the JTC bias is apparently not correlated with normal suspiciousness (e.g., "There might be negative comments being circulated about me") but rather with more psychopathological and psychosis-prone forms of paranoia (e.g., "My actions and thoughts might be controlled by others"). High scorers on the former dimension did not differ significantly from subjects in the normal range, whereas high scorers on the latter scale had a much greater JTC bias and lower decision threshold than those in the normal range. This finding corroborates recent research [68] that JTC is tied to psychotic themes: patients with obsessive compulsive disorders low on illness insight did not display a JTC bias.

A number of limitations need to be acknowledged. First, the study was conducted over the internet and none of the assessments was determined face-to-face. The sample consisted predominantly of females with higher education which markedly deviates from a clinical schizophrenia population (mainly male with low school achievements). While online research contains many advantages relating to economy and anonymity (e.g., subjects are perhaps more open to disclose psychological problems), results need verification in a conventional setting. However, prior results [69] and the fact that the Paranoia Checklist scores were in accord with mean values previously collected for nonclinical subjects [64, 65] tentatively speak for the validity of our findings. A more general problem with the probabilistic reasoning task is that it estimates the core parameter, JTC, by only a single item. The results of such "single shot" experiments are plagued by low reliability. This may be one reason why some studies using the traditional variant did not detect strong JTC in paranoid schizophrenia across all variants of the probabilistic reasoning task [68]. Alternative measures [25, 43, 70, 71] may be better in this regard and should at least complement the administration of the probabilistic reasoning task. One may also investigate whether another version of the beads task which separates ratings for the two choices [72] is more sensitive to paranoia. Finally, our study cannot fully answer the question why two studies using the extended variant failed to find strong support for JTC in schizophrenia. We can only speculate that perhaps levels of paranoia/delusions were lower in patients relative to the high-risk sample of the present study: paranoid symptoms wax and wane and patients with schizophrenia do not necessarily show high levels of positive symptoms throughout.

For future studies we recommend to test additional potential moderators. According to some studies patients with schizophrenia and even some controls have problems to grasp the task instruction [37] and several studies have found that a JTC bias is associated with lower intelligence [29]. It also remains unresolved whether JTC is associated with delusions in general or only special subtypes (see Introduction).

5. Conclusions

While our study showed that both versions of the probabilistic reasoning task are equally sensitive for JTC measurement per se, we argue that the extended version has an additional advantage: with the decision threshold it provides an important novel index that can pinpoint whether absence of differences on DTD or JTC may derive from differences on overall probability levels. As Table 2 shows, high-paranoid subjects display lower initial probability levels than those scoring in the normal range. Baseline differences can have a huge impact on the conventional JTC parameter. To illustrate, it is less incautious to decide after two fish if the subjective probability is estimated for example at 90% versus if the subjective probability for the same information is estimated at 70%. Here, the decision threshold is more sensitive than the conventional JTC index which may even obscure incautious decision making. Similar results were collected in a recent study [49] that employed a computerized beads task variant with sheep in two different colors as stimuli: schizophrenia patients assigned lower overall probability estimates than healthy subjects, but both groups yielded comparable results on JTC and DTD. This could have been mistaken as a normal decision making in task variants without concurrently collecting probability scores. However, the decision threshold was significantly lower in the patient sample suggesting risky decision making. Importantly and in support of this, the aforementioned study by Andreou et al. [41] found comparable JTC parameters between schizophrenia patients versus controls but a lower decision threshold in patients for the same reasons.

For future research we would like to encourage researchers interested in JTC to pay a closer look at specific task demands, context effects and patients' attitudes and expectancies. Across-task differences implicitly considered negligible and minor such as mode of presentation (computer, real jars) and test battery (e.g., task administered as a single test versus part of a larger battery that might have cautioned the patient from making hasty decisions) may well have a serious impact on performance. In our view the main question is not whether or not patients show jumping to conclusions but under which conditions this is the case and under which conditions it is not.

Acknowledgments

The authors declare no conflict of interests. The authors also thank Ulf Koether as well as Nora Blum for valuable contributions on a prior version of the paper.

References

[1] S. Moritz, F. Vitzthum, S. Randjbar, R. Veckenstedt, and T. S. Woodward, "Detecting and defusing cognitive traps: metacognitive intervention in schizophrenia," *Current Opinion in Psychiatry*, vol. 23, no. 6, pp. 561–569, 2010.

[2] M. van der Gaag, "A neuropsychiatric model of biological and psychological processes in the remission of delusions and auditory hallucinations," *Schizophrenia Bulletin*, vol. 32, pp. S113–122, 2006.

[3] D. Freeman, "Suspicious minds: the psychology of persecutory delusions," *Clinical Psychology Review*, vol. 27, no. 4, pp. 425–457, 2007.

[4] C. Fine, M. Gardner, J. Craigie, and I. Gold, "Hopping, skipping or jumping to conclusions? Clarifying the role of the JTC bias in delusions," *Cognitive Neuropsychiatry*, vol. 12, no. 1, pp. 46–77, 2007.

[5] M. J. V. Peters, M. J. Cima, T. Smeets, M. De Vos, M. Jelicic, and H. Merckelbach, "Did I say that word or did you? Executive dysfunctions in schizophrenic patients affect memory efficiency, but not source attributions," *Cognitive Neuropsychiatry*, vol. 12, no. 5, pp. 391–411, 2007.

[6] S. Moritz, T. S. Woodward, L. Jelinek, and R. Klinge, "Memory and metamemory in schizophrenia: a liberal acceptance account of psychosis," *Psychological Medicine*, vol. 38, no. 6, pp. 825–832, 2008.

[7] S. Moritz, T. S. Woodward, and R. Rodriguez-Raecke, "Patients with schizophrenia do not produce more false memories than controls but are more confident in them," *Psychological Medicine*, vol. 36, no. 5, pp. 659–667, 2006.

[8] S. Moritz and T. S. Woodward, "The contribution of metamemory deficits to schizophrenia," *Journal of Abnormal Psychology*, vol. 115, no. 1, pp. 15–25, 2006.

[9] Ł. Gaweda, S. Moritz, and A. Kokoszka, "Impaired discrimination between imagined and performed actions in schizophrenia," *Psychiatry Research*, vol. 195, no. 1-2, pp. 1–8, 2012.

[10] T. M. Lincoln, S. Mehl, C. Exner, J. Lindenmeyer, and W. Rief, "Attributional style and persecutory delusions. Evidence for an event independent and state specific external-personal attribution bias for social situations," *Cognitive Therapy and Research*, vol. 34, no. 3, pp. 297–302, 2010.

[11] R. P. Bentall, "Cognitive biases and abnormal beliefs: towards a model of persecutory delusions," in *The Neuropsychology of Schizophrenia*, A. S. David and J. Cutting, Eds., pp. 337–360, Erlbaum, London, UK, 1994.

[12] P. Kinderman and R. P. Bentall, "Causal attributions in paranoia and depression: internal, personal, and situational attributions for negative events," *Journal of Abnormal Psychology*, vol. 106, no. 2, pp. 341–345, 1997.

[13] S. Randjbar, R. Veckenstedt, F. Vitzthum, B. Hottenrott, and S. Moritz, "Attributional biases in paranoid schizophrenia: further evidence for a decreased sense of self-causation in paranoia," *Psychosis*, vol. 3, pp. 74–85, 2011.

[14] T. S. Woodward, W. J. Speechley, S. Moritz, T. Lecomte, and E. Ngan, "The contribution of integrating disconfirmatory evidence and jumping to conclusions to delusions in schizophrenia," *Schizophrenia Bulletin*, vol. 35, pp. 249–249, 2009.

[15] T. S. Woodward, L. Buchy, S. Moritz, and M. Liotti, "A bias against disconfirmatory evidence is associated with delusion proneness in a nonclinical sample," *Schizophrenia Bulletin*, vol. 33, no. 4, pp. 1023–1028, 2007.

[16] L. Buchy, T. S. Woodward, and M. Liotti, "A cognitive bias against disconfirmatory evidence (BADE) is associated with schizotypy," *Schizophrenia Research*, vol. 90, no. 1–3, pp. 334–337, 2007.

[17] S. Moritz and T. S. Woodward, "A generalized bias against disconfirmatory evidence in schizophrenia," *Psychiatry Research*, vol. 142, no. 2-3, pp. 157–165, 2006.

[18] T. S. Woodward, S. Moritz, C. Cuttler, and J. C. Whitman, "The contribution of a cognitive bias against disconfirmatory evidence (BADE) to delusions in schizophrenia," *Journal of Clinical and Experimental Neuropsychology*, vol. 28, no. 4, pp. 605–617, 2006.

[19] D. R. Combs, S. D. Adams, D. L. Penn, D. Roberts, J. Tiegreen, and P. Stem, "Social cognition and interaction training (SCIT) for schizophrenia," *Schizophrenia Bulletin*, vol. 33, no. 2, article 585, 2007.

[20] D. L. Roberts and D. L. Penn, "Social cognition and interaction training (SCIT) for outpatients with schizophrenia: a preliminary study," *Psychiatry Research*, vol. 166, no. 2-3, pp. 141–147, 2009.

[21] H. Waller, D. Freeman, S. Jolley, G. Dunn, and P. Garety, "Targeting reasoning biases in delusions: a pilot study of the Maudsley Review Training Programme for individuals with persistent, high conviction delusions," *Journal of Behavior Therapy and Experimental Psychiatry*, vol. 42, no. 3, pp. 414–421, 2011.

[22] S. Moritz, A. Kerstan, R. Veckenstedt et al., "Further evidence for the efficacy of a metacognitive group training in schizophrenia," *Behaviour Research and Therapy*, vol. 49, no. 3, pp. 151–157, 2011.

[23] S. Moritz, R. Veckenstedt, S. Randjbar, F. Vitzthum, and T. S. Woodward, "Antipsychotic treatment beyond antipsychotics: metacognitive intervention for schizophrenia patients improves delusional symptoms," *Psychological Medicine*, vol. 41, no. 09, pp. 1823–1832, 2011.

[24] P. A. Garety, D. R. Hemsley, and S. Wessely, "Reasoning in deluded schizophrenic and paranoid patients. Biases in performance on a probabilistic inference task," *Journal of Nervous and Mental Disease*, vol. 179, no. 4, pp. 194–201, 1991.

[25] M. Ziegler, W. Rief, S. M. Werner, S. Mehl, and T. M. Lincoln, "Hasty decision-making in a variety of tasks: does it contribute to the development of delusions?" *Psychology and Psychotherapy*, vol. 81, no. 3, pp. 237–245, 2008.

[26] P. A. Garety, D. Freeman, S. Jolley et al., "Reasoning, emotions, and delusional conviction in psychosis," *Journal of Abnormal Psychology*, vol. 114, no. 3, pp. 373–384, 2005.

[27] D. M. Warman, P. H. Lysaker, J. M. Martin, L. Davis, and S. L. Haudenschield, "Jumping to conclusions and the continuum of delusional beliefs," *Behaviour Research and Therapy*, vol. 45, no. 6, pp. 1255–1269, 2007.

[28] R. Langdon, P. B. Ward, and M. Coltheart, "Reasoning anomalies associated with delusions in schizophrenia," *Schizophrenia Bulletin*, vol. 36, no. 2, pp. 321–330, 2010.

[29] T. M. Lincoln, M. Ziegler, S. Mehl, and W. Rief, "The jumping to conclusions bias in delusions: specificity and changeability," *Journal of Abnormal Psychology*, vol. 119, no. 1, pp. 40–49, 2010.

[30] T. S. Woodward, M. Munz, C. LeClerc, and T. Lecomte, "Change in delusions is associated with change in 'jumping to conclusions'," *Psychiatry Research*, vol. 170, no. 2-3, pp. 124–127, 2009.

[31] S. H. So, D. Freeman, G. Dunn et al., "Jumping to conclusions, a lack of belief flexibility and delusional conviction in psychosis: a longitudinal investigation of the structure, frequency, and relatedness of reasoning biases," *Journal of Abnormal Psychology*, vol. 121, no. 1, pp. 129–139, 2012.

[32] M. Menon, R. Mizrahi, and S. Kapur, "'Jumping to conclusions' and delusions in psychosis: relationship and response to treatment," *Schizophrenia Research*, vol. 98, no. 1–3, pp. 225–231, 2008.

[33] T. S. Woodward, R. Mizrahi, M. Menon, and B. K. Christensen, "Correspondences between theory of mind, jumping to conclusions, neuropsychological measures and the symptoms of schizophrenia," *Psychiatry Research*, vol. 170, no. 2-3, pp. 119–123, 2009.

[34] R. Dudley, D. Shaftoe, K. Cavanagh et al., "'Jumping to conclusions' in first-episode psychosis," *Early Intervention in Psychiatry*, vol. 5, no. 1, pp. 50–56, 2011.

[35] D. Freeman, K. Pugh, N. Vorontsova, A. Antley, and M. Slater, "Testing the continuum of delusional beliefs: an experimental study using virtual reality," *Journal of Abnormal Psychology*, vol. 119, no. 1, pp. 83–92, 2010.

[36] F. Van Dael, D. Versmissen, I. Janssen, I. Myin-Germeys, J. Van Os, and L. Krabbendam, "Data gathering: biased in psychosis?" *Schizophrenia Bulletin*, vol. 32, no. 2, pp. 341–351, 2006.

[37] S. Moritz and T. S. Woodward, "Jumping to conclusions in delusional and non-delusional schizophrenic patients," *British Journal of Clinical Psychology*, vol. 44, no. 2, pp. 193–207, 2005.

[38] H. Startup, D. Freeman, and P. A. Garety, "Jumping to conclusions and persecutory delusions," *European Psychiatry*, vol. 23, no. 6, pp. 457–459, 2008.

[39] P. A. Garety, M. Gittins, S. Jolley et al., "Differences in cognitive and emotional processes between persecutory and grandiose delusions," *Schizophrenia Bulletin*. In press.

[40] C. Andreou, D. Roesch-Ely, R. Veckenstedt, F. Vitzthum, and S. Moritz, "Cognitive biases as predictors of symptomatic outcome in schizophrenia," in *Proceedings of the 20th European Conference of Psychiatry*, Prague, Czech Republic, 2012.

[41] C. Andreou, D. Roesch-Ely, R. Veckenstedt et al., "Predictors of symptomatic remission after an exacerbation of schizophrenia: the significance of symptoms, neuropsychological performance and cognitive biases," submitted.

[42] M. Wagner, M. Landsberg, S. Mehl et al., "Cognitive biases and cognitive deficits in patients with positive symptoms," in *European Conference on Schizophrenia Research*, Berlin, Germany, 2011.

[43] S. Moritz, R. Veckenstedt, B. Hottenrott, T. S. Woodward, S. Randjbar, and T. M. Lincoln, "Different sides of the same coin? Intercorrelations of cognitive biases in schizophrenia," *Cognitive Neuropsychiatry*, vol. 15, no. 4, pp. 406–421, 2010.

[44] S. Moritz, R. Veckenstedt, S. Randjbar et al., "Decision making under uncertainty and mood induction: further evidence for liberal acceptance in schizophrenia," *Psychological Medicine*, vol. 39, no. 11, pp. 1821–1829, 2009.

[45] S. Moritz, T. S. Woodward, and M. Lambert, "Under what circumtances do patients with schizophrenia jump to conclusions? A liberal acceptance account," *British Journal of Clinical Psychology*, vol. 46, no. 2, pp. 127–137, 2007.

[46] R. Miller, "Schizophrenic psychology, associative learning and the role of forebrain dopamine," *Medical Hypotheses*, vol. 2, no. 5, pp. 203–211, 1976.

[47] S. Moritz, T. S. Woodward, and D. Hausmann, "Incautious reasoning as a pathogenetic factor for the development of psychotic symptoms in schizophrenia," *Schizophrenia Bulletin*, vol. 32, no. 2, pp. 327–331, 2006.

[48] R. Veckenstedt, S. Randjbar, F. Vitzthum, B. Hottenrott, T. S. Woodward, and S. Moritz, "Incorrigibility, jumping to conclusions, and decision threshold in schizophrenia," *Cognitive Neuropsychiatry*, vol. 16, no. 2, pp. 174–192, 2011.

[49] F. Scheu, S. Moritz, J. Aghotor et al., "Liberal acceptance and jumping to conclusions in schizophrenia," in *International Schizophrenia Symposium Bern (ISSB '10)*, Bern, Switzerland, 2010.

[50] S. Moritz and T. S. Woodward, "Metacognitive control over false memories: a key determinant of delusional thinking," *Current Psychiatry Reports*, vol. 8, no. 3, pp. 184–190, 2006.

[51] S. R. Kay, L. A. Opler, and J. P. Lindenmayer, "The Positive and Negative Syndrome Scale (PANSS): rationale and standardisation," *British Journal of Psychiatry*, vol. 155, supplement 7, pp. 59–65, 1989.

[52] E. R. Peters, S. A. Joseph, and P. A. Garety, "Measurement of delusional ideation in the normal population: introducing the PDI (Peters et al. Delusions Inventory)," *Schizophrenia Bulletin*, vol. 25, no. 3, pp. 553–576, 1999.

[53] D. Freeman, P. A. Garety, P. E. Bebbington et al., "Psychological investigation of the structure of paranoia in a non-clinical population," *British Journal of Psychiatry*, vol. 186, pp. 427–435, 2005.

[54] G. Haddock, J. McCarron, N. Tarrier, and E. B. Faragher, "Scales to measure dimensions of hallucinations and delusions: the psychotic symptom rating scales (PSYRATS)," *Psychological Medicine*, vol. 29, no. 4, pp. 879–889, 1999.

[55] T. M. Lincoln, S. Salzmann, M. Ziegler, and S. Westermann, "When does jumping-to-conclusions reach its peak? the interaction of vulnerability and situation-characteristics in social reasoning," *Journal of Behavior Therapy and Experimental Psychiatry*, vol. 42, no. 2, pp. 185–191, 2011.

[56] L. J. Chapman and J. P. Chapman, "Psychosis proneness," in *Controversies in Schizophrenia: Changes and Constancies*, M. Alpert, Ed., pp. 157–174, Guilford Press, New York, NY, USA, 1985.

[57] M. F. Lenzenweger and L. Korfine, "Perceptual aberrations, schizotypy, and the Wisconsin Card Sorting Test," *Schizophrenia Bulletin*, vol. 20, no. 2, pp. 345–357, 1994.

[58] T. A. Judge, R. Ilies, and B. A. Scott, "Work-family conflict and emotions: effects at work and at home," *Personnel Psychology*, vol. 59, no. 4, pp. 779–814, 2006.

[59] A. S. Göritz, "Using online panels in psychological research," in *The Oxford Handbook of Internet Psychology*, A. N. Joinson, K. Y. A. McKenna, T. Postmes, and U.-D. Reips, Eds., pp. 473–485, Oxford University Press, Oxford, UK, 2007.

[60] R. F. Piccolo and J. A. Colquitt, "Transformational leadership and job behaviors: the mediating role of core job characteristics," *Academy of Management Journal*, vol. 49, no. 2, pp. 327–340, 2006.

[61] *EFS Survey Unipark Program* [computer program]. Version 8.1. Köln, Germany, 2011.

[62] T. M. Lincoln, N. Peter, M. Schäfer, and S. Moritz, "Research Letter: from stress to paranoia: an experimental investigation of the moderating and mediating role of reasoning biases," *Psychological Medicine*, vol. 40, no. 1, pp. 169–171, 2010.

[63] T. M. Lincoln, M. Ziegler, E. Lüllmann, M. J. Müller, and W. Rief, "Can delusions be self-assessed? Concordance between self- and observer-rated delusions in schizophrenia," *Psychiatry Research*, vol. 178, no. 2, pp. 249–254, 2010.

[64] S. Westermann, M.-L. Kesting, and T. M. Lincoln, "Being deluded after being excluded?—how emotion regulation deficits in paranoia-prone individuals impact on state paranoia during experimentally induced social stress," *Behavior Therapy*, vol. 43, no. 2, pp. 329–340.

[65] S. Westermann and T. M. Lincoln, "Using signal detection theory to test the impact of negative emotion on sub-clinical paranoia," *Journal of Behavior Therapy and Experimental Psychiatry*, vol. 41, no. 2, pp. 96–101, 2010.

[66] J. Lehrer, "The truth wears off—is there something wrong with the scientific method?" *Annals of Science, The New Yorker—Weekly Magazine*, 2010.

[67] C. E. L. Green, D. Freeman, E. Kuipers et al., "Measuring ideas of persecution and social reference: the Green et al. Paranoid Thought Scales (GPTS)," *Psychological Medicine*, vol. 38, no. 1, pp. 101–111, 2008.

[68] P. Jacobsen, D. Freeman, and P. Salkovskis, "Reasoning bias and belief conviction in obsessive-compulsive disorder and delusions: jumping to conclusions across disorders?" *British Journal of Clinical Psychology*, vol. 51, no. 1, pp. 84–99, 2012.

[69] S. Moritz, N. Van Quaquebeke, M. Hauschildt, L. Jelinek, and S. Gönner, "Good news for allegedly bad studies. Deception in psychopathological studies is less easy than it seems," *Journal of Obsessive-Compulsive and Related Disorders*, vol. 39, pp. 331–335, 2012.

[70] S. Moritz, R. Veckenstedt, S. Randjbar et al., "Decision making under uncertainty and mood induction: further evidence for liberal acceptance in schizophrenia," *Psychological Medicine*, vol. 39, no. 11, pp. 1821–1829, 2009.

[71] S. Westermann, S. Salzmann, X. Fuchs, and T. M. Lincoln, "Introducing a social beads task," *Journal of Experimental Psychopathology*. In press.

[72] W. J. Speechley, J. C. Whitman, and T. S. Woodward, "The contribution of hypersalience to the "jumping to conclusions" bias associated with delusions in schizophrenia," *Journal of Psychiatry and Neuroscience*, vol. 35, no. 1, pp. 7–17, 2010.

21

Neurocognitive and Social Cognitive Approaches for Improving Functional Outcome in Early Psychosis: Theoretical Considerations and Current State of Evidence

Cali F. Bartholomeusz[1] and Kelly Allott[2]

[1] *Melbourne Neuropsychiatry Centre, Department of Psychiatry, National Neuroscience Facility, The University of Melbourne, Level 2-3 Alan Gilbert Building, 161 Barry Street, Carlton South, VIC 3053, Australia*
[2] *Orygen Youth Health Research Centre, Centre for Youth Mental Health, The University of Melbourne, Locked Bag 10, Parkville, VIC 3052, Australia*

Correspondence should be addressed to Cali F. Bartholomeusz, barc@unimelb.edu.au

Academic Editor: César González-Blanch

Improving functional outcome, in addition to alleviating psychotic symptoms, is now a major treatment objective in schizophrenia research. Given the large body of evidence suggesting pharmacological treatments generally have minimal effects on indices of functioning, research has turned to psychosocial rehabilitation programs. Among these, neurocognitive and social cognitive interventions are at the forefront of this field and are argued to target core deficits inherent to the schizophrenia illness. However, to date, research trials have primarily focused on chronic schizophrenia populations, neglecting the early psychosis groups who are often as severely impaired in social and occupational functioning. This theoretical paper will outline the rationale for investigating adjunctive cognitive-based interventions in the early phases of psychotic illness, critically examine the current approach strategies used in these interventions, and assess the evidence supporting certain training programs for improving functional outcome in early psychosis. Potential pathways for future research will be discussed.

1. Introduction

The field of schizophrenia research and treatment is in a transitional phase, shifting from a focus on outcomes that are measured by symptomatic remission and basic illness management to an all-encompassing outlook on real-world functional recovery [1, 2]. This is an exciting time for researchers and consumers, as the improvement in social, occupational, and personally challenging activities that impact the individual's day-to-day living are now primary research objectives. In this research era it is also widely acknowledged that the early phase of a psychotic illness, known as the "critical period," is the most crucial in terms of limiting or even preventing the development of disability, with maximal levels of disability reached within the first 5 years after illness onset [3]. The first onset of psychosis typically occurs between the age of 18 and 24 [4], although prodromal symptoms are often detectable in the adolescent years [5]. There is a paucity of research that has focused investigation on the "functional" outcome of this early psychosis cohort. A systematic review of 37 early detection/intervention studies in first-episode psychosis (FEP) found that 42% of patients had "good" illness outcomes as opposed to 27% who had "poor" outcomes at an average of 3-year follow-up [6]. However, outcome was predominantly defined by hospital readmission or change in symptom severity, with only 4 of the 37 studies reporting functional recovery. Another review, which specifically focused on social, role/occupational, and community functioning, found long-term functional outcome to be poor for a substantial proportion of FEP patients [7]. Furthermore, two randomized controlled trials (RCTs) of intensive therapy, involving multidisciplinary teams offering a mixture of cognitive behavioural therapy (CBT), family therapy, vocational interventions, and social skills training, failed to find significant changes in the size of patients' social network [8, 9] or the amount of contact with existing friends [8]. In addition, although the latter study found more patients in the intensive therapy group (49%) to have spent at least 6 months in educational/vocational activities, a large percentage of patients who were considerably impaired in their role functioning at the 18-month follow-up remained. Overall, findings support early intervention strategies as key to the treatment and prevention of psychotic disorders, which has shown significant benefits over more traditional approaches [10]. However, this biopsychosocial approach [11] is largely ineffective for the treatment of social impairment, highlighting the need for innovative intervention strategies targeting functional outcome.

This paper will examine the evidence and potential for neurocognitive and social cognitive interventions in addressing the issue of functional recovery in early psychosis. With the impetus that cognitive deficits are at the core of schizophrenia [12], this paper will only include interventions that have a neurocognitive or social cognitive target; thus, interventions that focus primarily on changing behaviour, such as social skills training (SST) and cognitive behavioural therapy (CBT), will not be addressed here (for review of other interventions see [13]). For this review, the term "neurocognition" will be used to refer to elementary cognitive abilities (e.g., memory, attention, etc.) and remediation/therapies that are neurocognitive based. "Social cognition" which encompasses the perception, interpretation, and processing of social information, will refer to purely social cognitive abilities, primarily, emotion perception (recognition of facial and vocal affect); social perception and social knowledge (the ability to detect and comprehend social cues with respect to social context); Theory of Mind (ToM; the mental capacity to infer one's own and others' mental states); attributional style (tendencies in explaining the cause of events, i.e. to the self, others or the environment) [14]. The term "cognition" will be used to encompass both neurocognition and social cognition. We will first provide a rationale for focusing on cognition by drawing on evidence supporting the neurodevelopmental hypothesis and the link between cognition and functional outcome. This paper will then highlight the differences in the theoretical underpinnings of the available interventions, in addition to reviewing original research that has tested the effects of such interventions on functional outcome in FEP or ultra high-risk (UHR) of psychosis samples. Discussion surrounding future pathways for achieving real-world improvements in social and occupational functioning will be provided, within the context of the early phase of illness.

2. Why Focus on Cognitive-Based Interventions?

2.1. The Neurodevelopmental Hypothesis and Evidence from Neuroimaging Research. While basic cognitive skills are acquired by early childhood, research suggests higher-order cognitive abilities are refined during adolescence [15, 16]. This coincides with substantial changes in white and grey-matter volume as part of normal neurodevelopment [17]. Regions that appear to undergo substantial structural and functional changes are those particularly associated with response inhibition, evaluation of risk and reward, and emotion regulation [18], domains falling under the broader rubric of executive neurocognitive and social cognitive abilities. Notably, changes are occurring at a time when there is a corresponding shift in social behavior, given adolescence is typically a tumultuous period of life where an individual becomes more self-conscious, heavily influenced by peers, and begins to develop a personal identity [19]. Such brain and behavioural changes, along with pubertal hormonal changes, are thought to be causal factors for the higher rate of psychiatric illness onset observed during adolescence [20]. For example, in Australia, individuals aged between 14 and 25 have the highest prevalence (26%) of a current diagnosed mental disorder [21]. Approximately 65% of Australians who develop a psychotic disorder experience their first episode before the age of 25, with 23% experiencing psychosis onset between age of 25 and 34 [22]. Worth noting, almost 40% first experience psychotic symptoms in their teenage years. Taken together, the abnormal maturation of specific brain regions during this critical period may be related to cognitive deficits in schizophrenia and early psychosis. Furthermore, the chances of cognitive training/therapy being absorbed and retained is likely to be higher due to the greater brain plasticity associated with ongoing neurodevelopment in this adolescent/early-adult phase of life [23].

In FEP, impairments are present in all domains of neurocognition, with the most severe deficits observed in immediate verbal memory and speed of information processing [24, 25]. The profile and severity of neurocognitive impairment tends to be stable over time and is similar to that seen in chronic schizophrenia [26]. Findings regarding the UHR cohort are less consistent [27], but similarly tend to suggest general impairment with accentuated deficits specifically in verbal memory, working memory, and processing speed for individuals who later convert to full-threshold psychosis [28]. A recent meta-analysis of functional magnetic resonance imaging (fMRI) data has shown that both FEP and UHR patients display neurocognitive abnormalities most commonly related to the prefrontal and anterior cingulate cortices, the basal ganglia, hippocampus and cerebellum [29]. In FEP specifically, abnormal blood-oxygen-level-dependent (BOLD) responses were observed in the regions of interest (dorsolateral and ventrolateral prefrontal cortices and anterior prefrontal cortex) during tasks assessing working memory, verbal fluency, executive control, elementary information processing, context processing, and planning/logical reasoning, with medium to large effect sizes (ESs).

The study of social cognition in early psychosis is less advanced. Despite this, compelling evidence indicates that multiple social cognitive domains are dysfunctional in FEP, including emotion recognition [30–34], social perception [34–36], ToM [34, 37–39], and attributional style [40, 41]. Research into social cognition in UHR is scarce; however, review of the limited literature (see [42]) suggests deficits are present in emotion recognition [33, 34, 43–45], ToM [34, 46], and social perception/knowledge [34, 47], as well as bias in attributional style [41]. A recent cross-sectional study involving three patient groups at different developmental stages of the illness (i.e., prodromal, FEP, and chronic) provides further evidence for social cognitive deficits presenting early during the at-risk phase, which remain stable through the later illness phases [34]. Brain regions that are typically activated during social cognitive tasks include the medial prefrontal cortex (mPFC), orbitofrontal cortex (OFC), superior temporal sulcus (STS), temporoparietal junction (TPJ), cingulate cortex (CC), amygdala and anterior insula, collectively known as the "social brain" [48]. Numerous imaging studies have found these regions to be structurally abnormal in FEP and UHR (for review see [49, 50]). To date, only one study has examined brain activation during a social cognitive (emotion discrimination) task in adolescents with early-onset schizophrenia [51]. Although performance on the task was unimpaired, patients showed decreased activation in areas such as the CC and insula during facial emotion processing. Two studies in UHR patients have also found abnormal activation of social brain regions in relation to emotion processing [52] and ToM mental state attributions [53].

Evidence of abnormal anatomical and functional connectivity between frontal and temporal/parietal regions in early psychosis [54–57] further implicates dysfunctional brain networks that govern cognitive processes as central features in illness pathophysiology. Overall, neuroimaging evidence highlights cognitive deficits as being at the core of psychotic illness and supports general cognition, plus several specific domains, as good candidates for targeted interventions during the early phase of illness.

2.2. The Role of Neurocognition and Social Cognition in Functional Outcome. For well over a decade neurocognition has been acknowledged as having a significant impact on functioning and functional outcome [58]. We will use the term "functional outcome" in relation to prospective studies and follow-up trials, while the term "functioning" will generally refer to the current level of functioning at the time of testing. Functional outcome/functioning are usually measured by assessment of actual performance of activities of daily living/social activities (e.g., hours worked) or assessment of the ability to perform everyday functioning skills (e.g., using a role-play task). Systematic reviews in chronic schizophrenia suggest that cognitive deficits (especially in executive functioning, verbal learning, and memory and attention) have an equal or greater role than psychotic symptoms in predicting current and prospective functional impairment [58, 59]. Results are less consistent in FEP, most likely due to methodological issues; however, findings currently lean towards verbal/language skills most consistently predicting functional outcome [60].

While debate continues over the degree of overlap between neurocognitive (in particular attention/executive control, basic reasoning) and social cognitive processes, research supports these two domains as independent constructs that contribute unique variance to the prediction of functional outcome, social functioning, and interpersonal skills in both chronic schizophrenia and early psychosis [30, 61–65]. Social cognition, in addition to conferring direct effects, has been suggested to act as a mediator between neurocognition and social functioning [30, 66, 67]. Worth noting, social cognition has been argued to have a greater impact on work-related social skills and work outcomes than neurocognition [61, 68, 69]. A recent meta-analysis concluded that social cognition was a stronger predictor of overall community functioning, incorporating independent living skills plus social and work functioning, than general neurocognition [59]. The few studies that have examined the relationship between social cognition and functioning in FEP support the findings of chronic schizophrenia research. Specifically, emotion recognition [30, 66], emotional intelligence/social perception [65, 66, 70], and social knowledge [70] have all been shown to have direct or indirect effects on general social functioning, and in some cases interpersonal problem solving as well. Findings from a recent 12-month follow-up study further highlight the significant longitudinal impact of social cognitive deficits on work, independent living, and social functioning outcomes [71].

Despite some discrepancies in the literature and the limited studies in FEP, evidence from chronic schizophrenia research is robust in that cognition undeniably has a significant impact on functional outcome. In terms of neurocognition and social cognition, verbal fluency and ToM respectively, are shown to have the largest effects on community functioning [59]. Further research is needed to determine the impact of these two cognitive domains on alternative areas of functioning and functional outcome, such as social behaviour, social problem solving, and social skills.

Overall, behavioural findings coupled with neuroimaging evidence suggest that there is potential for significant improvement and even prevention of social and occupational decline for young people with emerging and first-onset psychosis and that interventions targeting cognitive processes are warranted.

3. Background of Cognitive Intervention Programs in Schizophrenia

Cognitive remediation is the most common form of the cognitive-based interventions used in schizophrenia and has recently been defined as "a behavioural training based intervention that aims to improve cognitive processes (attention, memory, executive function, social cognition or metacognition) with the goal of durability and generalization" [72, page 1]. This definition implies that although dysfunction in cognition, including social cognition, is the intervention target, improved and sustained functioning in the real world is the desired outcome [73]. It should be noted that, although social cognition is included in the above definition, the majority of cognitive remediation programs to date have predominantly targeted neurocognitive processes. The approaches used in cognitive remediation are highly variable, but a clear common element is repeated practice in exercises requiring effortful "thinking skills." The majority of programs also involve a trained facilitator (see [74] for exception). However, the frequency and duration of training sessions is inconsistent, as is whether the intervention is delivered one-on-one or involves a group-based component.

Numerous systematic reviews of neurocognitive remediation have been published, but the first quantitative meta-analysis (26 studies) to examine the effects of neurocognitive remediation on functional outcome found a small-to-medium mean ES of 0.36, which was only slightly lower than the improvement found in neurocognitive function (mean ES 0.41) [75]. Interestingly, the effect of neurocognitive remediation on functioning was significantly moderated by whether or not adjunctive psychosocial rehabilitation, such as vocational programs or SST, was provided, with the finding that provision of psychosocial rehabilitation led to significant improvements in social functioning (mean ES 0.47). In comparison, studies of neurocognitive remediation alone produced a meagre mean ES of 0.05. These findings were broadly replicated in an updated meta-analysis that included 40 RCTs, although the effect sizes were slightly larger [72]. The mechanism for this "synergistic" effect is hypothesised to be the improved neurocognitive functioning produced by neurocognitive remediation enhancing the capacity to learn new skills, which in turn leads to increased benefit from psychiatric rehabilitation [75]. However, this hypothesis requires further empirical investigation, such as examination of whether change in cognition is associated with change in functioning.

Because social cognitive neuropsychiatric research is in its infancy, social cognitive interventions are considered to be a relatively new line of treatment for improving social functioning. The primary goal of such interventions is to enhance social cognitive abilities, which as mentioned earlier, are considered to be largely independent constructs to neurocognitive processes. Social cognitive interventions typically employ a model that is bidirectional and flexible, where social cognitive processes, emotions, and actions are addressed in unison or in parallel, as opposed to a pure bottom-up information-processing framework characteristic of some neurocognitive interventions. Due to the limited research into social cognitive interventions, fewer reviews have been conducted. The most commanding review to date is a recent meta-analysis of 19 controlled trials of social cognitive training in established schizophrenia [76]. A large mean ES (0.78) was found for observer-rated indices of functional outcome (6 of the 19 studies), which in contrast to the neurocognition meta-analyses was larger than most of the ESs found for specific domains of social cognition. This finding is impressive given that the social cognitive interventions reviewed led to generalised improvements in functioning mostly in the absence of adjunctive psychosocial interventions. It has been suggested that the mediating role of social cognition between neurocognition and functional outcome implies that social cognition is more proximal to real-world functioning. Thus, targeting social cognition may produce greater effects on functioning than neurocognition [77].

Given that this paper is focused specifically on early psychosis, it is important to explore whether age or stage of illness may be a key moderator of outcome in trials of cognitive remediation. With respect to participant age as a moderator, the existing research is equivocal. The McGurk et al. [75] meta-analysis found that older patients (aged 38–50 years) benefited more from neurocognitive remediation in terms of functioning (mean ES 0.55) than younger patients (aged 15–37 years; mean ES 0.18). However, it should be noted that the younger patient group included a wide age range and likely included patients with a long duration of illness. The more recent meta-analysis by Wykes et al. [72] found that age did not moderate outcome, but it was unclear as to whether this included functional outcome. Conversely, the Kurtz and Richardson [76] meta-analysis found that age was negatively correlated with functional (and symptomatic) outcome, such that younger patients (youngest mean age was 25 years) benefited more from social cognition training than older patients, although exact age ranges were not stated. Some studies have suggested that illness stage (e.g., first-versus multiple-episode) or duration of illness affects responses to cognitive remediation, but again findings are mixed. Longer illness duration is associated with poorer response to neurocognitive remediation [78–82], but better response to social cognitive remediation [76]. Despite the majority of studies to date having recruited patients with longstanding psychotic disorders, evidence from neuroimaging and behavioural research discussed earlier suggests that intervening in the early stages of psychosis may provide greater potential for recovery to premorbid levels, when individuals are less removed from their original functional trajectories.

4. Current Approaches for Treating Cognitive Deficits

Having briefly reviewed the evidence for cognitive remediation in schizophrenia, the paper will now turn to describing the specific approaches used and their theoretical underpinnings.

4.1. Drill and Practice. Also referred to as the stimulation approach [83], drill and practice is the most common technique used in neurocognitive remediation programs for psychosis [72, 75]. Restoration or enhancement of cognitive function is the goal of drill and practice, and the underlying model presupposes neural plasticity and that cognitive impairment can be rectified, subsequently leading to improvements in performance in daily activities. In drill and practice, individuals are engaged in focused cognitive processing by repetitive training on progressively more difficult exercises. Usually these exercises are computerized, but may also be paper and pencil, and can be theoretically categorized as either "bottom-up" or "top-down." Bottom-up approaches presume that a basic deficit in signal-to-noise discrimination of auditory and visual information underlies higher-level cognitive dysfunction. An example of a bottom-up drill and practice approach is Targeted Cognitive Training (TCT) using the PositScience program [74, 84], which usually involves daily sessions totaling 50 to 100 hours [74, 84]. Top-down drill and practice approaches, such as the Neuropsychological Educational Approach to Cognitive

Remediation (NEAR) [85], target higher-order cognitive functions (executive, complex attention, memory) usually via exercises that simultaneously harness a broad range of cognitive abilities, believed to simulate one's cognitive engagement in real-world activities [73].

4.2. Strategy Coaching. Strategy coaching is a technique commonly used in cognitive remediation programs, usually in conjunction with drill and practice [72]. However, it is not well defined. There is some conjecture as to whether this approach involves transfer of remediated cognitive abilities to daily functioning (i.e., generalised restoration) or assists individuals to compensate for their cognitive deficits conferring improved functioning [75, 86]. Strategy coaching includes teaching individuals to use specific mental strategies to enhance performance on specific exercises or tasks, for instance, teaching a person to use visualisation/mental pictures to help them remember a list of words. An example of a program that relies heavily on strategy coaching (in addition to drill and practice) is Cognitive Remediation Therapy (CRT), adapted by Wykes and Reeder [87] from the work of Delahunty and Morice [88]. CRT is an individualised one-on-one 40-hour (3 times/week) teaching program aimed at enhancing working memory, planning, and problem solving (cognitive flexibility), with the goal of transferring cognitive skills to real-world functioning.

4.3. Compensation. Alternative approaches which are not traditionally used in cognitive remediation [72], but are used in other neurocognitive interventions, include compensation and adaptation [89–92]. The model underlying compensatory approaches assumes that developing alternative strategies will reduce cognitive load and minimize the impact of cognitive impairment on daily functioning, in much the same way as glasses reduce the impact of vision impairment [93]. Compensatory approaches can be broadly categorised into three techniques: self-management, environmental adaptation, and errorless learning.

Self-management techniques include internal (mental) and external (behavioural) strategies. An example of a self-management compensatory program is Cognitive Training (CT) [89]. CT is a manualised 12-week group-based intervention (although it can also be delivered individually) that focuses on four key cognitive domains: (1) prospective memory—remembering to remember (e.g., daily calendar use), (2) attention and vigilance (e.g., using self-talk to remain on task), (3) learning and memory (e.g., mnemonic strategies such as chunking or rhyming), and (4) executive functioning—problem solving and cognitive flexibility (e.g., six-step problem solving technique). Each 2-hour session includes didactic teaching, demonstration/observation, practice, and feedback as well as homework for further practice in daily life. The expectation is that the generic strategies taught in CT will be independently applied by participants to manage their individual day-to-day tasks [89, 94].

The second (not mutually exclusive) approach is *environmental adaptation*, which is applied by an individual and/or caregiver for the purpose of bypassing cognitive deficits. Environmental adaptation techniques generally aim to direct or capture a person's attention so as to prompt performance in goal-directed behaviour at the appropriate time. An exemplar of this approach is Cognitive Adaptation Training (CAT [91]). CAT is a manualised treatment involving the application of multiple external compensatory strategies (e.g., reducing distracting information at a work desk) and environmental supports (e.g., signs, alarms, checklists) that are individually tailored based on initial assessment of level of cognitive dysfunction, behavioural/learning type, and specific functional goals. A broad range of functional domains are targeted, ranging from grooming/personal care to leisure activities, and medication adherence. CAT is delivered in the community (usually at home) on a weekly basis for 9 months [95].

The final compensatory approach that warrants mention is *errorless learning*, which is a strategy used to compensate for a learning deficit in which there is difficulty distinguishing between correct performances and mistakes, even after feedback (which has been shown in schizophrenia [96–98]). Typically, a trainer prevents the individual from experiencing errors while learning a specific task, so that only correct responses are allowed [96]. The task in question (such as learning someone's name or performing a specific task at work) is learnt with a trainer via repetitive practice of smaller simpler task components, gradually working towards total task completion in a stepwise fashion without making any errors. Errorless learning approaches have been most extensively examined by Kern and colleagues with a strong focus on functional outcomes [96, 99, 100]. Like CAT, errorless learning is applied in a highly specific and individualised manner. This may be viewed as either a strength or limitation, depending on the desired outcome of the patient and the researcher/clinician.

4.4. Behavioural Learning. Behavioural learning approaches also form an important part of many cognitive rehabilitation interventions. One of the theories underlying behavioural learning is that motivation may impede performance in cognitive or functional tasks in schizophrenia [73, 83, 95, 101, 102]. These approaches are not usually used in isolation and are inherent to many cognitive rehabilitation programs, although often programs do not explicitly state this when describing their protocol. The simplest example is positive reinforcement via praise and encouragement delivered by cognitive specialists or therapists. Some programs explicitly target motivation to complete cognitive exercises via extrinsic monetary incentives [74, 103], while others target intrinsic motivation by using engaging and enjoyable tasks, allowing participant control over learning, and linking these tasks with individual goals [85, 104]. Other examples of behavioural learning approaches include setting tasks at the appropriate level to ensure the participant experiences success [74, 103, 104], shaping—rewarding successive approximations of the target goal [105], and scaffolding—instructional teaching and support in learning something new by building upon what is already known [106].

4.5. Metacognitive Learning. Metacognitive rehabilitation strategies, traditionally suggested as an adjunct to CBT for reducing negative beliefs about failure, stigmatization, and coping abilities, have more recently been integrated into cognitive intervention programs [107]. Metacognition can be defined as "thinking about one's thinking" [108], and more specifically knowing about one's own cognitive abilities, states of knowledge, and actual performance, which is distinct from the cognitive abilities, states of knowledge, and performance themselves [109]. Metacognition involves self-reflection, the ability to monitor decision-making and competence, and report-control (i.e., directing behaviour based on thought monitoring) [109]. Metacognitive strategies are almost always coupled with mediated learning and exposure to new experiences, and are therefore frequently incorporated with strategy coaching. For example, Metacognitive Skills Training (MCT) [108] is designed to facilitate participants' awareness of cognitive difficulties, to critically reflect on these difficulties, and to complement or change their current thinking styles accordingly. MCT addresses impairments in both neurocognitive and social cognitive domains by focusing on issues of self-serving bias, jumping to conclusions, bias against disconfirmatory evidence, deficits in ToM, overconfidence in memory errors, and depressive cognitive patterns.

4.6. Role-Play. Role-play, the acting out/simulation of one or more characters in a given social situation, has long been used in SST and as a way for assessing whether the desired behavioural skills were retained [110]. Within a cognitive-based model, role-play is used as a slightly different training tool in two particular ways. One is where cognitive skills are first taught (e.g., using Socratic questioning and metacognitive strategies), and participants are later asked to role-play a social scenario using the taught cognitive skills as practice for real-world application. Role-play is also helpful for the facilitator to determine what areas require further work and tailor the remaining training sessions accordingly. Secondly, similar to modeling, for interventions that involve more than one facilitator (such as Social Cognition and Interaction Training (SCIT) [111]), role-play may be conducted by the facilitators themselves and used as a demonstration tool. This, along with mimicry, is primarily used in social cognitive interventions, as it is thought to engage the simulation system of the brain [112], which has been linked to ToM, emotion perception, and empathic ability [113].

4.7. Exposure to Social Situations and Group-Based Therapy. Exposure therapy is fundamentally linked to behavioural learning approaches and is the most established psychosocial intervention for the treatment of social anxiety disorders [114]. Exposure therapy is based on the theory of experimental "extinction," which is the progressive weakening of a habit via the repeated evocation of the response without reinforcement [115, 116]. Use of exposure traditionally begins with identifying a hierarchy of the feared social situations, which the person then endures and works through starting with the least distressing situation to the point where the anxiety has decreased, before moving on to the next least anxiety-provoking situation [117]. This exposure therapy technique has predominantly been adapted for social cognitive interventions, where the technique is used in a less explicit way by means of group-based therapy and through administration of cognitive-based exercises requiring partner work. The design of SCIT, for example, integrates this technique in a subtle way by assuming social situations are inherently daunting for patients. As such, the level of participation required, and personal relevance to each individual, increases from week to week as group alliance grows [118]. The exposure technique, coupled with role-play, has also been used in Cognitive Enhancement Therapy (CET) [119], where patients are asked to give a 5–10 minute presentation on facts about themselves, qualities in themselves that they admire, examples of these qualities, and why they admire them. In addition, the participants take turns acting as "chairperson" during group discussions.

4.8. Theoretical Considerations. Many of the approaches and techniques described previously, particularly those used in social cognitive interventions, feature centrally in traditional CBT and SST. Although theoretically they differ in terms of their treatment target (cognition versus behaviour), it begs the question: how do cognitive interventions differ practically to CBT and SST? The main difference lies in the component of the technique that is emphasized or focused on. For example, in CBT clinicians will typically challenge the *logic* behind specific overvalued beliefs, while neurocognitive interventions conversely focus on the perceptual and interpretive *processes* that may have contributed to the development/maintenance of the delusional belief. SST on the other hand may, for example, use behavioural learning or role-play techniques to reinforce a certain socially appropriate behaviour. However, the underlying thought processes that relate to recognizing and interpreting when a social situation calls for a given emotional and subsequent behavioural response are not emphasized in SST, as they are in social cognitive programs. Lastly, the way in which particular approach strategies are combined will additionally distinguish cognitive interventions as unique from SST and CBT.

5. Effects of Neurocognitive Interventions on Functional Outcome in Early Psychosis

5.1. Ultra High-Risk. To the best of our knowledge there is only one published study of neurocognitive remediation in individuals at UHR for psychosis [79], with at least one other trial underway [120]. Functional outcome was not measured in the Rauchensteiner study, but given the novel application of cognitive remediation in this population, we will describe it briefly. Rauchensteiner et al. [79] conducted a small pilot study comparing the effects of 10 sessions of primarily drill and practice computer-based cognitive remediation (using Cogpack software) in UHR participants versus a schizophrenia control group. Only the UHR participants improved in cognitive performance following 4 weeks of training, specifically on tests of attention and verbal memory. Notwithstanding significant limitations, including the small sample size, possibility of practice effects, no measure of functioning, convenience sampling, and lack of a control condition, this study provides the first evidence of the potential advantages of delivering cognitive remediation at the putative earliest stage of schizophrenia. Given that cognitive deficits are significantly associated with functional outcome in ultra high-risk individuals [121, 122], there is clear rationale for further research into cognitive remediation in this population.

5.2. Recent-Onset Psychosis. Three research groups have published results on different cognitive remediation interventions in recent-onset psychosis and one other is underway [120]. Each of the completed trials will be described with a specific focus on functional outcome. In a small RCT, Ueland and Rund [123, 124] investigated whether 30 hours of individual neurocognitive remediation could enhance functional outcomes in inpatient adolescents (aged 12–18) with early-onset psychosis already receiving comprehensive psychoeducational treatment. Participants were randomized to receive cognitive remediation ($n = 14$) or treatment as usual (TAU; $n = 12$). Cognitive remediation comprised four modules: cognitive differentiation (basic conceptual cognitive skills), attention (enhanced instructions and monetary reinforcement), memory (practice and strategies on verbal and visual memory tasks), and social perception (training in encoding social stimuli). This program involved drill and practice, strategy coaching, and behavioural learning techniques. Both groups improved in cognition and functioning over time, with no significant between-group differences found in functional outcome (as measured by the Global Assessment Scale) at postintervention or 1-year follow-up. Furthermore, changes in cognition were not associated with changes in functioning.

The second study was an RCT of CRT (described previously) for patients with recently diagnosed adolescent-onset schizophrenia (aged 14–22) [125]. Participants were randomly allocated to CRT ($n = 21$) or TAU ($n = 19$). Despite CRT effecting improvement in cognitive flexibility relative to the control condition, there were no group differences in functioning as measured by the Social Behaviour Schedule. However, secondary analyses found that improvement in cognition was associated with improvements in social functioning in the context of CRT, providing preliminary evidence for restitution of cognitive function being associated with functional improvements.

Finally, the largest and longest RCT of cognitive remediation in recent-onset psychosis (defined as onset < 8 years prior) was conducted by Eack and colleagues [126]. Participants were randomized to receive CET ($n = 31$) or an active control condition: Enriched Supportive Therapy (EST; $n = 27$). CET [119] is a comprehensive program that integrates remediation in neurocognition and social cognition using multiple methods including 60 hours of computer-assisted exercises (attention, memory, and problem solving; PSSCogRehab program) conducted in pairs. It also includes 45 group-based weekly training sessions in social cognitive skills (perspective taking, social perception, managing emotions, and social context appraisal) taught and practiced *in vivo* via psychoeducation, role-play, and experimental and homework exercises. The program takes 2 years to complete. CET is unique in that it is the only cognitive remediation approach that comprehensively addresses both neurocognition and social cognition. EST is an individual therapy that focuses on psychoeducation and stress management, but is not matched to CET in session number or program duration. At 2 years (post-intervention), relative to EST, CET resulted in significantly greater improvements in almost all composite domains of neurocognitive and social cognitive function, as well as a composite index of social adjustment (Social Adjustment Scale-II, Major Role Adjustment Inventory, Global Assessment Scale, and Performance Potential Inventory) [126]. Further analyses revealed that CET participants achieved superior outcomes in terms of competitive employment (58% versus 19%), wages earned, work readiness, employment satisfaction, social relationships, social functioning, social leisure, role adjustment, activities of daily living, and instrumental task performance, as well as global functioning [126, 127]. These functional gains were largely maintained at 1-year follow-up [128]. One major caveat to these findings is that raters were not blind to treatment allocation.

An important question arising from this study is what are the active ingredients of CET catalysing the functional improvements observed? The largest effects were found in the domain of social cognition with over 60% improvement over 2 years compared to just over 10% improvement in neurocognition over the same period [126]. This possibly implicates the social cognitive training aspect of CET as the more active ingredient. Interestingly Eack et al. [128] found that improvement in neurocognition by treatment end was the only predictor of maintenance in social adjustment at 1-year follow-up. Subsequent analyses of specific employment outcomes found that improvements in both social cognition and neurocognition mediated the effects of CET on employment [127]. Notwithstanding these impressive findings, a second major caveat to this study is that the CET group received many more hours of therapist contact and socialization in pairs/groups compared to the control group, so it is possible that greater exposure to social situations and therapist support/guidance resulted in the improved functional outcomes. The issue of feasibility should also be questioned and whether CET can be supported within a clinical service given the additive level of input required by the treating clinical team and the sheer amount of time involved. It is also worth noting that, at baseline, participants had a mean age of 25.9 years (SD = 6.54 years) and a mean illness duration of 3.2 years (SD = 2.2) [126], with 22% of individuals having been unwell for more than 5 years (<8 years). Thus, findings may not be generalised to conventional definitions of early psychosis (which is typically within 2 years of first illness presentation). Further research is needed to tease out the active elements in CET as well as other remediation programs that are associated with improvements in functional outcome [73, 83, 129].

6. Effects of Social Cognitive Interventions on Functional Outcome in Early Psychosis

Due to the more recent inception of social cognition in the field of schizophrenia research, no published literature to date has investigated a social cognitive intervention program in a UHR or FEP cohort. Despite this, the meta-analysis of chronic schizophrenia studies mentioned earlier provides very promising findings [76]. We will briefly review the available interventions that have been trialed in established schizophrenia, with reference to their impact on functional outcome and applicability in early psychosis.

Social Cognition and Interaction Training (SCIT), developed by Penn et al. [130], is probably the most evidence-based stand-alone social cognitive intervention currently available. SCIT is a manualised 20-week (1 session/week) group-based intervention targeting multiple aspects of social cognition. SCIT employs a range of approaches including behavioural learning (and at times strategy coaching), metacognitive training, role-play, and exposure therapy techniques. There are three phases: (1) emotion training, which focuses on defining emotions, emotion mimicry, and understanding paranoia, (2) figuring out situations, which focuses on distinguishing facts from guesses, jumping to conclusions, and understanding bad events, and (3) integration, which encourages participants to "check it out" or apply their newly acquired social cognitive skills to personal real-life situations. A small trial that compared SCIT ($n = 18$) to a coping skills group ($n = 10$; which focused on problem-solving, symptom management, and relapse prevention) found SCIT to be significantly more effective at improving performance on measures of social and emotion perception, ToM, and attributional style [111]. Aggressive behaviour, patient's need for closure, and social relationships also improved with SCIT. Moreover, social functioning (as assessed with the Social Functioning Scales: engagement and interpersonal [131]) improved significantly, independent of changes in psychopathology. A more recent trial of SCIT in an outpatient setting has yielded similar positive results [132]. These successful trials led to the integration of the SCIT program into standard clinical practice within mental health services around New York [133]. Given the SCIT model emphasizes that performance varies as a function of the personal relevance and emotional tone of the social context and ultimately aims to improve day-to-day living, our research team has adapted SCIT to be suitable for young people with emerging psychosis. A pilot study in a FEP sample is currently underway.

Emotion and ToM Imitation Training (ETIT) [134] is one of the other few social cognition interventions that have been found to enhance functional outcome. This is a 12-week group-based program, involving participants imitating emotional facial expressions in the mirror, tracking eye-gaze of others, and observing pictures of art, sketches, and comic strips depicting social scenarios with the aim of enhancing the ability to infer mental states of others and attribution of intentions. ETIT stems from the mirror neuron theory of imitation [135], thus relies heavily on the mimicry approach, but also uses coaching and role-play techniques. A small RCT found that schizophrenia patients in the ETIT group ($n = 16$) improved significantly on multiple aspects of social cognition, but also on a global measure of personal and social functioning, in comparison to individuals in a problem solving skills training group ($n = 17$) [134]. To our knowledge no follow-up studies or trials in an early psychosis population have been published.

There are several other targeted and broad-based social cognitive interventions that have been developed and trialed in schizophrenia, but to date most have conducted limited assessment of functional outcome. However, as found by Kurtz and Richardson [76], significant effects on functioning are emerging. One of the programs available for possible use in FEP samples is Social Cognition Enhancement Training (SCET) developed by Kwon [136] and modified by Choi and Kwon [137]. This is a 6-month (36 session) group-based program consisting of three phases (elementary, middle, and advanced), each with 12 sessions. The use of cartoon stories is a central feature of SCET, which aid in the learning of social cue perception, context appraisal, and social knowledge. Additional techniques used are psychoeducation, behavioural learning approaches, and exposure to social situations via group work. Other programs include MCT (described earlier) and a similar intervention devised by Roncone et al. [138], Training of Affect Recognition (TAR) [139], and Ekman's Micro-Expression Training Tool (METT) [140], but comprehensive studies are lacking, even in established schizophrenia [76]. Nevertheless, these interventions and various techniques may still hold potential for enhancing social and other areas of functioning. However, larger studies that include functioning as a primary outcome across different illness stages are required before any inferences can be made.

7. Conclusions and Future Directions

The literature is clearly lacking in the area of early psychosis, with only four studies having trialed a cognitive intervention, and these were primarily focused on neurocognition as opposed social cognition. With respect to functional outcome, the most successful of these appeared to be CET. However, as discussed, the CET trial had significant limitations. These included the control group being unmatched for nonspecific treatment effects and raters not being blind to group allocation, making it difficult to draw firm conclusions regarding the potency of specific aspects of the intervention (i.e., neurocognitive versus social cognitive remediation). Furthermore, participants were not representative of traditional early psychosis samples.

Our review revealed that there are currently no published data available on the efficacy of an exclusive social cognitive intervention in an early psychosis sample. This is noteworthy, given that the behavioural evidence, discussed earlier, and the quantitative review revealing larger effects of social cognitive training on functioning relative to reviews of cognitive remediation in established schizophrenia [76], points towards social cognition as having a greater impact on functional outcome than neurocognition.

In summary, it is presently impossible to make any definitive conclusions regarding the usefulness of cognitive-based interventions in the treatment of functional disability for this early illness population.

While there is evidence that cognitive interventions lead to significant moderate improvements in specific cognitive abilities for individuals with established schizophrenia, residual cognitive deficits often remain [72, 75]. It has been previously suggested that there may be a ceiling to the effects of cognitive remediation at least when delivered in isolation [92]. At present, it is unclear how much improvement in cognition is enough to lead to significant functional improvements, whether stand-alone cognitive interventions are sufficient, or even whether improvement in cognition is essential for functional recovery. Furthermore, it is entirely possible that psychosocial programs that only target functioning may improve cognition, in the absence of a program specifically aimed at treating cognitive deficits [141]. These points open a number of important avenues for future research, with the overarching question being how do we optimize functional outcome?

Starting with evidence from neurocognitive interventions, the schizophrenia literature indicates that neurocognitive remediation combined with psychosocial rehabilitation is far superior with respect to functional outcome than when cognitive remediation is delivered alone [72, 75], yet apart from the Ueland and Rund [124] study, no other trials combining psychosocial with cognitive approaches have been completed in early psychosis, although at least two others are currently underway [142, 143]. One RCT proposes to combine Multifamily Group Psychoeducation with neurocognitive remediation using the PSSCogRehab computer program (drill and practice approach), with the primary outcome being relapse rates. Secondary outcomes include functioning in social, vocational, and activities of daily living domains and quality of life in patients with recent-onset psychosis [143]. Another RCT (NEUROCOM study) will recruit FEP patients and randomize them to receive a combination of cognitive training with a comprehensive psychosocial program (OPUS) or OPUS alone, with the primary outcome being everyday functional capacity [142]. In this study the cognitive training will comprise a combination of computer-assisted drill-and-practice exercises and strategy coaching as well as teaching compensatory strategies (e.g., calendar use). The outcomes of these studies will be very informative.

Despite the lack of early psychosis research into the combined intervention approach, Integrated Psychological Therapy (IPT) [144] has been extensively investigated in established schizophrenia and warrants discussion. IPT is a manualised group-based intervention that aims to ameliorate cognitive impairment and social behavioural deficits, with the ultimate goal of improving social competence [145]. It involves 30–60 min sessions three times per week for 3 months and comprises 5 hierarchically arranged subprograms targeting cognitive differentiation, social perception, verbal communication, social skills, and interpersonal problem solving. Meta-analysis of 30 IPT studies (7 of which were RCTs) showed that IPT compared to a control condition or TAU was more effective for enhancing neurocognition (mean ES 0.41), psychosocial functioning (mean ES 0.31), and psychopathology (mean 0.31) [146]. The largest effect was on neurocognition, which is not surprising given IPT is heavily focused on this domain. Not only do the findings support the combined approach as putatively superior to stand-alone interventions, but further implicate the importance of early intervention, given that duration of illness was the only negative predictor on the global therapy outcome of IPT.

One question that cannot be answered from these combination studies is whether targeting neurocognition or social cognition will be more fruitful regarding functional outcome, and furthermore, which approach strategies/techniques or combination of techniques are likely to have the biggest impact on functioning. We suggest that social cognitive interventions, which typically rely on approaches such as metacognitive learning, didactic teaching and exposure techniques via group-based therapy, hold promise for producing robust effects on functional outcome, but to reiterate they are yet to be trialed in early psychosis. Furthermore, while some neurocognitive approaches have been trialed in early psychosis, others have not. For example, evidence suggests that compensatory approaches may play an important role in maximizing functional recovery, and indeed, large effects (>0.80) have been found in individual studies of chronic schizophrenia populations [89, 91, 147]. Head-to-head studies of the various cognitive interventions are required to tease out the most effective techniques.

A recent elegant study by Horan and colleagues [77] attempted to address this. After trialing a modified version of SCIT [148], Horan et al. developed the Social Cognitive Skills Training (SCST) program comprising 24 sessions. This program is similar to SCIT in that it targets emotional processing, social perception, attributional bias and mentalising skills with the primary aim of enabling participants to become more proficient in social interacting. Schizophrenia outpatients were randomized to receive either SCST (n = 16), computerized neurocognitive remediation (n = 19; exercises developed by PositScience), standard skills training (n = 19), or a hybrid of SCST and neurocognitive remediation (n = 14) [77]. Groups were matched for session number and time with the therapist. This was the first study to directly examine the effects of combining a social cognitive with a neurocognitive intervention and is also the first study to conduct a well-controlled head-to-head comparison of neurocognitive versus social cognitive remediation. The SCST was more successful in treating deficits in facial affect recognition, when compared to the neurocognitive remediation and standard skills training groups, as well as emotion management, when compared to the neurocognitive remediation and the hybrid groups. The hybrid group, in comparison to the three other groups, improved significantly on the measure of attributional bias. For other social cognitive and neurocognitive measures there were general improvements, but these did not differ between treatment groups. There were no significant improvements on the measures of functional outcome in any group, although a positive trend was observed for both the SCST and the neurocognitive remediation groups on a measure of social competence. The findings suggest SCST as a stand-alone treatment can enhance emotion processing, but functioning was unaffected. However, group numbers were small, and authors suggested that integration sessions conducted within the community may lead to better skill retention and generalisation, but this requires further investigation. It should also be noted that the neurocognitive remediation program was a prototype and appeared to use only the drill and practice approach without utilizing complimentary techniques such as strategy coaching. Furthermore, participants were compensated for attending training sessions, making it difficult to determine the true participant acceptability of the different approaches.

While Horan et al. [77] provide evidence to support the SCST as a successful stand-alone intervention for treating emotional processing deficits, the finding that the hybrid intervention had a significant effect on attributional bias also suggests a combined approach may be useful. This line of work warrants further research, especially given that the hybrid training was matched in number of hours to the other interventions, meaning the amount of time spent on social cognitive training was half that of the SCST group and similarly for the neurocognitive component. However, to reiterate, functioning, which is the outcome of primary interest, was not significantly affected by either the SCST alone or the combined approach. The results from the CET trial [126–128], an intervention that encompasses both neurocognitive and social cognitive training, add further weight to the idea that a combined/hybrid approach appears complimentary and may work synergistically to enhance social and occupational functioning.

Finally, coming back to the neurodevelopmental hypothesis and biological basis of schizophrenia, it would be advantageous for future clinical trials to utilise modern brain imaging techniques not only to explore the origins of cognitive impairment but to evaluate the effects of intervention programs on the illness at its source. Indeed, Eack and colleagues [149] found CET to have a neuroprotective effect against grey matter volume reductions and that CET was a significant mediator between grey matter volume changes in the parahippocampus, fusiform gyrus, and amygdala and improved cognitive performance. Normalization of brain activation [150] and serum brain-derived neurotrophic factor [151] have also been demonstrated in chronic schizophrenia following neurocognitive remediation.

In conclusion, given the evidence for debilitating cognitive and functional difficulties occurring at or even before onset of psychosis and the clear relationship between these two constructs, we argue that the maximal benefits of cognitive remediation are likely to occur early in the course of illness, even in the putative prodromal phase. This is based on the premise that the "ceiling" for potential recovery may be higher in early psychosis due to ongoing neurodevelopment in this phase of life. Needless to say there is a great deal more research to be done in this area; however, preliminary findings suggest there are a number of potential avenues that may alleviate functional impairments of young people with psychotic disorders.

Acknowledgments

Dr. C. F. Bartholomeusz and Dr. K. Allott are each supported by a National Health and Medical Research Council Australian-based Clinical Research Fellowship (567042 and 628884, resp.).

References

[1] R. W. Buchanan, M. Davis, D. Goff et al., "A summary of the FDA-NIMH-MATRICS workshop on clinical trial design for neurocognitive drugs for schizophrenia," *Schizophrenia Bulletin*, vol. 31, no. 1, pp. 5–19, 2005.

[2] P. D. Harvey and A. S. Bellack, "Toward a terminology for functional recovery in schizophrenia: is functional remission a viable concept?" *Schizophrenia Bulletin*, vol. 35, no. 2, pp. 300–306, 2009.

[3] M. Birchwood, P. Todd, and C. Jackson, "Early intervention in psychosis: the critical period hypothesis," *British Journal of Psychiatry*, vol. 172, no. 33, pp. 53–59, 1998.

[4] A. Jablensky, "Epidemiology of schizophrenia: the global burden of disease and disability," *European Archives of Psychiatry and Clinical Neuroscience*, vol. 250, no. 6, pp. 274–285, 2000.

[5] A. R. Yung, L. J. Phillips, H. P. Yuen et al., "Psychosis prediction: 12-Month follow up of a high-risk ("prodromal") group," *Schizophrenia Research*, vol. 60, no. 1, pp. 21–32, 2003.

[6] N. M. Menezes, T. Arenovich, and R. B. Zipursky, "A systematic review of longitudinal outcome studies of first-episode psychosis," *Psychological Medicine*, vol. 36, no. 10, pp. 1349–1362, 2006.

[7] A. Malla and J. Payne, "First-episode psychosis: psychopathology, quality of life, and functional outcome," *Schizophrenia Bulletin*, vol. 31, no. 3, pp. 650–671, 2005.

[8] P. A. Garety, T. K. J. Craig, G. Dunn et al., "Specialised care for early psychosis: symptoms, social functioning and patient satisfaction—randomised controlled trial," *British Journal of Psychiatry*, vol. 188, pp. 37–45, 2006.

[9] A. Thorup, L. Petersen, P. Jeppesen et al., "Integrated treatment ameliorates negative symptoms in first episode psychosis—results from the Danish OPUS trial," *Schizophrenia Research*, vol. 79, no. 1, pp. 95–105, 2005.

[10] E. Killackey and A. R. Yung, "Effectiveness of early intervention in psychosis," *Current Opinion in Psychiatry*, vol. 20, no. 2, pp. 121–125, 2007.

[11] P. D. McGorry, J. Edwards, C. Mihalopoulos, S. M. Harrigan, and H. J. Jackson, "EPPIC: an evolving system of early detection and optimal management," *Schizophrenia Bulletin*, vol. 22, no. 2, pp. 305–326, 1996.

[12] R. M. Bilder, "The neuropsychology of schizophrenia circa 2009," *Neuropsychology Review*, vol. 19, no. 3, pp. 277–279, 2009.

[13] C. F. Bartholomeusz, E. Killackey, A. Thompson et al., "Interventions targeting social and vocational dysfunction in individuals with a schizophrenia spectrum disorder," in *Handbook of Schizophrenia Spectrum Disorders*, M. Ritsner, Ed., vol. 3, Springer, New York, NY, USA, 2011.

[14] S. M. Couture, D. L. Penn, and D. L. Roberts, "The functional significance of social cognition in schizophrenia: a review," *Schizophrenia bulletin*, vol. 32, pp. S44–S63, 2006.

[15] S. J. Blakemore, "Development of the social brain during adolescence," *Quarterly Journal of Experimental Psychology*, vol. 61, no. 1, pp. 40–49, 2008.

[16] T. Paus, "Mapping brain maturation and cognitive development during adolescence," *Trends in Cognitive Sciences*, vol. 9, no. 2, pp. 60–68, 2005.

[17] N. Gogtay, J. N. Giedd, L. Lusk et al., "Dynamic mapping of human cortical development during childhood through early adulthood," *Proceedings of the National Academy of Sciences of the United States of America*, vol. 101, no. 21, pp. 8174–8179, 2004.

[18] L. Steinberg, "Cognitive and affective development in adolescence," *Trends in Cognitive Sciences*, vol. 9, no. 2, pp. 69–74, 2005.

[19] L. Steinberg and A. S. Morris, "Adolescent development," *Annual Review of Psychology*, vol. 52, pp. 83–110, 2001.

[20] T. Paus, M. Keshavan, and J. N. Giedd, "Why do many psychiatric disorders emerge during adolescence?" *Nature Reviews Neuroscience*, vol. 9, no. 12, pp. 947–957, 2008.

[21] Australian Bureau of Statistics, *National survey of mental health and wellbeing: summary of results*, Australain Bureau of Statistics,, Sydney, Australia, 2007.

[22] V. Morgan, A. Waterreus, A. Jablensky et al., *People living with psychotic illness 2010: report on the second Australian national survey*, Department of Health and Aging, Canberra, Australia, 2011.

[23] C. Pantelis, M. Yücel, E. Bora et al., "Neurobiological markers of illness onset in psychosis and schizophrenia: the search for a moving target," *Neuropsychology Review*, vol. 19, no. 3, pp. 385–398, 2009.

[24] R. I. Mesholam-Gately, A. J. Giuliano, K. P. Goff, S. V. Faraone, and L. J. Seidman, "Neurocognition in first-episode Schizophrenia: a meta-analytic review," *Neuropsychology*, vol. 23, no. 3, pp. 315–336, 2009.

[25] D. Dickinson, J. D. Ragland, J. M. Gold, and R. C. Gur, "General and specific cognitive deficits in schizophrenia: Goliath defeats David?" *Biological Psychiatry*, vol. 64, no. 9, pp. 823–827, 2008.

[26] V. P. Bozikas and C. Andreou, "Longitudinal studies of cognition in first episode psychosis: a systematic review of the literature," *Australian and New Zealand Journal of Psychiatry*, vol. 45, no. 2, pp. 93–108, 2011.

[27] W. J. Brewer, S. J. Wood, L. J. Phillips et al., "Generalized and specific cognitive performance in clinical high-risk cohorts: a review highlighting potential vulnerability markers for psychosis," *Schizophrenia Bulletin*, vol. 32, no. 3, pp. 538–555, 2006.

[28] C. U. Correll, M. Hauser, A. M. Auther, and B. A. Cornblatt, "Research in people with psychosis risk syndrome: a review of the current evidence and future directions," *Journal of Child Psychology and Psychiatry and Allied Disciplines*, vol. 51, no. 4, pp. 390–431, 2010.

[29] P. Fusar-Poli, J. Perez, M. Broome et al., "Neurofunctional correlates of vulnerability to psychosis: a systematic review and meta-analysis," *Neuroscience and Biobehavioral Reviews*, vol. 31, no. 4, pp. 465–484, 2007.

[30] J. Addington, H. Saeedi, and D. Addington, "Facial affect recognition: a mediator between cognitive and social functioning in psychosis?" *Schizophrenia Research*, vol. 85, no. 1–3, pp. 142–150, 2006.

[31] J. Edwards, P. E. Pattison, H. J. Jackson, and R. J. Wales, "Facial affect and affective prosody recognition in first-episode schizophrenia," *Schizophrenia Research*, vol. 48, no. 2-3, pp. 235–253, 2001.

[32] A. E. Pinkham, D. L. Penn, D. O. Perkins, K. A. Graham, and M. Siegel, "Emotion perception and social skill over the course of psychosis: a comparison of individuals "at-risk" for psychosis and individuals with early and chronic schizophrenia spectrum illness," *Cognitive Neuropsychiatry*, vol. 12, no. 3, pp. 198–212, 2007.

[33] G. P. Amminger, M. R. Schafer, K. Papageorgiou et al., "Emotion recognition in individuals at clinical high-risk for Schizophrenia," *Schizophrenia Bulletin*. In press.

[34] M. F. Green, C. E. Bearden, T. D. Cannon et al., "Social cognition in Schizophrenia, Part 1: performance across phase of illness," *Schizophrenia Bulletin*. In press.

[35] M. C. Bertrand, H. Sutton, A. M. Achim, A. K. Malla, and M. Lepage, "Social cognitive impairments in first episode psychosis," *Schizophrenia Research*, vol. 95, no. 1–3, pp. 124–133, 2007.

[36] T. Montreuil, M. Bodnar, M. C. Bertrand, A. K. Malla, R. Joober, and M. Lepage, "Social cognitive markers of short-term clinical outcome in first-episode psychosis," *Clinical Schizophrenia and Related Psychoses*, vol. 4, no. 2, pp. 105–114, 2010.

[37] Y. Inoue, K. Yamada, M. Hirano et al., "Impairment of theory of mind in patients in remission following first episode of schizophrenia," *European Archives of Psychiatry and Clinical Neuroscience*, vol. 256, no. 5, pp. 326–328, 2006.

[38] J. W. L. Kettle, L. O'Brien-Simpson, and N. B. Allen, "Impaired theory of mind in first-episode schizophrenia: comparison with community, university and depressed controls," *Schizophrenia Research*, vol. 99, no. 1–3, pp. 96–102, 2008.

[39] K. Koelkebeck, A. Pedersen, T. Suslow, K. A. Kueppers, V. Arolt, and P. Ohrmann, "Theory of Mind in first-episode schizophrenia patients: correlations with cognition and personality traits," *Schizophrenia Research*, vol. 119, no. 1–3, pp. 115–123, 2010.

[40] H. Krstev, H. Jackson, and D. Maude, "An investigation of attributional style in first-episode psychosis," *British Journal of Clinical Psychology*, vol. 38, no. 2, pp. 181–194, 1999.

[41] S. K. An, J. I. Kang, J. Y. Park, K. R. Kim, S. Y. Lee, and E. Lee, "Attribution bias in ultra-high risk for psychosis and first-episode schizophrenia," *Schizophrenia Research*, vol. 118, no. 1–3, pp. 54–61, 2010.

[42] A. D. Thompson, C. Bartholomeusz, and A. R. Yung, "Social cognition deficits and the 'ultra high risk' for psychosis population: a review of literature," *Early Intervention in Psychiatry*, vol. 5, no. 3, pp. 192–202, 2011.

[43] J. Addington, D. Penn, S. W. Woods, D. Addington, and D. O. Perkins, "Facial affect recognition in individuals at clinical high risk for psychosis," *British Journal of Psychiatry*, vol. 192, no. 1, pp. 67–68, 2008.

[44] M. Schloegelhofer, M. Schaefer, K. Papageorgiou et al., "Emotion recognition in individuals at Ultra High Risk for psychosis," *Schizophrenia Bulletin*, vol. 86, pp. S94–S95, 2006.

[45] S. van Rijn, A. Aleman, L. de Sonneville et al., "Misattribution of facial expressions of emotion in adolescents at increased risk of psychosis: the role of inhibitory control," *Psychological Medicine*, vol. 41, pp. 499–508, 2011.

[46] Y. S. Chung, D. H. Kang, N. Y. Shin, S. Y. Yoo, and J. S. Kwon, "Deficit of theory of mind in individuals at ultra-high-risk for schizophrenia," *Schizophrenia Research*, vol. 99, no. 1–3, pp. 111–118, 2008.

[47] S. M. Couture, D. L. Penn, J. Addington, S. W. Woods, and D. O. Perkins, "Assessment of social judgments and complex mental states in the early phases of psychosis," *Schizophrenia Research*, vol. 100, no. 1–3, pp. 237–241, 2008.

[48] S. J. Blakemore, "The social brain in adolescence," *Nature Reviews Neuroscience*, vol. 9, no. 4, pp. 267–277, 2008.

[49] C. Pantelis, D. Velakoulis, S. J. Wood et al., "Neuroimaging and emerging psychotic disorders: the Melbourne ultra-high risk studies," *International Review of Psychiatry*, vol. 19, no. 4, pp. 373–381, 2007.

[50] W. H. Jung, J. H. Jang, M. S. Byun, S. K. An, and J. S. Kwon, "Structural brain alterations in individuals at ultra-high risk for psychosis: a review of magnetic resonance imaging studies and future directions," *Journal of Korean Medical Science*, vol. 25, no. 12, pp. 1700–1709, 2010.

[51] N. Y. Seiferth, K. Pauly, T. Kellermann et al., "Neuronal correlates of facial emotion discrimination in early onset schizophrenia," *Neuropsychopharmacology*, vol. 34, no. 2, pp. 477–487, 2009.

[52] N. Y. Seiferth, K. Pauly, U. Habel et al., "Increased neural response related to neutral faces in individuals at risk for psychosis," *NeuroImage*, vol. 40, no. 1, pp. 289–297, 2008.

[53] M. Brüne, S. Özgürdal, N. Ansorge et al., "An fMRI study of "theory of mind" in at-risk states of psychosis: comparison with manifest schizophrenia and healthy controls," *NeuroImage*, vol. 55, no. 1, pp. 329–337, 2011.

[54] K. Boksman, J. Théberge, P. Williamson et al., "A 4.0-T fMRI study of brain connectivity during word fluency in first-episode schizophrenia," *Schizophrenia Research*, vol. 75, no. 2-3, pp. 247–263, 2005.

[55] N. D. Woodward, B. Waldie, B. Rogers, P. Tibbo, P. Seres, and S. E. Purdon, "Abnormal prefrontal cortical activity and connectivity during response selection in first episode psychosis, chronic schizophrenia, and unaffected siblings of individuals with schizophrenia," *Schizophrenia Research*, vol. 109, no. 1–3, pp. 182–190, 2009.

[56] D. Luck, L. Buchy, Y. Czechowska et al., "Fronto-temporal disconnectivity and clinical short-term outcome in first episode psychosis: a DTI-tractography study," *Journal of Psychiatric Research*, vol. 45, no. 3, pp. 369–377, 2011.

[57] N. A. Crossley, A. Mechelli, P. Fusar-Poli et al., "Superior temporal lobe dysfunction and frontotemporal dysconnectivity in subjects at risk of psychosis and in first-episode psychosis," *Human Brain Mapping*, vol. 30, no. 12, pp. 4129–4137, 2009.

[58] M. F. Green, R. S. Kern, D. L. Braff, and J. Mintz, "Neurocognitive deficits and functional outcome in schizophrenia: are we measuring the "right stuff"?" *Schizophrenia Bulletin*, vol. 26, no. 1, pp. 119–136, 2000.

[59] A. K. J. Fett, W. Viechtbauer, M. D. G. Dominguez, D. L. Penn, J. van Os, and L. Krabbendam, "The relationship between neurocognition and social cognition with functional outcomes in schizophrenia: a meta-analysis," *Neuroscience and Biobehavioral Reviews*, vol. 35, no. 3, pp. 573–588, 2011.

[60] K. Allott, P. Liu, T. M. Proffitt, and E. Killackey, "Cognition at illness onset as a predictor of later functional outcome in early psychosis: systematic review and methodological critique," *Schizophrenia Research*, vol. 125, pp. 221–235, 2011.

[61] M. Bell, H. W. H. Tsang, T. C. Greig, and G. J. Bryson, "Neurocognition, social cognition, perceived social discomfort, and vocational outcomes in schizophrenia," *Schizophrenia Bulletin*, vol. 35, no. 4, pp. 738–747, 2009.

[62] M. Brüne, "Emotion recognition, "theory of mind," and social behavior in schizophrenia," *Psychiatry Research*, vol. 133, no. 2-3, pp. 135–147, 2005.

[63] A. E. Pinkham and D. L. Penn, "Neurocognitive and social cognitive predictors of interpersonal skill in schizophrenia," *Psychiatry Research*, vol. 143, no. 2-3, pp. 167–178, 2006.

[64] D. N. Allen, G. P. Strauss, B. Donohue, and D. P. van Kammen, "Factor analytic support for social cognition as a separable cognitive domain in schizophrenia," *Schizophrenia Research*, vol. 93, no. 1–3, pp. 325–333, 2007.

[65] L. M. Williams, T. J. Whitford, G. Flynn et al., "General and social cognition in first episode schizophrenia: identification of separable factors and prediction of functional outcome using the IntegNeuro test battery," *Schizophrenia Research*, vol. 99, no. 1–3, pp. 182–191, 2008.

[66] J. Addington, T. A. Girard, B. K. Christensen, and D. Addington, "Social cognition mediates illness-related and cognitive influences on social function in patients with schizophrenia-spectrum disorders," *Journal of Psychiatry and Neuroscience*, vol. 35, no. 1, pp. 49–54, 2010.

[67] M. J. Sergi, Y. Rassovsky, K. H. Nuechterlein, and M. F. Green, "Social perception as a mediator of the influence of early visual processing on functional status in schizophrenia," *American Journal of Psychiatry*, vol. 163, no. 3, pp. 448–454, 2006.

[68] R. Vauth, N. Rüsch, M. Wirtz, and P. W. Corrigan, "Does social cognition influence the relation between neurocognitive deficits and vocational functioning in schizophrenia?" *Psychiatry Research*, vol. 128, no. 2, pp. 155–165, 2004.

[69] J. Brekke, D. D. Kay, K. S. Lee, and M. F. Green, "Biosocial pathways to functional outcome in schizophrenia," *Schizophrenia Research*, vol. 80, no. 2-3, pp. 213–225, 2005.

[70] J. Addington, H. Saeedi, and D. Addington, "Influence of social perception and social knowledge on cognitive and social functioning in early psychosis," *British Journal of Psychiatry*, vol. 189, pp. 373–378, 2006.

[71] W. P. Horan, M. F. Green, M. Degroot et al., "Social cognition in Schizophrenia, Part 2: 12-month stability and prediction of functional outcome in first-episode patients," *Schizophrenia Bulletin*. In press.

[72] T. Wykes, V. Huddy, C. Cellard, S. R. McGurk, and P. Czobor, "A meta-analysis of cognitive remediation for schizophrenia: methodology and effect sizes," *American Journal of Psychiatry*, vol. 168, no. 5, pp. 472–485, 2011.

[73] A. Medalia and J. Choi, "Cognitive remediation in schizophrenia," *Neuropsychology Review*, vol. 19, no. 3, pp. 353–364, 2009.

[74] M. Fisher, C. Holland, M. M. Merzenich, and S. Vinogradov, "Using neuroplasticity-based auditory training to improve verbal memory in schizophrenia," *American Journal of Psychiatry*, vol. 166, no. 7, pp. 805–811, 2009.

[75] S. R. McGurk, E. W. Twamley, D. I. Sitzer, G. J. McHugo, and K. T. Mueser, "A meta-analysis of cognitive remediation in schizophrenia," *American Journal of Psychiatry*, vol. 164, no. 12, pp. 1791–1802, 2007.

[76] M. M. Kurtz and C. L. Richardson, "Social cognitive training for schizophrenia: a meta-analytic investigation of controlled research," *Schizophrenia Bulletin*. In press.

[77] W. P. Horan, R. S. Kern, C. Tripp et al., "Efficacy and specificity of social cognitive skills training for outpatients with psychotic disorders," *Journal of Psychiatric Research*, vol. 45, no. 8, pp. 1113–1122, 2011.

[78] V. Roder, D. R. Mueller, K. T. Mueser, and H. D. Brenner, "Integrated psychological therapy (IPT) for schizophrenia: is it effective?" *Schizophrenia bulletin*, vol. 32, pp. S81–S93, 2006.

[79] S. Rauchensteiner, W. Kawohl, S. Ozgurdal et al., "Test-performance after cognitive training in persons at risk mental state of schizophrenia and patients with schizophrenia," *Psychiatry Research*, vol. 185, pp. 334–339, 2011.

[80] S. R. McGurk and K. T. Mueser, "Response to cognitive rehabilitation in older versus younger persons with severe mental illness," *American Journal of Psychiatric Rehabilitation*, vol. 11, no. 1, pp. 90–105, 2008.

[81] T. Wykes, C. Reeder, S. Landau, P. Matthiasson, E. Haworth, and C. Hutchinson, "Does age matter? Effects of cognitive rehabilitation across the age span," *Schizophrenia Research*, vol. 113, no. 2-3, pp. 252–258, 2009.

[82] G. E. Hogarty, S. Flesher, R. Ulrich et al., "Cognitive enhancement therapy for schizophrenia: effects of a 2-year randomized trial on cognition and behavior," *Archives of General Psychiatry*, vol. 61, no. 9, pp. 866–876, 2004.

[83] M. F. Green, "Cognitive remediation in schizophrenia: is it time yet?" *American Journal of Psychiatry*, vol. 150, no. 2, pp. 178–187, 1993.

[84] M. Fisher, C. Holland, K. Subramaniam, and S. Vinogradov, "Neuroplasticity-based cognitive training in schizophrenia: an interim report on the effects 6 months later," *Schizophrenia Bulletin*, vol. 36, no. 4, pp. 869–879, 2010.

[85] A. Medalia and B. Freilich, "The Neuropsychological Educational Approach to Cognitive Remediation (NEAR) model: practice principles and outcome studies," *American Journal of Psychiatric Rehabilitation*, vol. 11, no. 2, pp. 123–143, 2008.

[86] E. W. Twamley, D. V. Jeste, and A. S. Bellack, "A review of cognitive training in schizophrenia," *Schizophrenia Bulletin*, vol. 29, no. 2, pp. 359–382, 2003.

[87] T. Wykes and C. Reeder, *Cognitive Remediation Therapy for Schizophrenia: Theory and Practice*, Routledge, London, UK, 2005.

[88] A. Delahunty and R. Morice, *A training programme for the remediation of cognitive deficits in schizophrenia*, Department of Health, Albury, Australia, 1993.

[89] E. W. Twamley, G. N. Savla, C. H. Zurhellen, R. K. Heaton, and D. V. Jeste, "Development and pilot testing of a novel compensatory cognitive training intervention for people with psychosis," *American Journal of Psychiatric Rehabilitation*, vol. 11, no. 2, pp. 144–163, 2008.

[90] G. H. M. Pijnenborg, F. K. Withaar, J. J. Evans, R. J. Van Den Bosch, and W. H. Brouwer, "SMS text messages as a prosthetic aid in the cognitive rehabilitation of schizophrenia," *Rehabilitation Psychology*, vol. 52, no. 2, pp. 236–240, 2007.

[91] D. I. Velligan, C. C. Bow-Thomas, C. Huntzinger et al., "Randomized controlled trial of the use of compensatory strategies to enhance adaptive functioning in outpatients with schizophrenia," *American Journal of Psychiatry*, vol. 157, no. 8, pp. 1317–1323, 2000.

[92] A. S. Bellack, J. M. Gold, and R. W. Buchanan, "Cognitive rehabilitation for schizophrenia: problems, prospects, and strategies," *Schizophrenia Bulletin*, vol. 25, no. 2, pp. 257–274, 1999.

[93] D. I. Velligan, J. L. Ritch, and N. J. Maples, *Cognitive Adaptation Training: The Use of Compensatory Strategies in the Psychosocial Rehabilitation of Patients with Schizophrenia*, UTHSC, Department of Psychiatry, San Antonio, Tex, USA, 2nd edition, 2010.

[94] E. W. Twamley, C. Z. Burton, and L. Vella, "Compensatory cognitive training for psychosis: who benefits? who stays in treatment?" *Schizophrenia Bulletin*, vol. 37, supplement 2, pp. S55–S62, 2011.

[95] D. I. Velligan, R. S. Kern, and J. M. Gold, "Cognitive rehabilitation for schizophrenia and the putative role of motivation and expectancies," *Schizophrenia Bulletin*, vol. 32, no. 3, pp. 474–485, 2006.

[96] R. S. Kern, M. F. Green, J. Mintz, and R. P. Liberman, "Does "errorless learning" compensate for neurocognitive impairments in the work rehabilitation of persons with schizophrenia?" *Psychological Medicine*, vol. 33, no. 3, pp. 433–442, 2003.

[97] J. W. Pope and R. S. Kern, "An "errorful" learning deficit in schizophrenia?" *Journal of Clinical and Experimental Neuropsychology*, vol. 28, no. 1, pp. 101–110, 2006.

[98] R. E. O'Carroll, H. H. Russell, S. M. Lawrie, and E. C. Johnstone, "Errorless learning and the cognitive rehabilitation of memory-impaired schizophrenic patients," *Psychological Medicine*, vol. 29, no. 1, pp. 105–112, 1999.

[99] R. S. Kern, M. F. Green, S. Mitchell, A. Kopelowicz, J. Mintz, and R. P. Liberman, "Extensions of errorless learning for social problem-solving deficits in schizophrenia," *American Journal of Psychiatry*, vol. 162, no. 3, pp. 513–519, 2005.

[100] R. S. Kern, R. P. Liberman, D. R. Becker, R. E. Drake, C. A. Sugar, and M. F. Green, "Errorless learning for training individuals with schizophrenia at a community mental health setting providing work experience," *Schizophrenia Bulletin*, vol. 35, no. 4, pp. 807–815, 2009.

[101] S. M. Silverstein, "Bridging the gap between extrinsic and intrinsic motivation in the cognitive remediation of schizophrenia," *Schizophrenia Bulletin*, vol. 36, no. 5, pp. 949–956, 2010.

[102] L. Krabbendam and A. Aleman, "Cognitive rehabilitation in schizophrenia: a quantitative analysis of controlled studies," *Psychopharmacology*, vol. 169, no. 3-4, pp. 376–382, 2003.

[103] M. Bell, G. Bryson, T. Greig, C. Corcoran, and B. E. Wexler, "Neurocognitive enhancement therapy with work therapy: effects on neuropsychological test performance," *Archives of General Psychiatry*, vol. 58, no. 8, pp. 763–768, 2001.

[104] S. R. McGurk, K. T. Mueser, and A. Pascaris, "Cognitive training and supported employment for persons with severe mental illness: one-year results from a randomized controlled trial," *Schizophrenia Bulletin*, vol. 31, no. 4, pp. 898–909, 2005.

[105] S. M. Silverstein, W. D. Spaulding, A. A. Menditto et al., "Attention shaping: a reward-based learning method to enhance skills training outcomes in schizophrenia," *Schizophrenia Bulletin*, vol. 35, no. 1, pp. 222–232, 2009.

[106] T. Wykes, C. Reeder, C. Williams, J. Corner, C. Rice, and B. Everitt, "Are the effects of cognitive remediation therapy (CRT) durable? Results from an exploratory trial in schizophrenia," *Schizophrenia Research*, vol. 61, no. 2-3, pp. 163–174, 2003.

[107] L. W. Davis and P. H. Lysaker, "Cognitive behavioral therapy and functional and metacognitive outcomes in schizophrenia: a single case study," *Cognitive and Behavioral Practice*, vol. 12, no. 4, pp. 468–478, 2005.

[108] S. Moritz, M. Burlon, and T. S. Woodward, *Metacognitive Skills Training for Patients with Schizophrenia (MCT). Version 3.2*, VanHam Campus Press, Hamburg, Germany, 2005.

[109] D. Koren, L. J. Seidman, M. Goldsmith, and P. D. Harvey, "Real-world cognitive—and metacognitive—dysfunction in schizophrenia: a new approach for measuring (and remediating) more 'right stuff'," *Schizophrenia Bulletin*, vol. 32, no. 2, pp. 310–326, 2006.

[110] A. S. Bellack, C. H. Brown, and S. Thomas-Lohrman, "Psychometric characteristics of role-play assessments of social skill in schizophrenia," *Behavior Therapy*, vol. 37, no. 4, pp. 339–352, 2006.

[111] D. R. Combs, S. D. Adams, D. L. Penn, D. Roberts, J. Tiegreen, and P. Stem, "Social Cognition and Interaction Training

(SCIT) for inpatients with schizophrenia spectrum disorders: preliminary findings," *Schizophrenia Research*, vol. 91, no. 1–3, pp. 112–116, 2007.
[112] L. Carr, M. Iacoboni, M. C. Dubeaut, J. C. Mazziotta, and G. L. Lenzi, "Neural mechanisms of empathy in humans: a relay from neural systems for imitation to limbic areas," *Proceedings of the National Academy of Sciences of the United States of America*, vol. 100, no. 9, pp. 5497–5502, 2003.
[113] L. M. Oberman and V. S. Ramachandran, "The simulating social mind: the role of the mirror neuron system and simulation in the social and communicative deficits of autism spectrum disorders," *Psychological Bulletin*, vol. 133, no. 2, pp. 310–327, 2007.
[114] J. S. Singh and D. A. Hope, "Cognitive-behavioral approaches to the treatment of social anxiety disorder," *Israel Journal of Psychiatry and Related Sciences*, vol. 46, no. 1, pp. 62–69, 2009.
[115] J. Wolpe, *The Practice of Behaviour Therapy*, Pergamon, New York, NY, USA, 2nd edition, 1969.
[116] K. Ponniah and S. D. Hollon, "Empirically supported psychological interventions for social phobia in adults: a qualitative review of randomized controlled trials," *Psychological Medicine*, vol. 38, no. 1, pp. 3–14, 2008.
[117] K. Ponniah and S. D. Hollon, "Empirically supported psychological interventions for social phobia in adults: a qualitative review of randomized controlled trials," *Psychological Medicine*, vol. 38, no. 1, pp. 3–14, 2008.
[118] D. Roberts, D. Penn, and D. Combs, "Social Cognition and Interaction Training (SCIT) Treatment Manual," 2010.
[119] G. E. Hogarty and D. P. Greenwald, *Cognitive Enhancement Therapy: The Training Manual*, University of Pittsburgh Medical Center, Pittsburgh, Pa, USA, 2006.
[120] S. Vinogradov, R. Loewy, M. Fisher et al., "Neuroplasticity-based cognitive training in early psychosis (Abstract)," *Biological Psychiatry*, vol. 67, pp. S188–S189, 2010.
[121] A. Lin, S. J. Wood, B. Nelson et al., "Neurocognitive predictors of functional outcome two to 13 years after identification as ultra-high risk for psychosis," *Schizophrenia Research*, vol. 132, no. 1, pp. 1–7, 2011.
[122] T. A. Niendam, C. E. Bearden, J. K. Johnson et al., "Neurocognitive performance and functional disability in the psychosis prodrome," *Schizophrenia Research*, vol. 84, no. 1, pp. 100–111, 2006.
[123] T. Ueland and B. R. Rund, "A controlled randomized treatment study: the effects of a cognitive remediation program on adolescents with early onset psychosis," *Acta Psychiatrica Scandinavica*, vol. 109, no. 1, pp. 70–74, 2004.
[124] T. Ueland and B. R. Rund, "Cognitive remediation for adolescents with early onset psychosis: a 1-year follow-up study," *Acta Psychiatrica Scandinavica*, vol. 111, no. 3, pp. 193–201, 2005.
[125] T. Wykes, E. Newton, S. Landau, C. Rice, N. Thompson, and S. Frangou, "Cognitive remediation therapy (CRT) for young early onset patients with schizophrenia: an exploratory randomized controlled trial," *Schizophrenia Research*, vol. 94, no. 1–3, pp. 221–230, 2007.
[126] S. M. Eack, D. P. Greenwald, S. S. Hogarty et al., "Cognitive enhancement therapy for early-course schizophrenia: effects of a two-year randomized controlled trial," *Psychiatric Services*, vol. 60, no. 11, pp. 1468–1476, 2009.
[127] S. M. Eack, G. E. Hogarty, D. P. Greenwald, S. S. Hogarty, and M. S. Keshavan, "Effects of cognitive enhancement therapy on employment outcomes in early schizophrenia: results from a 2-year randomized trial," *Research on Social Work Practice*, vol. 21, no. 1, pp. 32–42, 2011.
[128] S. M. Eack, D. P. Greenwald, S. S. Hogarty, and M. S. Keshavan, "One-year durability of the effects of cognitive enhancement therapy on functional outcome in early schizophrenia," *Schizophrenia Research*, vol. 120, no. 1–3, pp. 210–216, 2010.
[129] T. Wykes and W. D. Spaulding, "Thinking about the future cognitive remediation therapy-what works and could we do better?" *Schizophrenia Bulletin*, vol. 37, supplement 2, pp. S80–S90, 2011.
[130] D. L. Penn, D. L. Roberts, D. Combs, and A. Sterne, "The development of the social cognition and interaction training program for schizophrenia spectrum disorders," *Psychiatric Services*, vol. 58, no. 4, pp. 449–451, 2007.
[131] M. Birchwood, J. Smith, R. Cochrane, S. Wetton, and S. Copestake, "The Social Functioning Scale. The development and validation of a new scale of social adjustment for use in family intervention programmes with schizophrenic patients," *British Journal of Psychiatry*, vol. 157, pp. 853–859, 1990.
[132] D. L. Roberts and D. L. Penn, "Social cognition and interaction training (SCIT) for outpatients with schizophrenia: a preliminary study," *Psychiatry Research*, vol. 166, no. 2-3, pp. 141–147, 2009.
[133] D. L. Roberts, D. L. Penn, D. Labate, S. A. Margolis, and A. Sterne, "Transportability and feasibility of Social Cognition and Interaction Training (SCIT) in community settings," *Behavioural and Cognitive Psychotherapy*, vol. 38, no. 1, pp. 35–47, 2010.
[134] M. Mazza, G. Lucci, F. Pacitti et al., "Could schizophrenic subjects improve their social cognition abilities only with observation and imitation of social situations?" *Neuropsychological Rehabilitation*, vol. 20, no. 5, pp. 675–703, 2010.
[135] V. Gallese, "Mirror neurons, embodied simulation, and the neural basis of social identification," *Psychoanalytic Dialogues*, vol. 19, no. 5, pp. 519–536, 2009.
[136] J. H. Kwon, *Social Cognition Enhancement Rehabilitation Program*, Hakjisa, Seoul, Korea, 2003.
[137] K. H. Choi and J. H. Kwon, "Social cognition enhancement training for schizophrenia: a preliminary randomized controlled trial," *Community Mental Health Journal*, vol. 42, no. 2, pp. 177–187, 2006.
[138] R. Roncone, M. Mazza, I. Frangou et al., "Rehabilitation of theory of mind deficit in schizophrenia: a pilot study of metacognitive strategies in group treatment," *Neuropsychological Rehabilitation*, vol. 14, no. 4, pp. 421–435, 2004.
[139] W. Wölwer, N. Frommann, S. Halfmann, A. Piaszek, M. Streit, and W. Gaebel, "Remediation of impairments in facial affect recognition in schizophrenia: efficacy and specificity of a new training program," *Schizophrenia Research*, vol. 80, no. 2-3, pp. 295–303, 2005.
[140] T. A. Russell, M. J. Green, I. Simpson, and M. Coltheart, "Remediation of facial emotion perception in schizophrenia: concomitant changes in visual attention," *Schizophrenia Research*, vol. 103, no. 1–3, pp. 248–256, 2008.
[141] D. S. Bio and W. F. Gattaz, "Vocational rehabilitation improves cognition and negative symptoms in schizophrenia," *Schizophrenia Research*, vol. 126, no. 1–3, pp. 265–269, 2011.
[142] L. Vesterager, T. T. Christensen, B. B. Olsen et al., "Cognitive training plus a comprehensive psychosocial programme (OPUS) versus the comprehensive psychosocial programme

alone for patients with first-episode schizophrenia (the NEUROCOM trial): a study protocol for a centrally randomised, observer-blinded multi-centre clinical trial," *Trials*, vol. 12, article 35, 2011.

[143] N. J. K. Breitborde, F. A. Moreno, N. Mai-Dixon et al., "Multifamily group psychoeducation and cognitive remediation for first-episode psychosis: a randomized controlled trial," *BMC Psychiatry*, vol. 11, article 9, 2011.

[144] H. D. Brenner, "The treatment of basic psychological dysfunctions from a systemic point of view," *British Journal of Psychiatry*, vol. 155, no. 5, pp. 74–83, 1989.

[145] H. D. Brenner, B. Hodel, V. Roder, and P. Corrigan, "Treatment of cognitive dysfunctions and behavioral deficits in schizophrenia," *Schizophrenia Bulletin*, vol. 18, no. 1, pp. 21–26, 1992.

[146] V. Roder, D. R. Mueller, K. T. Mueser, and H. D. Brenner, "Integrated psychological therapy (IPT) for schizophrenia: is it effective?" *Schizophrenia bulletin*, vol. 32, supplement1, pp. S81–93, 2006.

[147] D. I. Velligan, P. M. Diamond, J. Mintz et al., "The use of individually tailored environmental supports to improve medication adherence and outcomes in schizophrenia," *Schizophrenia Bulletin*, vol. 34, no. 3, pp. 483–493, 2008.

[148] W. P. Horan, R. S. Kern, K. Shokat-Fadai, M. J. Sergi, J. K. Wynn, and M. F. Green, "Social cognitive skills training in schizophrenia: an initial efficacy study of stabilized outpatients," *Schizophrenia Research*, vol. 107, no. 1, pp. 47–54, 2009.

[149] S. M. Eack, G. E. Hogarty, R. Y. Cho et al., "Neuroprotective effects of cognitive enhancement therapy against gray matter loss in early schizophrenia: results from a 2-year randomized controlled trial," *Archives of General Psychiatry*, vol. 67, no. 7, pp. 674–682, 2010.

[150] B. E. Wexler, M. Anderson, R. K. Fulbright, and J. C. Gore, "Preliminary evidence of improved verbal working memory performance and normalization of task-related frontal lobe activation in schizophrenia following cognitive exercises," *American Journal of Psychiatry*, vol. 157, no. 10, pp. 1694–1697, 2000.

[151] S. Vinogradov, M. Fisher, C. Holland, W. Shelly, O. Wolkowitz, and S. H. Mellon, "Is serum brain-derived neurotrophic factor a biomarker for cognitive enhancement in schizophrenia?" *Biological Psychiatry*, vol. 66, no. 6, pp. 549–553, 2009.

22

Intervention to Prevent Child Custody Loss in Mothers with Schizophrenia

Mary V. Seeman

Department of Psychiatry, Institute of Medical Science, University of Toronto, One King's College Circle, 7213 Medical Sciences Building, Toronto, ON, Canada M5S 1A8

Correspondence should be addressed to Mary V. Seeman, mary.seeman@utoronto.ca

Academic Editor: Susana Ochoa

Depending on jurisdiction, time period studied, and specifics of the population, approximately 50 percent of mothers who suffer from schizophrenia lose custody of their children. The aim of this paper is to recommend interventions aimed at preventing unnecessary custody loss. This paper reviews the social work, nursing, psychology, psychiatry, and law literature on mental illness and custody loss, 2000–2011. Recommendations to mothers are to (a) ensure family health (b) prevent psychotic relapse, (c) prepare in advance for crisis, (d) document daily parenting activities, (e) take advantage of available parenting resources, and f) become knowledgeable about legal issues that pertain to mental health and custody. From a policy perspective, child protection and adult mental health agencies need to dissolve administrative barriers and collaborate. Access to appropriate services will help mothers with schizophrenia to care appropriately for their children and allow these children to grow and develop within their family and community.

1. Intervention to Prevent Child Custody Loss in Mothers with Schizophrenia

A psychotic illness can, but does not need to, interfere with an individual's ability to be a good parent. Given well-timed, appropriate, and adequate education and resources, many individuals with psychotic illness succeed in parenting their children. This is not always recognized by child welfare workers who may continue to be influenced by outdated views of psychotic illness as intractable and parenting with schizophrenia as impossible [1]. Without effective intervention, parents who suffer from psychotic illness too often lose custody of their children [2], an unfortunate outcome that can be avoided by early intervention [3–5]. The emphasis in this clinical review is on *mothers* with a diagnosis of schizophrenia (because there is very little literature on fathers and effects on children merit a separate paper).

2. Method

This paper used the following grouped search terms in Google Scholar (which includes MEDLINE, EMBASE, PsycINFO, and SOCINDEX, as well as the nursing and legal literature) for the years 2000–2011: schizophrenia/diagnosis/custody; schizophrenia/impact/custody; schizophrenia/postpartum/custody; schizophrenia/termination parental rights. Following the literature review and case illustrations (from which identifying facts have been removed), recommendations are made for mothers, care providers, and policy makers.

3. Prevalence of Custody Loss in Mothers with Psychosis

Studying reports published in the last ten years, it appears that approximately 50% of women with schizophrenia who are mothers lose custody of their children, either temporarily or permanently, although the percentage varies by jurisdiction. For instance, a report from Canada indicates that 84% of parents treated for schizophrenia by a community treatment team were not living with their children at the time of interview [6], but this figure includes both male and female parents, so is probably higher than it would be for women alone. In London, UK, Howard and colleagues [7] established that 63% of women with psychosis (but only 26% of men) were parents. Hollingsworth [8] studied 322 women with serious mental illness and found that 26% had lost custody at some point in the child's life. A survey of mothers in psychiatric rehabilitative services [9] reported that 68% had been permanently separated from at least one child under the age of 18, often with little subsequent contact. The number of women with schizophrenia who experience custodial loss of their children is probably diminishing with time, as stigma lessens and interventions improve. Nevertheless, it remains high and effective intervention at the earliest stage of psychosis is warranted.

4. The Impact of Diagnosis on Custody Loss

Mothers with serious mental illness, as a group, fear that schizophrenia is equated in the mind of the public with parental incompetence or, worse, with parental neglect or violence [10]. This may well be the case because mothers with schizophrenia are often given relatively little opportunity to prove their parenting competence. Ackerson [11] has commented that parents with a diagnosis of psychosis are victimized twice first, by psychotic illness, then by protective removal of their children.

5. The Impact of Custody Loss on Mothers

Removing a child from a mother's care causes grief and distress to both. It is especially difficult for the mother when she has had little say in the process or when the event occurs at a time when she is too ill to understand what is happening. Diaz-Caneja and Johnson [12], in their qualitative study of 22 women with schizophrenia who were mothers, conclude that fear of losing child custody or access is always uppermost in the minds of severely mentally ill women, making it problematic to disclose to their care providers parenting difficulties that they may experience. Sands and colleagues [13] have reported that mothers with mental illness whose children are apprehended by child protection agencies are usually bewildered by events and confused about what steps to take in order to regain custody. Without psychiatric and legal guidance, they find it difficult to maintain contact with their children.

6. Postpartum Vulnerability to Custody Loss

The postpartum period is a particularly vulnerable time for women at risk of losing custody. Psychotic symptoms may emerge for the first time during this period and, for mothers with a prior history of mental illness, the risk of relapse is high during this reproductive phase [14, 15], bringing with it a very real threat of protective removal of children from the mother's care. Newborns are the most vulnerable members of society, and child protection legislation is therefore biased, as it needs to be, towards their needs rather than to the needs of the mother, however vulnerable she may also be. In order to meet the demands of competent infant care and retain custody of their infants, young mothers with severe postpartum psychiatric illness require substantial support and advocacy [16].

7. Composite Case Example of Unnecessary Children's Aid Involvement in Postpartum Psychosis

Patient A. was admitted to hospital for a postpartum psychotic episode. She had never been ill before. While she was in hospital, her infant was looked after at home by her parents. The baby's father was also involved in the child's care. Before the patient's hospital discharge, the psychiatric resident contacted Children's Aid, as a preventive measure, in order to notify the agency that Ms. A. might need help with mothering. Ms. A. had by then recovered and was functioning well. Psychiatric followup had been arranged, in addition to which several adults at home expressed willingness and availability to help look after the baby. The decision to call Children's Aid was solely determined by the fact that the patient had suffered a psychosis, placing her "on the books" of Children's Aid. While this could be perceived as a safety precaution for the family, it could also become a problem for the mother should, for example, the baby's father decide in the future to sue for sole custody of the child.

8. Causes of Termination of Parental Rights

The central moral and legal issue involved in temporary or permanent cessation of parental rights is the child's safety. When an environment is unsafe, the child must be removed until the situation changes [17, 18]. For small children, the safety of the environment is generally judged on the presence/absence of abuse and neglect. The parent must be able to provide basic care (shelter, nutrition, hygiene, clothing, and medical care) and security (protection from dangers, including unsafe people). As the child grows older, other domains of the parental environment take precedence. Brockington et al. [18] categorize these as the parent's ability to provide: *emotional warmth* (comfort, praise, and affection), *encouragement of learning* (through play, language, support of schooling, and social opportunities), *guidance and setting consistent limits (teaching consideration of others, self-discipline,* and *internal moral values),* and *a stable family base* for engagement with the wider world.

Assessing competent parenting requires skill and experience. While it is relatively easy to ascertain the presence of gross neglect or abuse, the more subtle qualities of parenting are harder to evaluate. Parent competency instruments are imperfect; they tend to focus on deficits rather than on strengths, and they are subject to cultural biases, since parental norms differ among cultures [19, 20].

9. Overrepresentation of Psychiatric Patients in Parental Termination Hearings

Besides parental competence, conditions such as physical and mental disability, side effects of medications, hospitalization history, quality and permanence of living arrangements, employment record, and socioeconomic status enter into decision making about custody. These variables are all intimately associated with mental illness, and, as a result, parents with psychiatric diagnoses are overrepresented in parental termination proceedings. In an Australian study, parental psychiatric illness was the most prevalent condition at such court hearings [21]. Marital status is also important—unmarried women (and this describes the majority of women with a diagnosis of schizophrenia) are more likely to lose custody than their married peers [22]. Social integration in a network of family, friends, and community members, often deficient in women with schizophrenia, is also relevant [8]. The more dense a social network is, the less likely it is for children to be apprehended by child protection services. The diagnosis of schizophrenia in itself undermines a woman's chances of retaining custody, so does the substance abuse that frequently accompanies mental illness [7]. Recent studies have shown that substance abuse is perhaps the most important contributory factor [23, 24], although there are many interacting factors that determine out-of-home placements. Young mothers suffering from psychosis find it very hard to disentangle themselves and their children from the web of problems in which they become caught.

10. Preventing Custody Loss: Recommendations for Mothers and Care Providers

There are several ways in which mothers with severe mental illness can reduce the risk of child apprehension. It is the responsibility of care providers to provide mothers with this information and training in order to help them to preserve the integrity of their family [25].

10.1. Maintaining Mental Health. In trying to provide for their children, mothers often neglect their own health and yet maintenance of personal health is a crucial first step toward ensuring child custody. This includes proper diet, a healthy sleep schedule, an exercise program, regular physician and mental health visits, and adherence to a prescribed regimen of medication. When questioned, most mothers with schizophrenia do understand that custody can be lost if prescribed treatment for their condition is not adhered to [26].

When women deny psychiatric illness, the intense desire to retain custody of their children can be used as a form of leverage, a controversial but effective strategy [26–28].

11. Case Example

Patient B., the sole caregiver of a 5-year old son, sought treatment for psychotic symptoms but refused antipsychotic medication. She was hospitalized against her will after she was verbally abusive to another mother at her son's school. During her hospitalization, her son was placed in the care of a cousin. In hospital, Ms. B. continued to refuse medication. She asked for a lawyer to represent her so that she could leave hospital and return to her son. The lawyer advocated for her with hospital staff and persuaded Ms. B. to agree to community treatment orders (outpatient commitment), which included monthly depot antipsychotic injections. The lawyer convinced her that this would be her best recourse in order to regain custody of her son. Ms. B. had an excellent therapeutic response to the antipsychotic and soon went home. Her son returned to her care, and, when the 6-month community treatment order expired, Ms. B. continued the injections voluntarily because she felt so much better. Child protection worked collaboratively with legal and mental health agencies to help this family stay together. Followup after many years showed that Ms. B. has succeeded as a parent. She has had no further hospitalizations, and her son remains in good health.

As symptoms of psychosis decline, parenting stress is reduced and the quality of parenting inevitably improves [29]. Addressing symptoms alone is never sufficient [30], but does show the court that mothers are taking responsibility for this aspect of their recovery.

11.1. Self-Monitoring for Signs of Relapse. Avoiding recurrence of symptoms and the possibility of hospitalization is important for continuity of parental care, which means that psychiatric crises need to be avoided through anticipatory planning and self-monitoring. Mothers can be advised to maintain a written list of personal relapse triggers and early warning signs (sleeplessness, lapsed hygiene, increased suspiciousness, and so on) and to be knowledgeable about their medications. A requirement for dose changes whenever relapse threatens should be thoroughly discussed between mothers and care providers; the mother needs to know when and how she can increase (or decrease) her prescription to prevent a crisis. She needs to document what has worked in previous predicaments of a similar nature and what she can do to avert them. She needs ready access to crisis help. Evidence of self-monitoring convinces the court that mothers recognize that they suffer from a potentially relapsing illness and are doing their best to prevent recurrence.

11.2. Developing a Crisis Plan. Should hospitalization become necessary, it is important for mothers to be prepared for this disruption in their ability to care for their children. Several crisis plan templates are available electronically for parents with mental illness, none of which have as yet been evaluated for effectiveness [31]. It is best for all family members and all care providers to be involved in developing the crisis plan. The aim is to negotiate what needs to occur in an emergency and to clarify the responsibility of each member of the support network. Older children need to be part of the response team as they may be the first to notice their mother's early illness symptoms and they need to know whom to turn to under such circumstances. It is important, however, not to overburden children with the responsibility of looking after an ill parent.

The phone numbers and addresses of surrogate caregivers must be made available to children and also to care providers. Thought should be given to establishing backup caregivers in case of the unavailability of first choices.

The plan should be written down, shared, and periodically updated because names and details will change. It should include critical information about the children's needs: their doctor, dentist, teachers, allergies, food and activity preferences, favorite toys, bedtime routines, and physical and psychological history. Plans for family pets should be included. Reupert and colleagues [31] report that it typically takes 6–12 months to develop a comprehensive crisis plan because all the necessary interagency meetings take that long to organize. Such a plan indicates to the court that mothers place their parental responsibilities above all else.

11.3. Taking Advantage of Parenting Resources. Depending on the community, parenting skills classes, parenting mutual aid or support groups, parent coaches, parenting warm lines, home visiting, and respite services may all be available resources [32–34]. An online parenting course has even been developed in The Netherlands [35]. Well-trained care providers should be able to point mothers in the right directions to access the best resources [36]. Upgrading parental skills demonstrates to the court that mothers are trying their best to be responsible parents.

11.4. Documenting Household and Child Care Routines. When asked by a judge to give evidence of good parenting, many mothers do not know what to say, especially because such questions are not usually asked of mothers unless they suffer from mental illness. The judge, however, is entitled to ask about safety issues and about issues pertaining to domains of parenting competence similar to those outlined by Brockington et al. [18] Mothers can be helped to document the day to day manner in which they address their child's instrumental and emotional problems, how they help their children resolve conflicts, how they set limits, and how they help to socialize their children. They need to build a record detailing their parenting strengths and the quality of the bonds that exist with their children. Care providers should be able to provide guidance for the mother so that she is not at a loss when questions about her parenting emerge in court.

11.5. Navigating the Legal System. Mothers need to understand the mandated child abuse reporting laws of their jurisdictions. They need to connect with attorneys who understand mental illness and family law and the family court system and who can act as strong advocates. Policies intended to promote a speedy resolution for children in out-of-home care may unintentionally discriminate against parents with mental illness because they fast-track the termination of parental rights, allowing only a brief time period for new parents to meet the goals set by child protection agencies. Attorneys and care providers need to help mothers achieve these goals as quickly as possible by ensuring access and legal rights to the necessary supports and services. Collaboration is important between child protection and lawyers who represent parents in custody and termination proceedings. It is not an easy collaboration, however, because child welfare professionals and court professionals come from two distinct cultures, the first a culture of care and concern, the second an adversarial system that, above all else, values individual rights [37]. There is a definite need for mental health education of judges and court professionals.

12. Recommendations for Policy Makers

Early intervention services, adult mental health services, and child protection services often act in competition rather than in cooperation [38]. It is crucial to develop a philosophy and care system that cooperatively addresses the needs of the whole family. There is now a promising evidence base of effectiveness of wraparound services for families impacted by serious mental illness [39].

The term, "wraparound," is increasingly being used to describe a family-driven, strengths-based approach that uses an array of both formal services and natural supports [40]. Another phrase often used is "system of care." A system of care is a network of structures and relationships that is held together by shared values and that operates across administrative and funding jurisdictions [41, 42]. A family-driven system of care is based on the needs of children, parents, and extended family. It supports choice, ongoing evaluation, and accountability and promotes partnerships between families and professionals, collaboration between multiple agencies and service sectors, and individualized services that are sensitive to cultural differences. The cultural sensitivity of a service refers to the ability of its staff to understand, value, and incorporate the perspective of the family into service provision and, whenever possible, provide services in the family's language of choice.

In a wraparound system, there is a single point of entry for the many services that are provided. Among these are early identification and prevention strategies, attention to reproductive and child health, substance abuse counseling, case management, liaison with schools and the legal system, financial support, crisis management, housing, transportation aid, vocational help, spiritual, cultural, and recreational guidance, and respite care. Ideally, the services are open ended and sensitive to the stigma associated with mental illness. Cook and Steigman [43] advocate supports specifically designed to preserve the parental relationship. They identify assessment of parenting strengths and needs, birth control counseling, pregnancy decision-making support, trauma and abuse counseling, peer support, parent mentoring, self-help, support groups for children, and medication management as important aspects of a system of care for families with a mentally ill member. Specific counseling around benefits and entitlements is also critical for low-income mothers, some of whom may be intermittently homeless and require housing support [44]. Administrative policies, training opportunities for service providers, and hard work on the part of mothers themselves are all needed to ensure that children of mentally ill parents grow up, whenever possible, in their family of origin.

References

[1] S. E. Mason and R. Miller, "Stigma and schizophrenia: directions in student training," *Journal of Teaching in Social Work*, vol. 26, no. 1-2, pp. 73–91, 2006.

[2] C. Mason, S. Subedi, and R. B. Davis, "Clients with mental illness and their children: Iimplications for clinical practice," *Issues in Mental Health Nursing*, vol. 28, no. 10, pp. 1105–1123, 2007.

[3] A. Reupert and D. Maybery, "Programmes for parents with a mental illness," *Journal of Psychiatric and Mental Health Nursing*, vol. 18, pp. 257–264, 2011.

[4] C. A. Clark, P. R. Smith, and P. Smith, "Promoting collaborative practice for children of parents with mental illness and their families," *Psychiatric Rehabilitation Journal*, vol. 33, no. 2, pp. 95–97, 2009.

[5] B. R. Hinden, K. Biebel, J. Nicholson, A. Henry, and J. Katz-Leavy, "A survey of programs for parents with mental illness and their families: identifying common elements to build the evidence base," *Journal of Behavioral Health Services and Research*, vol. 33, no. 1, pp. 21–38, 2006.

[6] R. Gewurtz, T. Krupa, S. Eastabrook, and S. Horgan, "Prevalence and characteristics of parenting among people served by assertive community treatment," *Psychiatric Rehabilitation Journal*, vol. 28, no. 1, pp. 63–65, 2004.

[7] L. M. Howard, R. Kumar, and G. Thornicroft, "Psychosocial characteristics and needs of mothers with psychotic disorders," *British Journal of Psychiatry*, vol. 178, pp. 427–432, 2001.

[8] L. D. Hollingsworth, "Child custody loss among women with persistent severe mental illness," *Social Work Research*, vol. 28, no. 4, pp. 199–209, 2004.

[9] H. Dipple, S. Smith, H. Andrews, and B. Evans, "The experience of motherhood in women with severe and enduring mental illness," *Social Psychiatry and Psychiatric Epidemiology*, vol. 37, no. 7, pp. 336–340, 2002.

[10] I. Savvidou, V. P. Bozikas, S. Hatzigeleki, and A. Karavatos, "Narratives about their children by mothers hospitalized on a psychiatric unit," *Family Process*, vol. 42, no. 3, pp. 391–402, 2003.

[11] B. J. Ackerson, "Parents with serious and persistent mental illness: Issues in assessment and services," *Social Work*, vol. 48, no. 2, pp. 187–195, 2003.

[12] A. Diaz-Caneja and S. Johnson, "The views and experiences of severely mentally ill mothers—a qualitative study," *Social Psychiatry and Psychiatric Epidemiology*, vol. 39, no. 6, pp. 472–482, 2004.

[13] R. G. Sands, N. Koppelman, and P. Solomon, "Maternal custody status and living arrangements of children of women with severe mental illness," *Health and Social Work*, vol. 29, no. 4, pp. 317–325, 2004.

[14] N. R. Matevosyan, "Pregnancy and postpartum specifics in women with schizophrenia: a meta-study," *Archives of Gynecology and Obstetrics*, vol. 283, no. 2, pp. 141–147, 2011.

[15] S. N. Vigod and L. E. Ross, "Epidemiology of psychotic symptoms during pregnancy and postpartum in women with schizophrenia," *Current Women's Health Reviews*, vol. 6, no. 1, pp. 17–21, 2010.

[16] M. Lagan, K. Knights, J. Barton, and P. M. Boyce, "Advocacy for mothers with psychiatric illness: a clinical perspective," *International Journal of Mental Health Nursing*, vol. 18, no. 1, pp. 53–61, 2009.

[17] A. Monds-Watson, R. Manktelow, and M. McColgan, "Social work with children when parents have mental health difficulties: acknowledging vulnerability and maintaining the 'rights of the child'," *Child Care in Practice*, vol. 16, no. 1, pp. 35–55, 2010.

[18] I. Brockington, P. Chandra, H. Dubowitz et al., "WPA guidance on the protection and promotion of mental health in children of persons with severe mental disorders," *World Psychiatry*, vol. 10, pp. 1–10, 2011.

[19] R. Kuersten-Hogan, C. Benjet, and S. T. Azar, "Evaluating the parental fitness of psychiatrically diagnosed individuals: advocating a functional-contextual analysis of parenting," *Journal of Family Psychology*, vol. 17, no. 2, pp. 238–251, 2003.

[20] M. V. Seeman, "Cross-cultural evaluation of maternal competence in a culturally diverse society," *American Journal of Psychiatry*, vol. 165, no. 5, pp. 565–568, 2008.

[21] G. Llewellyn, D. McConnell, and L. Ferronato, "Prevalence and outcomes for parents with disabilities and their children in an Australian court sample," *Child Abuse and Neglect*, vol. 27, no. 3, pp. 235–251, 2003.

[22] S. Strega, C. Fleet, L. Brown, L. Dominelli, M. Callahan, and C. Walmsley, "Connecting father absence and mother blame in child welfare policies and practice," *Children & Youth Services Review*, vol. 30, no. 7, pp. 705–716, 2008.

[23] D. Jones, R. L. Macias, P. B. Gold, P. Barreira, and W. Fisher, "When parents with severe mental illness lose contact with their children: are psychiatric symptoms or substance use to blame?" *Journal of Loss and Trauma*, vol. 13, no. 4, pp. 261–287, 2008.

[24] L. Lewin and A. Abdrbo, "Mothers with self-reported axis I diagnoses and child protection," *Archives of Psychiatric Nursing*, vol. 23, no. 3, pp. 200–209, 2009.

[25] L. B. Kundra and L. B. Alexander, "Termination of parental rights proceedings: legal considerations and practical strategies for parents with psychiatric disabilities and the practitioners who serve them," *Psychiatric Rehabilitation Journal*, vol. 33, no. 2, pp. 142–149, 2009.

[26] A. Busch and A. D. Redlich, "Patients' perception of possible child custody or visitation loss for nonadherence to psychiatric treatment," *Psychiatric Services*, vol. 58, no. 7, pp. 999–1002, 2007.

[27] J. Monahan, A. D. Redlich, J. Swanson et al., "Use of leverage to improve adherence to psychiatric treatment in the community," *Psychiatric Services*, vol. 56, no. 1, pp. 37–44, 2005.

[28] J. Nicholson, "Use of child custody as leverage to improve treatment adherence," *Psychiatric Services*, vol. 56, no. 3, pp. 357–358, 2005.

[29] S. K. Kahng, D. Oyserman, D. Bybee, and C. Mowbray, "Mothers with serious mental illness: when symptoms decline does parenting improve? " *Journal of Family Psychology*, vol. 22, no. 1, pp. 162–166, 2008.

[30] M. W. Wan, S. Moulton, and K. M. Abel, "A review of mother-child relational interventions and their usefulness for mothers with schizophrenia," *Archives of Women's Mental Health*, vol. 11, no. 3, pp. 171–179, 2008.

[31] A. E. Reupert, K. T. Green, and D. J. Maybery, "Care plans for families affected by parental mental illness," *Families in Society*, vol. 89, no. 1, pp. 39–43, 2008.

[32] E. A. Craig, "Parenting programs for women with mental illness who have young children: a review," *Australian and New Zealand Journal of Psychiatry*, vol. 38, no. 11-12, pp. 923–928, 2004.

[33] M. V. Seeman, "Parenting issues in mothers with schizophrenia," *Current Women's Health Reviews*, vol. 6, no. 1, pp. 51–57, 2010.
[34] P. D. Zeanah, J. A. Larrieu, N. W. Boris, and G. A. Nagle, "Nurse home visiting: perspectives from nurses," *Infant Mental Health Journal*, vol. 27, no. 1, pp. 41–54, 2006.
[35] R. A. P. van der Zanden, P. A. M. Speetjens, K. S. E. Arntz, and S. A. Onrust, "Online group course for parents with mental illness: development and pilot study," *Journal of Medical Internet Research*, vol. 12, no. 5, article e50, 2010.
[36] A. Reupert and D. Maybery, "Families affected by parental mental illness: a multiperspective account of issues and interventions," *American Journal of Orthopsychiatry*, vol. 77, no. 3, pp. 362–369, 2007.
[37] M. Han, S. Carnochan, and M. J. Austin, "The challenges to promoting collaboration between child protection services workers and court professionals: an exploratory study of case records," *Journal of Public Child Welfare*, vol. 1, no. 3, pp. 115–131, 2007.
[38] Y. Darlington, J. A. Feeney, and K. Rixon, "Practice challenges at the intersection of child protection and mental health," *Child and Family Social Work*, vol. 10, no. 3, pp. 239–247, 2005.
[39] M. L. Kessler and B. J. Ackerson, "Wraparound services: an effective intervention for families impacted by severe mental illness," *Journal of Family Social Work*, vol. 8, no. 4, pp. 29–45, 2005.
[40] N. C. Winters and W. P. Metz, "The wraparound approach in systems of care," *Psychiatric Clinics of North America*, vol. 32, no. 1, pp. 135–151, 2009.
[41] E. J. Bruns and J. S. Walker, "Defining practice: flexibility, legitimacy, and the nature of systems of care and wraparound," *Evaluation and Program Planning*, vol. 33, no. 1, pp. 45–48, 2010.
[42] S. Hodges, K. Ferreira, N. Israel, and J. Mazza, "Systems of care, featherless bipeds, and the measure of all things," *Evaluation and Program Planning*, vol. 33, no. 1, pp. 4–10, 2010.
[43] J. Cook and P. Steigman, "Experiences of parents with mental illnesses and their services needs," *Journal of National Association for the Mentally (NAMI) California*, vol. 11, no. 2, pp. 21–23, 2000.
[44] L. Weinreb, J. Nicholson, V. Williams, and F. Anthes, "Integrating behavioral health services for homeless mothers and children in primary care," *American Journal of Orthopsychiatry*, vol. 77, no. 1, pp. 142–152, 2007.

23

Second Generation Antipsychotics Improve Sexual Dysfunction in Schizophrenia: A Randomised Controlled Trial

Ahmed Mahmoud,[1] Karen P. Hayhurst,[2] Richard J. Drake,[1] and Shôn W. Lewis[1]

[1] *Mental Health and Neurodegeneration Research Group, The University of Manchester, Manchester M13 9PL, UK*
[2] *National Drug Evidence Centre (NDEC), School of Community Based Medicine, The University of Manchester, Manchester M15 6SZ, UK*

Correspondence should be addressed to Karen P. Hayhurst, karen.hayhurst@manchester.ac.uk

Academic Editor: D. Naber

The impact of antipsychotic drug treatment on sexual function was investigated during a randomised trial comparing first generation antipsychotics (FGAs) to (nonclozapine) second generation antipsychotics (SGAs). Sexual function and quality of life were (rater-blind) assessed in 42 patients with DSM-IV schizophrenia (aged 18–65) using the self-report version of the Derogatis Interview for Sexual Function (DISF-SR) and the Heinrichs Quality of Life Scale (QLS), prior to, and 12 weeks following, a change in medication from an FGA drug to either an FGA or SGA drug. SGAs significantly improved sexual function compared to FGAs. Change in sexual function was associated with change in quality of life. Where impaired sexual functioning is a distressing adverse effect of treatment with an FGA agent, consideration should be given to switching to an SGA.

1. Introduction

Sexual dysfunction is common in people with schizophrenia [1] affecting around a half of all patients [2–4] and likely to contribute to impaired quality of life [5–7]. Little systematic research has been carried out to date on the sexual behaviour of schizophrenic patients and a Cochrane review recently called for further research on the management of antipsychotic treatment-related sexual dysfunction [8].

Patients themselves report that the sexual side effects of medication are distressing [9]. For example, Finn and colleagues [10] found that patients with schizophrenia rated impotence, as a treatment side effect, as worse than any symptoms of the illness itself. Men may perceive sexual dysfunction as more distressing than women [11], but the experience of sexual dysfunction in women with schizophrenia has been underresearched. Sexual dysfunction can be a significant reason for nonadherence to prescribed antipsychotic treatment [1, 2, 12–15].

The relationship between antipsychotic drugs and sexual dysfunction is mediated in part by antipsychotic blockade of pituitary D2 receptors increasing prolactin secretion, although direct correlations have not been established between raised prolactin levels and clinical symptoms [16–18]. More recent studies highlight that a variety of mechanisms are likely to contribute to antipsychotic-related sexual dysfunction, including hyperprolactinaemia, sedation, and antagonism of a number of neurotransmitter receptors ($\alpha-$adrenergic, dopaminergic, histaminic, and muscarinic) [19, 20].

Conventional, or first generation antipsychotic (FGA) drugs are associated with sexual side effects. Ghadirian and colleagues [21] found that up to 60% of men and 33% of women on FGAs reported changes in the quality of orgasm. A further study reported that chlorpromazine was associated with problems of orgasm and sulpiride with problems of arousal in female patients [3]. A Cochrane review highlights increased prolactin levels seen with sulpiride treatment [22]. Recent research demonstrates that as sulpiride is less lipophilic than other antipsychotics it has relatively high concentrations in the pituitary (outside the blood-brain barrier) compared to brain parenchyma [23]. This means that hyperprolactinaemia is more likely to occur at clinical doses of sulpiride.

Individual second generation antipsychotic (SGA) drugs appear to be associated with less sexual dysfunction than that attributable to FGAs. One recent review concluded that risperidone had the largest impact on sexual dysfunction, followed by FGA drugs, then olanzapine, then clozapine, then quetiapine and, finally, aripiprazole [19]. Antipsychotic drugs with high D2-binding affinity have been identified as more likely to cause sexual dysfunction [1, 24] and risperidone may be associated with higher prolactin elevation than other SGAs [25–27]. Amisulpride is less lipophilic than risperidone or other SGAs and this may (as for sulpiride) explain why it is particularly identified with hyperprolactinaemia [26]. Bearing in mind the limitations associated with its design, data from the SOHO study, a large observational study funded by Lilly, indicates an advantage to both olanzapine and quetiapine, compared with risperidone and FGA drugs, across areas of sexual dysfunction [28–30]. A previous European study concluded that there were no real benefits of any of the SGAs over FGA treatment, apart from that seen with quetiapine in short-term trials [31]. Further studies have confirmed the association of both quetiapine [1, 32, 33] and aripiprazole [34, 35] with less severe sexual dysfunction.

Sexual dysfunction is a difficult area to investigate. Sexual problems may be underreported to clinicians who, in turn, may underestimate the sexual side effects of antipsychotic treatment [1, 2, 6, 7, 13, 29, 31]. Researchers in the field have used a variety of assessment tools to measure sexual function, leading to difficulty when reviewing the published literature.

We set out to examine sexual dysfunction in a subgroup of participants in a large trial. Patients already taking, but unresponsive to, an FGA were randomised to change to either another FGA or a non-clozapine SGA for 12 weeks while sexual function and quality of life were assessed.

We tested two hypotheses. Firstly, that sexual dysfunction contributes measurably to reduced health-related quality of life in patients with schizophrenia. Secondly, that sexual function and hence quality of life is better in patients with schizophrenia on SGAs than FGAs.

2. Materials and Methods

Patients ($N = 42$) were treated with an FGA drug prior to randomisation into the study. The study was conducted alongside CUtLASS (Cost Utility of the Latest Antipsychotics in Severe Schizophrenia [36–38]: a multicentre RCT that compared FGAs with SGA drugs. All participants of the sub-study were recruited from one centre. The North West Multi-Centre Research Ethics Committee granted ethical approval with local approval obtained from each participating district.

2.1. Inclusion Criteria. Patients had a diagnosis of DSM-IV schizophrenia (and related disorders). The sample comprised patients recruited to CUtLASS ($N = 20$) and additional patients recruited from clinical practice ($N = 22$). All participants entered the study because of an identified need for a change to their FGA treatment, either because of ineffectiveness or intolerable side effects. No participants were referred because of sexual side effects. Patients were aged 18 to 65 years of both sexes. Patients receiving anticholinergic drugs were included.

2.2. Exclusion Criteria. Excluded patients included those with a diagnosis of schizoaffective disorder, patients with a comorbid history of alcohol or drug misuse within the last 12 months, and patients receiving treatment with more than one antipsychotic drug at baseline.

2.3. Randomisation. Randomisation, of all included patients, took place via a remote telephone service provided by the Medical Statistics Department at the Paterson Institute, Christie Hospital, Manchester, UK. The method of allocation was permuted blocks within strata with block sizes varying at random between four and 12. Arrangements were in place to ensure that the patient commenced their new antipsychotic drug treatment within hours of randomisation to either an FGA or an SGA drug. All subjects had a change to their antipsychotic drug and all completed the 12-week period on their assigned treatment. Randomised treatment allocation was revealed to the responsible clinician, the CUtLASS trial manager and the participant's GP.

2.4. Measures. Primary and secondary outcome measures used, respectively, were the self-report Derogatis Interview for Sexual Function (DISF-SR) [39] and the (rater-blinded) Quality of Life Scale (QLS) [40]. The Derogatis interview is a widely used, brief, self report, multidimensional and gender-keyed instrument designed to measure quality of current sexual functioning across five primary domains: sexual cognition and fantasy (5 items); sexual arousal (5 items); sexual behaviour and experiences (5 items); orgasm (6 items); sexual drive and relationship (4 items). The first three of these key domains are scored using a nine-point scale (from "0" as "not at all" through to "8" as "4 or more times per day"); orgasm is scored using a five-point scale (from "0" as "not at all" to "4" as "extremely"); the fifth domain, sexual drive, and relationship, is scored using a combination of nine- and five-point scales. The aggregate total score can be used repeatedly throughout efficacy or effectiveness studies without any significant practice effects or loss of validity [39].

The QLS [40] is the most widely used quality of life scale in the evaluation of psychopharmacological treatments for schizophrenia [41]. The 21-item scale covers four domains: social relationships; instrumental role functioning; intrapsychic foundations; activities of daily life. The QLS has been shown to be both sensitive to change and of clinical relevance [42].

2.5. Statistical Analysis and Power. Results were analysed using SPSS version 15 to carry out analyses of covariance (ANCOVAs) and correlational analyses (Pearson's r and Spearman's rho). An *a priori* power calculation suggested that the sample size obtained would have 90% power to detect a difference of 30 points on the DISF-SR between the two treatment groups, which was selected as a difference

TABLE 1: Demographic Characteristics.

	FGA Arm ($N = 22$)	SGA Arm ($N = 20$)	P	test
Age				
Mean/SD	38.4 (10.0)	43.0 (11.7)	.173	*t* test
Median/Range	39.6/18–53	45.9/19–57		
Illness duration				
Mean/SD	14.4 (8.7)	18.6 (11.9)		
Median/Range	13.0/0.5–34	24.6/1–33	.182	Mann-Whitney
Gender				
Male (%)	19 (86%)	12 (60%)	.052	Chi Square
Ethnicity				
White (%)	20 (91%)	18 (90%)	1.000	Chi Square

TABLE 2: This table shows antipsychotic drug treatment received by the two groups.

FGA Arm ($N = 22$)			SGA Arm ($N = 20$)		
N	Drug	Dose range	*N*	Drug	Dose range
2	Flupentixol	3–6 mg	2	Amisulpride	400 mg
1	Haloperidol	3 mg	7	Olanzapine	5–15 mg
3	Sulpiride	400–2000 mg	7	Quetiapine	100–700 mg
1	Trifluoperazine	15 mg	4	Risperidone	3–4 mg
7	Zuclopenthixol	4–20 mg			
1	Flupentixol depot	40 2/52			
1	Fluphenazine depot	25 2/52			
1	Pipotiazine palm.	50 3/52			
5	Zuclopenthixol depot	200 4/52–400 2/52			

that both appeared clinically relevant and related to previous findings of differences between treatment groups [43].

3. Results

Table 1 shows demographic characteristics of the two treatment groups. Thirty-one men and 11 women with a mean age of 41 years (range 18 to 57 years) were randomised.

The two groups were statistically comparable in terms of their ethnicity and age. The FGA arm had a lower median duration of illness and a higher proportion of males, compared with the SGA arm, although neither measure differed significantly between the two groups.

Table 2 shows antipsychotic drug treatment received by the two groups.

Table 3 shows sexual function scores of the two treatment groups over the two assessment time points.

Mean baseline total and subsection scores on the DISF-SR differed between the two groups (Table 3), but not significantly. Table 3 also shows that mean DISF-SR scores of the FGA-treated group worsened somewhat between the two time points.

There was no significant correlation between DISF SR total score and QLS total score at baseline ($r = 0.167$, $P = .290$) and a weak (nonsignificant) correlation at week 12 ($r = 0.293$, $P = .063$). The trend relationship seen by week 12 of the study resulted from a significant correlation between score on QLS subscale 1 (interpersonal relations & social network) and score on Section 3 of the DISF-SR (sexual behaviour & experience: Spearman's rho = 0.356, $P = .022$). There was a significant correlation between change in DISF-SR total score and change in QLS total score from baseline to week 12 (Spearman's rho = 0.627, $P < .001$).

Twelve week DISF-SR total was modelled with an analysis of covariance. Final sexual function was significantly better ($F = 7.45$, $P = .010$) for patients randomised to an SGA ($N = 20$), compared to patients receiving an FGA ($N = 22$), covarying for baseline score and gender. Adjusted 12-week marginal mean DISF-SR score was 58.0 in the SGA group and 37.7 in the FGA group (difference 20.3, 95% confidence interval 5.2, 35.4). Age was dropped as a covariate as it was not independently significant. There was no significant difference between groups in final QLS total ($F = 0.421$, $P =$

Table 3: DISF-SR score.

DISF-SR Mean (SD)	FGA Group (N = 22)		SGA Group (N = 20)		
	Baseline	Week 12	Baseline	Week 12	*Baseline comparison*
Section 1: sexual cognition/fantasy	15.5 (12.7)	13.8 (10.6)	10.4 (9.3)	16.2 (11.0)	P = .130[†]
Section 2: sexual arousal	10.2 (8.2)	9.3 (8.9)	7.0 (8.4)	9.5 (9.0)	P = .202[†]
Section 3: sexual behaviour/experience	6.7 (5.8)	6.4 (5.9)	4.6 (6.8)	6.8 (8.5)	P = .085[‡]
Section 4: orgasm	9.1 (7.2)	8.0 (6.8)	5.6 (8.0)	9.0 (8.0)	P = .128[†]
Section 5: sexual drive	10.6 (4.5)	9.6 (5.0)	9.0 (4.6)	11.1 (5.0)	P = .236[†]
Total Score	52.6 (32.7)	47.5 (32.3)	36.4 (33.7)	52.6 (37.3)	P = .121[†]

[†] *t*-test.
[‡] Mann-Whitney.
NB: A higher score on the DISF-SR scale is indicative of better sexual functioning.

.521) or QLS subscales, covarying for gender and baseline score.

4. Discussion

Regarding the first hypothesis, sexual dysfunction did not have a straightforward relationship with reduced quality of life. It was unrelated at baseline but improvement in sexual function had a weak to moderate relationship with improving quality of life. This drove a trend-level association at final assessment. It may be that changes in sexual function have a more direct effect on quality of life than static sexual function, perhaps because over time there is a degree of adjustment to dysfunction. It is also worth noting that the QLS is an objective measure of quality of life, influenced by social function as well as participants' subjective experience; subjective quality of life may be more strongly related.

Previous studies have linked male sexual dysfunction with poor quality of life in schizophrenia [6]. Although our results do not confirm this, again, the QLS may not be the best type of measure to detect a relationship. Total score on the QLS may not have sufficient sensitivity to detect sexual functioning-related changes in quality of life, and there is an argument for examining subscales of the QLS and DISF-SR.

In terms of the second of our hypotheses, those who were in the SGA group had significantly better sexual function by the end of the trial. This suggests that switching from an FGA to an SGA can improve sexual function significantly. Note that none of the participants were referred into the study because of the sexual side effects of antipsychotic drug treatment. Sexual side effects can lessen with time following a treatment switch [44]. This reduction over time could, in part, explain the improvement in sexual function seen in the SGA group but fails to account for the deterioration seen in the FGA group.

The study had a number of limitations. As stated earlier, the nature of the QLS, being determined largely by the deficit symptoms of schizophrenia [45], may explain the lack of effect of drug type on measured quality of life. Other treatment-related side effects, such as parkinsonism or sedation, which may also affect sexual function, were not measured in the study. The relatively small sample size did not permit an analysis of individual drugs. At the time of the study, some SGA drugs, such as ziprasidone and paliperidone, were not available in the UK, whilst others, such as zotepine, were little used. Female patients made up a relatively small proportion of those recruited limiting the generalisability of the findings. The study did, however, have the advantage of being a prospective, randomised comparison, one of a few to assess sexual function comprehensively. The self-report Derogatis scale was selected for this study because of its high validity and reliability.

These findings add to the evidence that SGA drugs, as a group, have less adverse sexual side effects than those associated with FGA treatment. As an RCT of a change in medication it confirms the implication of existing non-randomised survey data that switching antipsychotics can reduce the risk of treatment-associated sexual dysfunction [12, 19, 25]. Of course, it is not clear what effect switching within SGAs or from SGA to FGA would be, so it is uncertain whether this is an effect of switching class.

5. Conclusions

Switching from FGAs to SGAs improved sexual function compared to switching within FGAs. The relationship between the self-report measure of sexual function and the assessor-rated, objective quality of life measure used was complex, but it appeared that change in sexual function was associated with change in quality of life. Where impaired sexual functioning is a distressing adverse effect of treatment with an FGA agent consideration should be given to switching to an SGA.

Acknowledgments

This study was conducted alongside the CUtLASS trials (Cost utility of the latest antipsychotics in severe schizophrenia, [36–38]) which were funded by NHS R&D Health Technology Assessment. The authors are grateful to reviewers for their comments on an earlier draft of this paper.

References

[1] D. L. Kelly and R. R. Conley, "A randomized double-blind 12-week study of quetiapine, risperidone or fluphenazine on sexual functioning in people with schizophrenia," *Psychoneuroendocrinology*, vol. 31, no. 3, pp. 340–346, 2006.

[2] M. Dossenbach, A. Hodge, M. Anders et al., "Prevalence of sexual dysfunction in patients with schizophrenia: international variation and underestimation," *International Journal of Neuropsychopharmacology*, vol. 8, no. 2, pp. 195–201, 2005.

[3] S. M. Smith, V. O'Keane, and R. Murray, "Sexual dysfunction in patients taking conventional antipsychotic medication," *British Journal of Psychiatry*, vol. 181, pp. 49–55, 2002.

[4] A. Üçok, C. İncesu, T. Aker, and Ş. Erkoç, "Sexual dysfunction in patients with schizophrenia on antipsychotic medication," *European Psychiatry*, vol. 22, no. 5, pp. 328–333, 2007.

[5] P. Assalian, R. Fraser, R. Tempier, and D. Cohen, "Sexuality and quality of life of patients with schizophrenia," *International Journal of Psychiatry in Clinical Practice*, vol. 4, no. 1, pp. 29–33, 2000.

[6] M. Olfson, T. Uttaro, W. H. Carson, and E. Tafesse, "Male sexual dysfunction and quality of life in schizophrenia," *Journal of Clinical Psychiatry*, vol. 66, no. 3, pp. 331–338, 2005.

[7] J. Peuskens, P. Sienaert, and M. De Hert, "Sexual dysfunction: the unspoken side effect of antipsychotics," *European Psychiatry*, vol. 13, supplement 1, pp. 23s–30s, 1998.

[8] M. M. Berner, M. Hagen, and L. Kriston, "Management of sexual dysfunction due to antipsychotic drug therapy," *Cochrane Database of Systematic Reviews*, no. 1, Article ID CD003546, 2007.

[9] M. Lambert, P. Conus, P. Eide et al., "Impact of present and past antipsychotic side effects on attitude toward typical antipsychotic treatment and adherence," *European Psychiatry*, vol. 19, no. 7, pp. 415–422, 2004.

[10] S. E. Finn, J. M. Bailey, R. T. Schultz, and R. Faber, "Subjective utility ratings of neuroleptics in treating schizophrenia," *Psychological Medicine*, vol. 20, no. 4, pp. 843–848, 1990.

[11] W. K. H. Fakhoury, D. Wright, and M. Wallace, "Prevalence and extent of distress of adverse effects of antipsychotics among callers to a United Kingdom national mental health helpline," *International Clinical Psychopharmacology*, vol. 16, no. 3, pp. 153–162, 2001.

[12] A. J. Cutler, "Sexual dysfunction and antipsychotic treatment," *Psychoneuroendocrinology*, vol. 28, supplement 1, pp. 69–82, 2003.

[13] D. L. Kelly and R. R. Conley, "Sexuality and schizophrenia: a review," *Schizophrenia Bulletin*, vol. 30, no. 4, pp. 767–779, 2004.

[14] D. O. Perkins, "Predictors of noncompliance in patients with schizophrenia," *Journal of Clinical Psychiatry*, vol. 63, no. 12, pp. 1121–1128, 2002.

[15] S. Smith, "Effects of antipsychotics on sexual and endocrine function in women: implications for clinical practice," *Journal of Clinical Psychopharmacology*, vol. 23, no. 3, pp. S27–S32, 2003.

[16] M. Hamner, "The effects of atypical antipsychotics on serum prolactin levels," *Annals of Clinical Psychiatry*, vol. 14, no. 3, pp. 163–173, 2002.

[17] H. Knegtering, R. van den Bosch, S. Castelein, R. Bruggeman, S. Sytema, and J. van Os, "Are sexual side effects of prolactin-raising antipsychotics reducible to serum prolactin?" *Psychoneuroendocrinology*, vol. 33, no. 6, pp. 711–717, 2008.

[18] P. Malik, "Sexual dysfunction in schizophrenia," *Current Opinion in Psychiatry*, vol. 20, no. 2, pp. 138–142, 2007.

[19] M. Baggaley, "Sexual dysfunction in schizophrenia: focus on recent evidence," *Human Psychopharmacology*, vol. 23, no. 3, pp. 201–209, 2008.

[20] P. M. Haddad and S. G. Sharma, "Adverse effects of atypical antipsychotics: differential risk and clinical implications," *CNS Drugs*, vol. 21, no. 11, pp. 911–936, 2007.

[21] A. M. Ghadirian, G. Chouinard, and L. Annable, "Sexual dysfunction and plasma prolactin levels in neuroleptic-treated schizophrenic outpatients," *Journal of Nervous and Mental Disease*, vol. 170, no. 8, pp. 463–467, 1982.

[22] B. G. Soares, M. Fenton, and P. Chue, "Sulpiride for schizophrenia," *Cochrane Database of Systematic Reviews*, no. 1, Article ID CD001162, 2000.

[23] R. Arakawa, M. Okumura, H. Ito et al., "Positron emission tomography measurement of dopamine D_2 receptor occupancy in the pituitary and cerebral cortex: relation to antipsychotic-induced hyperprolactinemia," *Journal of Clinical Psychiatry*, vol. 71, no. 9, pp. 1131–1137, 2010.

[24] P. M. Haddad and A. Wieck, "Antipsychotic-induced hyperprolactinaemia: mechanisms, clinical features and management," *Drugs*, vol. 64, no. 20, pp. 2291–2314, 2004.

[25] C. Bushe, D. Yeomans, T. Floyd, and S. M. Smith, "Categorical prevalence and severity of hyperprolactinaemia in two UK cohorts of patients with severe mental illness during treatment with antipsychotics," *Journal of Psychopharmacology*, vol. 22, supplement 2, pp. 56–62, 2008.

[26] P. Falkai, T. Wobrock, J. Lieberman et al., "World Federation of Societies of Biological Psychiatry (WFSBP) guidelines for biological treatment of schizophrenia—part 1: acute treatment of schizophrenia," *World Journal of Biological Psychiatry*, vol. 6, no. 3, pp. 132–191, 2005.

[27] M. Hummer and J. Huber, "Hyperprolactinaemia and antipsychotic therapy in schizophrenia," *Current Medical Research and Opinion*, vol. 20, no. 2, pp. 189–197, 2004.

[28] I. Bitter, B. R. Basson, and M. R. Dossenbach, "Antipsychotic treatment and sexual functioning in first-time neuroleptic-treated schizophrenic patients," *International Clinical Psychopharmacology*, vol. 20, no. 1, pp. 19–21, 2005.

[29] M. Dossenbach, Y. Dyachkova, S. Pirildar et al., "Effects of atypical and typical antipsychotic treatments on sexual function in patients with schizophrenia: 12-month results from the Intercontinental Schizophrenia Outpatient Health Outcomes (IC-SOHO) study," *European Psychiatry*, vol. 21, no. 4, pp. 251–258, 2006.

[30] M. Lambert, J. M. Haro, D. Novick et al., "Olanzapine vs. other antipsychotics in actual out-patient settings: six months tolerability results from the European schizophrenia out-patient health outcomes study," *Acta Psychiatrica Scandinavica*, vol. 111, no. 3, pp. 232–243, 2005.

[31] J. Bobes, M. P. García-Portilla, J. Rejas et al., "Frequency of sexual dysfunction and other reproductive side-effects in patients with schizophrenia treated with risperidone, olanzapine, quetiapine, or haloperidol: the results of the EIRE study," *Journal of Sex and Marital Therapy*, vol. 29, no. 2, pp. 125–147, 2003.

[32] M. J. Byerly, P. A. Nakonezny, B. M. Bettcher, T. Carmody,

R. Fisher, and A. J. Rush, "Sexual dysfunction associated with second-generation antipsychotics in outpatients with schizophrenia or schizoaffective disorder: an empirical evaluation of olanzapine, risperidone, and quetiapine," *Schizophrenia Research*, vol. 86, no. 1–3, pp. 244–250, 2006.

[33] R. Knegtering, S. Castelein, H. Bous et al., "A randomized open-label study of the impact of quetiapine versus risperidone on sexual functioning," *Journal of Clinical Psychopharmacology*, vol. 24, no. 1, pp. 56–61, 2004.

[34] L. Hanssens, G. L'Italien, J. Y. Loze, R. N. Marcus, M. Pans, and W. Kerselaers, "The effect of antipsychotic medication on sexual function and serum prolactin levels in community-treated schizophrenic patients: results from the Schizophrenia Trial of Aripiprazole (STAR) study (NCT00237913)," *BMC Psychiatry*, vol. 8, article no. 95, 2008.

[35] A. Mir, K. Shivakumar, R. J. Williamson, V. McAllister, V. O'Keane, and K. J. Aitchison, "Change in sexual dysfunction with aripiprazole: a switching or add-on study," *Journal of Psychopharmacology*, vol. 22, no. 3, pp. 244–253, 2008.

[36] P. B. Jones, T. R. E. Barnes, L. Davies et al., "Randomized controlled trial of the effect on quality of life of second- vs first-generation antipsychotic drugs in schizophrenia: cost utility of the latest antipsychotic drugs in schizophrenia study (CUtLASS 1)," *Archives of General Psychiatry*, vol. 63, no. 10, pp. 1079–1087, 2006.

[37] S. W. Lewis, T. R. E. Barnes, L. Davies et al., "Randomized controlled trial of effect of prescription of clozapine versus other second-generation antipsychotic drugs in resistant schizophrenia," *Schizophrenia Bulletin*, vol. 32, no. 4, pp. 715–723, 2006.

[38] S. W. Lewis, L. Davies, P. B. Jones et al., "Randomised controlled trials of conventional antipsychotic versus new atypical drugs, and new atypical drugs versus clozapine, in people with schizophrenia responding poorly to, or intolerant of, current drug treatment," *Health Technology Assessment*, vol. 10, no. 17, 2006.

[39] L. R. Derogatis, "The Derogatis Interview for Sexual Functioning (DISF/DISF-SR): an introductory report," *Journal of Sex and Marital Therapy*, vol. 23, no. 4, pp. 291–304, 1997.

[40] D. W. Heinrichs, T. E. Hanlon, and W. T. Carpenter, "The quality of life scale: an instrument for rating the schizophrenic deficit syndrome," *Schizophrenia Bulletin*, vol. 10, no. 3, pp. 388–398, 1984.

[41] A. F. Lehman, "Measures of quality of life among persons with severe and persistent mental disorders," *Social Psychiatry and Psychiatric Epidemiology*, vol. 31, no. 2, pp. 78–88, 1996.

[42] J. Cramer, R. Rosenheck, W. Xu, W. Henderson, J. Thomas, and D. Charney, "Detecting improvement in quality of life and symptomatology in schizophrenia," *Schizophrenia Bulletin*, vol. 27, pp. 227–234, 2001.

[43] D. Aizenberg, Z. Zemishlany, P. Dorfman-Etrog, and A. Weizman, "Sexual dysfunction in male schizophrenic patients," *Journal of Clinical Psychiatry*, vol. 56, no. 4, pp. 137–141, 1995.

[44] D. Novick, J. M. Haro, E. Perrin, D. Suarez, and J. M. Texeira, "Tolerability of outpatient antipsychotic treatment: 36-month results from the European Schizophrenia Outpatient Health Outcomes (SOHO) study," *European Neuropsychopharmacology*, vol. 19, no. 8, pp. 542–550, 2009.

[45] R. Gourevitch, S. Abbadi, and J. D. Guelfi, "Quality of life in schizophrenics with and without the deficit syndrome," *European Psychiatry*, vol. 19, no. 3, pp. 172–174, 2004.

Permissions

All chapters in this book were first published in SCHIZORT, by BioMed Central; hereby published with permission under the Creative Commons Attribution License or equivalent. Every chapter published in this book has been scrutinized by our experts. Their significance has been extensively debated. The topics covered herein carry significant findings which will fuel the growth of the discipline. They may even be implemented as practical applications or may be referred to as a beginning point for another development.

The contributors of this book come from diverse backgrounds, making this book a truly international effort. This book will bring forth new frontiers with its revolutionizing research information and detailed analysis of the nascent developments around the world.

We would like to thank all the contributing authors for lending their expertise to make the book truly unique. They have played a crucial role in the development of this book. Without their invaluable contributions this book wouldn't have been possible. They have made vital efforts to compile up to date information on the varied aspects of this subject to make this book a valuable addition to the collection of many professionals and students.

This book was conceptualized with the vision of imparting up-to-date information and advanced data in this field. To ensure the same, a matchless editorial board was set up. Every individual on the board went through rigorous rounds of assessment to prove their worth. After which they invested a large part of their time researching and compiling the most relevant data for our readers.

The editorial board has been involved in producing this book since its inception. They have spent rigorous hours researching and exploring the diverse topics which have resulted in the successful publishing of this book. They have passed on their knowledge of decades through this book. To expedite this challenging task, the publisher supported the team at every step. A small team of assistant editors was also appointed to further simplify the editing procedure and attain best results for the readers.

Apart from the editorial board, the designing team has also invested a significant amount of their time in understanding the subject and creating the most relevant covers. They scrutinized every image to scout for the most suitable representation of the subject and create an appropriate cover for the book.

The publishing team has been an ardent support to the editorial, designing and production team. Their endless efforts to recruit the best for this project, has resulted in the accomplishment of this book. They are a veteran in the field of academics and their pool of knowledge is as vast as their experience in printing. Their expertise and guidance has proved useful at every step. Their uncompromising quality standards have made this book an exceptional effort. Their encouragement from time to time has been an inspiration for everyone.

The publisher and the editorial board hope that this book will prove to be a valuable piece of knowledge for researchers, students, practitioners and scholars across the globe.

List of Contributors

Victor Vostrikov and Natalya Uranova
Laboratory of Clinical Neuropathology, Mental Health Research Center, Moscow 115522, Russia

Matthias J.Müller
Clinic for Psychiatry and Psychotherapy Giessen and Marburg, Vitos Clinical Centre Giessen-Marburg, Academic Teaching Hospital, University of Giessen, Licher Strasse 106, 35392 Giessen, Germany

Carissa M. Coulston and Gin S.Malhi
Discipline of Psychiatry, Sydney Medical School, University of Sydney, NSW 2006, Australia
Department of Psychiatry, CADE Clinic, Royal North Shore Hospital, St. Leonards, Sydney, NSW 2065, Australia

Michael Perdices
Discipline of Psychiatry, Sydney Medical School, University of Sydney, NSW 2006, Australia
Department of Neurology, Royal North Shore Hospital, St. Leonards, Sydney, NSW 2065, Australia

Antony F. Henderson
Discipline of Psychiatry, Sydney Medical School, University of Sydney, NSW 2006, Australia
Department of Psychiatry, CADE Clinic, Royal North Shore Hospital, St. Leonards, Sydney, NSW 2065, Australia

Amy L. Barnes,Meghan E.Murphy, Christopher A. Fowler and Melisa V. Rempfer
Department of Psychology, University of Missouri-Kansas City, 5030 Cherry Hall, Kansas City, MO 64110, USA

Radovan Přikryl, Hana Přikrylová Kučerová and Eva Češková
Central European Institute of Technology, Masaryk University (CEITEC-MU), Kamenice 753/5, 62500 Brno, Czech Republic
Department of Psychiatry, Faculty of Medicine Masaryk University, University Hospital Brno, Jihlavska 20, 62500 Brno, Czech Republic

Michaela Vrzalová
Department of Psychiatry, Faculty of Medicine Masaryk University, University Hospital Brno, Jihlavska 20, 62500 Brno, Czech Republic

Brian Dean
The Rebecca L. Cooper Research Laboratories, The Mental Health Research Institute, Locked bag 11, Parkville, VIC 3052, Australia
The Department of Psychiatry, The University of Melbourne, Parkville, VIC 3052, Australia

Murat Yildiz
Department of Neurology, Cantonal Hospital St. Gallen, 9007 St. Gallen, Switzerland

Stefan J. Borgwardt
Psychiatric Outpatient Clinic, University Hospital Basel, 4031 Basel, Switzerland

Gregor E. Berger
Integrierte Psychiatrie Winterthur, Zurich Unterland, 8408 Winterthur, Switzerland

Borah Kim and Sang-Hyuk Lee
Department of Psychiatry, CHA Bundang Medical Center, CHA University, 59 Yatap-ro, Bundang-gu, Seongnam-si 463-712, Gyeonggi-do, Republic of Korea

Yen Kuang Yang
Department of Psychiatry, National Cheng Kung University Hospital, College of Medicine, National Cheng Kung University, 138 Sheng Li Road, Tainan 70428, Taiwan

Jong-Il Park
Department of Psychiatry, Chonbuk National University Medical School, 567 Baekje-daero, Deokjin-gu,
Jeonju-si 561-756, Jeollabuk-do, Republic of Korea

Young-Chul Chung
Department of Psychiatry, Chonbuk National University Medical School, 567 Baekje-daero, Deokjin-gu,
Jeonju-si 561-756, Jeollabuk-do, Republic of Korea
Research Institute of ClinicalMedicine of Chonbuk National University, Biomedical Research Institute of Chonbuk National University Hospital, 20 Geonjiro, Deokjin-gu, Jeonju-si 561-712, Jeollabuk-do, Republic of Korea

Christian Asseburg
ESiOR Oy, Tulliportinkatu 2, 70100 Kuopio, Finland

MichaelWillis and Ulf Persson
The Swedish Institute for Health Economics (IHE), 22002 Lund, Sweden

Mickael Löthgren
Amgen (Europe) GmbH Dammstrasse 23, P.O. Box 1557, CH-6301 Zug, Switzerland

Niko Seppälä and Mika Hakala,
Department of Psychiatry, Satakunta Hospital District, 29200 Harjavalta, Finland

Carolyn S. Dewa
Centre for Research on Employment and Workplace Health, Centre for Addition and Mental Health, 455 Spadina Avenue, Suite` 300, Toronto, ON, Canada M5S 2G8
Department of Psychiatry, University of Toronto, 250 College Street, Toronto, ON, Canada M5T 1R8

Lucy Trojanowski and Desmond Loong
Centre for Research on Employment and Workplace Health, Centre for Addition and Mental Health, 455 Spadina Avenue, Suite 300, Toronto, ON, Canada M5S 2G8

Chiachen Cheng
Centre for Research on Employment and Workplace Health, Centre for Addition and Mental Health, 455 Spadina Avenue, Suite 300, Toronto, ON, Canada M5S 2G8
Clinic & Resource Centre, Canadian Mental Health Association, 272 Park Avenue, Thunder Bay, ON, Canada P7B 1C5

Sara Dawson and Lisa Kettler
School of Psychology, The University of Adelaide, Adelaide, SA 5000, Australia

Cassandra Burton
The Adelaide Clinic, Ramsay Health Care (SA) Mental Health Services, Gilberton, SA 5000, Australia

Cherrie Galletly
The Adelaide Clinic, Ramsay Health Care (SA) Mental Health Services, Gilberton, SA 5000, Australia
Discipline of Psychiatry, School of Medicine, The University of Adelaide, Adelaide, SA 5000, Australia
Northern Mental Health, Adelaide Metro Mental Health Directorate, Adelaide, SA 5000, Australia
The Adelaide Clinic Consulting Suites, 33 Park Terrace, Gilberton, SA 5081, Australia

Esme Fuller-Thomson and Bailey Hollister
Factor-Inwentash Faculty of Social Work, University of Toronto, Toronto, ON, Canada M5S 1V4

Cynthia GayleWible
Laboratory of Neuroscience, Department of Psychiatry VA Boston Healthcare System, Harvard Medical School, Psychiatry 116A, 940 Belmont Street, Brockton, MA 02301, USA

OliverMason and DominicWakerley
Research Department of Clinical, Educational and Health Psychology, 1-19 Torrington Place, University College London, London WC1N 6BT, UK

Takayoshi Koide, Branko Aleksic, Masahiro Banno, Kunihiro Kohmura, Yasunori Adachi, Naoko Kawano, Tetsuya Iidaka and Norio Ozaki
Department of Psychiatry, Nagoya University Graduate School of Medicine, 65 Tsurumai-cho, Showa-ku, Nagoya 466-8550, Japan

Tsutomu Kikuchi
Department of Psychiatry, Nagoya University Graduate School of Medicine, 65 Tsurumai-cho, Showa-ku, Nagoya 466-8550, Japan
Department of Psychiatry, Matsuzaki Hospital, 67 Azamotosanbongi, Sanbongi-cho, Aichi, Toyohashi 441-8152, Japan

S. M. Arcuri
Department of Psychosis Studies, Institute of Psychiatry, King's College London, London, UK
NIF, Functional Neuroimaging, Lab/LIM 44, Instituto de Radiologia, University of Sao Paulo, Sao
Paulo, Brazil

M. R. Broome
Department of Psychosis Studies, Institute of Psychiatry, King's College London, London, UK
Coventry, UK
Warwick Medical School, University of Warwick, Coventry UK and Psychosis Clinical Academic Group

V. Giampietro, S. C. R. Williams, C. M. Andrew and M. Brammer
Department of Neuroimaging, Institute of Psychiatry, King's College London, London, UK

P. K. McGuire
Department of Psychosis Studies, Institute of Psychiatry, King's College London, London, UK

E. Amaro Jr.
NIF, Functional Neuroimaging, Lab/LIM 44, Instituto de Radiologia, University of Sao Paulo, Sao Paulo, Brazil

T. T. J. Kircher
Marburg University, Marburg, Germany

R. G. Morris
Department of Psychology, Institute of Psychiatry, King's College London, London, UK

Annie Viala, Franc¸oise Cornic and Marie-Nöelle Vacheron
SM 13, Centre Hospitalier Sainte-Anne, 1 Rue Cabanis, 75014 Paris, France

Fabio Panariellom and Vincenzo De Luca
Department of Psychiatry, Centre for Addiction and Mental Health, University of Toronto, 250 College Street, Room 30, Toronto, ON, Canada M5T 1R8

Andrea de Bartolomeis
Dipartimento di Neuroscienze, Sezione di Psichiatria, Laboratorio di Psichiatria Molecolare University of Napoli "Federico II", Via Pansini 5, 80131 Napoli, Italy

Julieta Ramos-Loyo and LeonorMora-Reynoso
Instituto de Neurociencias, CUCBA, Universidad de Guadalajara, 44130 Guadalajara, JAL, Mexico

LuisMiguel S´anchez-Loyo
Departamento de Neurociencias, CUCS, Universidad de Guadalajara, 44130 Guadalajara, JAL, Mexico

VirginiaMedina-Heráandez
Centro Comunitario de Salud Mental No. 1, Guadalajara, 45150 Zapopan, JAL, Mexico

Steffen Moritz
Department of Psychiatry and Psychotherapy, University Medical Center Hamburg-Eppendorf, Martinistraße 52, 20246 Hamburg, Germany

Niels Van Quaquebeke
Department of Management and Economics, Kuehne Logistics University, Hamburg, Germany

Tania M. Lincoln
Department of Psychology, University of Hamburg, Hamburg, Germany

Cali F. Bartholomeusz
Melbourne Neuropsychiatry Centre, Department of Psychiatry, National Neuroscience Facility, The University of Melbourne, Level 2-3 Alan Gilbert Building, 161 Barry Street, Carlton South, VIC 3053, Australia

Kelly Allott
Orygen Youth Health Research Centre, Centre for Youth Mental Health, The University of Melbourne, Locked Bag 10, Parkville, VIC 3052, Australia

Mary V. Seeman
Department of Psychiatry, Institute of Medical Science, University of Toronto, One King's College Circle, 7213 Medical Sciences Building, Toronto, ON, Canada M5S 1A8

AhmedMahmoud, Richard J. Drake and ShônW. Lewis
Mental Health and Neurodegeneration Research Group, The University of Manchester, Manchester M13 9PL, UK

Karen P. Hayhurst
National Drug Evidence Centre (NDEC), School of Community Based Medicine, The University of Manchester, Manchester M15 6SZ, UK

Index